The Science of Food

The Science of Food

Fourth edition

P. M. Gaman and K. B. Sherrington

Routledge
Taylor & Francis Group
LONDON AND NEW YORK

First published by Butterworth-Heinemann

This edition published 2011 by Routledge
2 Park Square, Milton Park, Abingdon, Oxfordshire OX14 4RN
711 Third Avenue, New York, NY 10017, USA

First issued in hardback 2015

Routledge is an imprint of the Taylor & Francis Group, an informa business

First published 1977
Second edition 1981
Third edition 1990
Fourth edition 1996

British Library Cataloguing in Publication Data
Gaman, P. M.
The science of food – 4th ed.
1. Nutrition 2. Food – Analysis 3. Food – Composition
I. Title II. Sherrington, K. B.
641.1

Library of Congress Cataloguing in Publication Data
Gaman, P. M.
The science of food/P. M. Gaman and K. B. Sherrington – 4th ed.
p. cm.
Includes bibliographical references and index.
ISBN 0 7506 2373 X
1. Food – Composition. 2. Food – Microbiology 3. Nutrition
I. Sherrington, K. B. II. Title
TX531.G35
641.1—dc20 96-5933
CIP

ISBN 13: 978-1-138-17083-4 (hbk)
ISBN 13: 978-0-750-62373-5 (pbk)

Contents

Preface to fourth edition

In the course of teaching applied science to catering students, we came to realize the need for a textbook which dealt with the various scientific aspects of food preparation at an intermediate level.

In this book we have covered three different subject areas: food science, nutrition and microbiology. Microbiology has been given more emphasis than is usual in books on food science and nutrition, since we feel that this is an area which is often overlooked.

This book is intended to fill the gap between elementary books, containing little scientific explanation, and advanced books which examine the subjects in detail but are only suitable for those students who have a comprehensive scientific training. We have assumed little prior scientific knowledge on the part of the reader. An attempt has been made to convey basic scientific facts and principles, necessary for the understanding of food science, nutrition and microbiology, which are dealt with in some depth.

This book is intended primarily for students following GNVQ and HND courses in Catering and Hospitality Management. It should also be of value to Home Economics students and students taking courses in Food Science, Food Technology, Dietetics and Nutrition. It will serve as an introduction for undergraduates following degree courses in food related subjects. Science teachers in secondary schools may find it useful for developing courses in applied science. There may also be many other people, wishing to find out more about food and health, who would find this book both informative and interesting.

The fourth edition contains revised and updated information and figures. Since the publication of the third edition there have been many changes in relation to nutrition and health, and in the field of food hygiene and food safety. In this latest edition we have included details of the latest government guidelines on healthy eating and the new recommended intakes of nutrients (Dietary Reference Values). We have attempted to explain some of the new ideas and terminology in relation to nutrition. This edition also has up-to-date information on food poisoning and food hygiene. The chapter on food hygiene has been extended and revised to include more practical advice. It also includes details of current legislation including the Food Safety (General Food Hygiene) Regulations 1995. We have covered quality control aspects of food safety by including a section on HACCP, a system of quality control based on hazard analysis.

Acknowledgements

We wish to acknowledge the help and encouragement given to us by family, friends and colleagues during the writing of this book. Particular thanks go to Valerie Ward and David Sale for their very valuable assistance with proof reading.

Some of the statistical data in the book has come from copyright material. Figures relating to the nutrient content of foods are taken from *McCance and Widdowson's The Composition of Foods* (The Royal Society of Chemistry and Ministry of Agriculture, Fisheries and Food). Data from *The Composition of Foods*, 5th edition, are reproduced with the permission of The Royal Society of Chemistry and the Controller of Her Majesty's Stationery Office.

Crown copyright material has been used in various parts of the book. The table in Appendix I which shows the contributions made by groups of foods to the nutritional value of the average household diet is an abridged version of data from the *National Food Survey, compendium of results, 1992* (Ministry of Agriculture, Fisheries and Food). The tables in Appendix II showing recommended energy and nutrient intakes are modified versions of those published in *Dietary Reference Values for Food Energy and Nutrients for the United Kingdom*, 1991 (Department of Health). Crown copyright is reproduced with the permission of the Controller of Her Majesty's Stationery Office.

Introduction

Many people do not associate science with food. Even though they are aware of the rapid development of technology and of the applications of science to many aspects of everyday life, they remain unaware of the importance of science in the preparation of the food on their tables.

Scientific study related to the food we eat can be roughly divided into three broad categories: food science, nutrition and microbiology.

Food science involves the study of all aspects of science related to food. A major part of this book deals with the chemistry of food, since this is an important aspect. An understanding of the chemical nature of food is essential if one is to achieve an understanding of the composition of food and the reactions which take place in food when conditions are changed. A study of food science will explain, for example, why baking powder makes cakes rise or why freshly cut apples go brown when exposed to the air.

Food, like oxygen, is a necessity of life. The human body requires food as a source of energy and for the growth and replacement of tissues. Food also supplies substances which help to regulate the reactions involved in these processes. Nutrition is the study of the composition of food and the utilization of food by the body. Foods are mixtures of substances known as nutrients. Each nutrient has a particular type of chemical composition and performs at least one specific function in the body.

The five groups of nutrients are:

1	Carbohydrates	provide energy and dietary fibre.
2	Fats and oils	provide energy.
3	Proteins	used for the growth and replacement of tissue, may also provide energy.
4	Vitamins	regulate body processes.
5	Minerals	regulate body processes; some are used for growth and replacement of tissue.

Most foods also contain water. Few foods contain only one nutrient. Most consist of mixtures of nutrients, together with water.

A well-balanced diet is necessary for the maintenance of good health. This means that the food a person consumes should provide adequate, but not excessive, amounts of essential nutrients and energy. A poor diet leads to malnutrition, which literally means 'bad nutrition'. There are many types of malnutrition. Malnutrition may be caused by a lack of one or more of the essential nutrients in the diet. For example, a prolonged lack of vitamin C will give rise to a deficiency disease known as scurvy.

Not only is malnutrition caused by the consumption of foods with an incorrect nutrient balance but also by the consumption of either too little or too much food. Insufficient food will lead to starvation, a form of malnutrition which, if prolonged, will lead to death. In some poorer, less developed parts of the world in recent years natural disasters, such as drought and flooding, have caused famines in which many people have died.

In wealthy, industrialized countries malnutrition occurs either as a result of eating too much food, or by the consumption of a diet with an unbalanced nutrient intake. Excesses and deficiencies of some components of the diet are associated with certain 'diseases of affluence'. For example, an excessive intake of fat is linked with heart disease, too little dietary fibre with cancer of the bowel, too much sugar with tooth decay and too much food (energy) with obesity (overweight). Advice is now available on how the diet should be altered in order to make it more healthy. It is recommended that the amounts of fat, sugar and salt in the diet should be reduced, while the amounts of starch and dietary fibre should be increased.

Microbiology is the study of micro-organisms; these are very small, simple forms of life, such as bacteria and yeasts. Some species of micro-organisms are beneficial and are used extensively in food production. Other types are responsible for many undesirable effects in food. Certain bacteria, if present in food in large enough numbers, will cause food poisoning. Currently there is widespread concern over the rapid increase in cases of food poisoning in England and Wales in recent years. Micro-organisms can also cause food spoilage, e.g. the souring of milk, the growth of moulds on foods such as bread and cheese. A knowledge of the nature of micro-organisms, their growth requirements and how growth can be prevented, is necessary if one is to understand correct procedures of hygiene and the principles involved in the various methods of food preservation.

In order to obtain adequate food supplies in urbanized societies, we depend very greatly on food technology. It is no longer possible for people to depend on locally grown, fresh foods. Food is now transported, often over very great distances, from rural areas, where it is produced, to urban areas. Unless food is processed or preserved in some way, much of it would be unfit for human consumption by the time it reaches the consumer. Food can be canned, frozen, chilled or dried in order to extend its shelf life. Preservation of food may also reduce the preparation and cooking time and is advantageous from the point of view of convenience. Many foods are 'manufactured' with convenience and acceptability in mind. Food technologists have developed a large variety of products ranging from frozen complete meals, dried soups, pie fillings and cake mixes to breakfast cereals. Food technology is an important part of modern society.

1 Measurement

All scientific study involves accurate measurement. This applies to food science, nutrition and microbiology as much as to any other scientific discipline. For example, in order to assess the nutritional value of a food it is necessary to be able to state its nutrient content in precise terms.

The metric system has, for a long time, been the universal system of measurement in pure science. Being a decimal system it is logical and easy to use. Some people in Britain may still be more familiar with Imperial units (inches, pints, pounds, etc.) than with metric units (metres, litres, kilograms, etc.) but Imperial units are being phased out.

SI units

SI is an abbreviation for Système International d'Unités (International System of Units). It is an extension and refinement of the traditional metric system and it has been adopted in the United Kingdom for all scientific measurement. There are six basic SI units; each is used for measuring a different physical quantity and each is represented by a different symbol. These basic units are shown in Table 1.1.

Table 1.1 *Basic SI units*

Physical quantity	*Name of unit*	*Symbol*
Length	metre	m
Mass	kilogram	kg
Time	second	s
Electric current	ampere	A
Thermodynamic temperature	degree Kelvin	K
Luminous intensity	candela	cd

In addition there are other units, derived from these basic quantities, and also some non-SI units, still in common use, which are allowed in conjunction with SI. Units which are relevant to this book are shown in Table 1.2.

Table 1.2 *Other units*

Physical quantity	*Name of unit*	*Symbol*	
Energy	joule	J	derived units
Customary temperature	degree Celsius	°C	
Area	square metre	m^2	
Volume	cubic metre	m^3	
Density	kilogram per cubic metre	$kg\ m^{-3}$	
Force	newton	N	
Pressure	pascal	Pa	
Volume	litre	l	allowed in conjunction with SI

It is sometimes more convenient for practical purposes to use a unit considerably larger or smaller than the standard unit. In order to make the units larger or smaller, words can be used in front of the unit. These prefixes increase or decrease the basic units by multiples or fractions of ten. Each multiple or fraction has a symbol which is placed in front of the symbol of the unit (Table 1.3).

The following examples illustrate the use of prefixes:

5 kJ = five kilojoules = five thousand joules
12 mm = twelve millimetres = twelve thousandths of a metre
8 μg = eight micrograms = eight millionths of a gram

NB Symbols never take a plural form; 12 mms would be incorrect.

Table 1.3 *Metric prefixes*

Multiple	*Prefix*	*Symbol*
10 (ten)	deci-	da
10^2 (hundred)	hecto-	h
10^3 (thousand)	kilo-	k
10^6 (million)	mega-	M
Fraction	*Prefix*	*Symbol*
10^{-1} (tenth)	deci-	d
10^{-2} (hundredth)	centi-	c
10^{-3} (thousandth)	milli-	m
10^{-6} (millionth)	micro-	μ
10^{-9} (thousand millionth)	nano-	n

Length

The basic unit for the measurement of length is the metre. Large distances are now measured in kilometres rather than miles, and small distances in centimetres or millimetres. Very short lengths, such as the wavelength of light and the size of microorganisms, are measured in micrometres or nanometres.

$$1 \text{ kilometre (km)} = 1000 \text{ metres } (10^3 \text{ m})$$

$$1 \text{ centimetre (cm)} = \frac{1}{100} \text{ metre } (10^{-2} \text{ m})$$

$$1 \text{ millimetre (mm)} = \frac{1}{1000} \text{ metre } (10^{-3} \text{ m})$$

$$1 \text{ micrometre } (\mu\text{m}) = \frac{1}{1{,}000{,}000} \text{ metre } (10^{-6} \text{ m})$$

$$1 \text{ nanometre (nm)} = \frac{1}{1{,}000{,}000{,}000} \text{ metre } (10^{-9} \text{ m})$$

Some of the factors used for converting Imperial units to SI units are as follows:

1 inch = 2.54 cm (approximately $2\frac{1}{2}$)
1 mile = 1.61 km (approximately $\frac{8}{5}$)

Area

Area is a physical quantity derived from the measurement of length.

Area = length × breadth

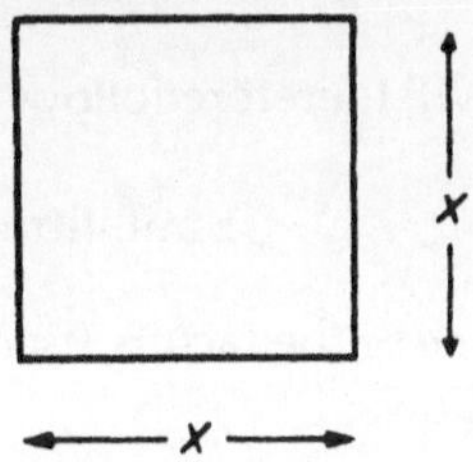

The area of a square of side x is x^2

The SI unit of area is the square metre.

$$1 \text{ square metre } (\text{m}^2) = 100 \text{ cm} \times 100 \text{ cm}$$
$$= 10{,}000 \text{ square centimetres } (10^4 \text{ cm}^2)$$

Volume and capacity

Volume is also derived from the measurement of length.

Volume = length × breadth × height

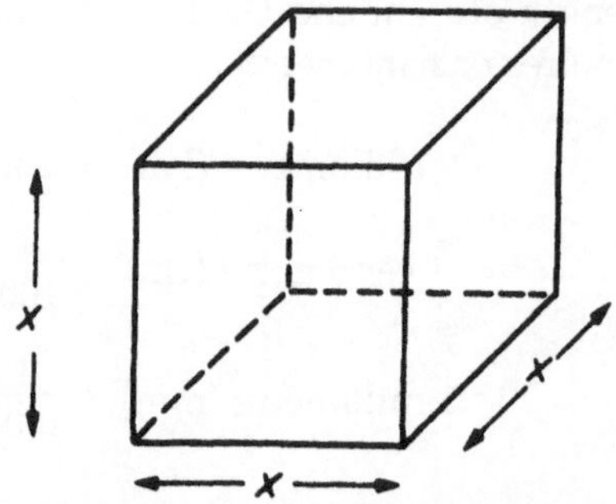

The volume of a cube of side x is x^3

The SI unit of volume is the cubic metre.

$$\begin{aligned} 1 \text{ cubic metre } (m^3) &= 100 \text{ cm} \times 100 \text{ cm} \times 100 \text{ cm} \\ &= 1{,}000{,}000 \text{ cubic centimetres } (10^6 \text{ cm}^3) \end{aligned}$$

For liquid measure or capacity the litre is the unit most often used. Quantities of wine are often measured in centilitres. The litre is derived from the measurement of volume, since it was originally defined as the volume occupied by 1 kg of water at its temperature of maximum density and under a pressure of one standard atmosphere.

$$\begin{aligned} 1 \text{ litre (l)} &= 1000 \text{ cm}^3 \\ 1 \text{ millilitre (ml)} &= \frac{1}{1000} \text{ litre } (10^{-3} \text{ l}) \end{aligned}$$

It will therefore follow that

$$1 \text{ millilitre (ml)} = 1 \text{ cubic centimetre } (\text{cm}^3)$$

Some of the factors used for converting Imperial units to SI units are as follows:

$$\begin{aligned} 1 \text{ fluid ounce} &= 28.4 \text{ ml} \\ 1 \text{ pint} &= 568 \text{ ml } (0.568 \text{ l}) \\ 1 \text{ gallon} &= 4.55 \text{ l} \end{aligned}$$

For some purposes it is convenient to know that

1 litre = 1.76 pints (approximately 1¾)

Mass and weight

For practical purposes mass and weight are the same and the terms are interchangeable, although the scientific definitions of mass and weight are different.

The basic SI unit of mass is the kilogram, which is now used instead of the pound. It has been suggested that a new name be found for the kilogram, since it is the only basic unit which is a multiple and has a prefix in its name. Quantities formerly measured in ounces are now measured in grams. Very small quantities of substances found in foods, such as vitamins and mineral elements, are measured in milligrams or micrograms. For large weights the tonne is used.

$$\begin{aligned}\text{1 tonne (t)} &= \text{1,000,000 grams } (10^6 \text{ g})\\ \text{1 kilogram (kg)} &= \text{1000 grams } (10^3 \text{ g})\\ \text{1 milligram (mg)} &= \frac{1}{1000} \text{ gram } (10^{-3} \text{ g})\\ \text{1 microgram } (\mu\text{g}) &= \frac{1}{1{,}000{,}000} \text{ gram } (10^{-6} \text{ g})\end{aligned}$$

Some of the factors used for converting Imperial units to SI units are as follows:

1 ounce = 28.4 g (approximately 30)
1 pound = 454 g (0.454 kg – approximately ½)
1 stone = 6.35 kg
1 ton = 1.016 t (metric tonnes)

For some purposes it is useful to remember that

$$1 \text{ kg} = 2.2 \text{ pounds}$$

Density

Density is derived from volume and weight. The density of a substance is a measure of its 'heaviness'. The popular expressions 'as heavy as lead' and 'as light as a feather' imply correctly that lead has a high density and feathers a very low density. A given weight of feathers will occupy a much greater volume than the same weight of lead.

$$\text{Density} = \frac{\text{Weight}}{\text{Volume}}$$

Since the SI unit of weight is the kilogram and the unit of volume is the cubic metre, the SI unit of density is the kilogram per cubic metre (kg/m^3 or more correctly $kg\ m^{-3}$). Density is also measured in grams per cubic centimetre ($g\ cm^{-3}$). The density of water is $1.0\ g\ cm^{-3}$. The

relative density (RD) of a substance is the number of times a substance is heavier than an equal volume of water, i.e. its density relative to water.

$$\text{Relative Density} = \frac{\text{Density of substance}}{\text{Density of water}}$$

NB Relative density is a ratio and therefore has no unit.

If a substance is dissolved in water to form a solution, the density is altered. The density varies directly with the concentration of the solution. Most substances, e.g. sugar and salt, cause the density to increase but sometimes the density may be lowered, e.g. by the presence of fat or alcohol.

A quick method of determining the concentration of pure solutions in water is to measure the density of the solution, using an instrument known as a **hydrometer.**

A hydrometer consists of a glass bulb weighted with lead shot; attached to this is a thin glass stem bearing a scale (see Figure 1.1).

The hydrometer is placed in the solution so that it floats freely. The further it sinks into the solution the lower the density. The scale may give the density of the solution or it may be calibrated to give a direct reading of the concentration of a substance. Some examples of hydrometers used to give direct readings of concentration are saccharometers, used to measure sugar in solution, and salinometers, which measure the concentration of brine (salt solutions). Lactometers are used in dairies to give a rapid measurement of the density of milk, giving an indication of its quality. Normal milk should have a relative density of 1.030. In the wine industry hydrometers are used to show how much alcohol has been produced during fermentation.

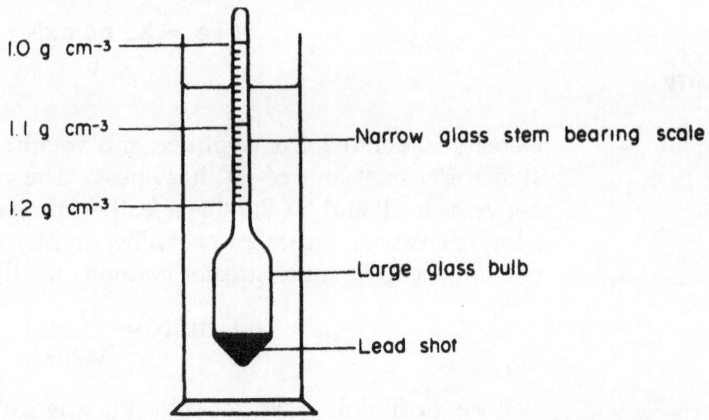

Figure 1.1 *Diagram of a hydrometer used to measure densities in the range 1.0 g cm*$^{-3}$ *to 1.2 g cm*$^{-3}$.

Energy

The measurement of the energy released when a nutrient or food is oxidized is of importance in nutrition. The energy value of a food can be assessed by burning the food in oxygen and measuring the amount of heat energy produced.

The SI unit of energy is the joule and this has replaced the calorie. In nutrition the kilojoule has replaced the kilocalorie.

1 kilojoule (kJ) = 1000 joules

The factor used for conversion is

1 kilocalorie (kcal) = 4.18 kilojoules (kJ)

Kilocalories are often written as Calories (using a capital letter).

1 kilocalorie = 1 Calorie (Cal) = 1000 calories (cal)

The use of the same word for two units of widely differing magnitudes causes a lot of confusion and term kilocalorie is preferred.

Temperature

The customary unit of temperature is the degree Celsius (°C). The Celsius (or Centigrade) scale is a temperature scale in which the melting point of ice is 0° and the boiling point of water is 100°. On the Fahrenheit scale the melting point of ice is 32° and the boiling point of water is 212°.

Fixed point	*Celsius scale*	*Fahrenheit scale*
Melting point of ice	0°	32°
Boiling point of water	100°	212°

On the Celsius scale it can be seen that there are 100 degrees between the two fixed points, whereas on the Fahrenheit scale there are 180 degrees. The ratio 100 : 180 is equal to 5 : 9 and therefore 5 Celsius degrees are equal to 9 Fahrenheit degrees.

To convert °C to °F
(a) Multiply by 9 then
(b) Divide by 5 then
(c) Add 32

Example: to convert 10°C to °F
(a) $10 \times 9 = 90$
(b) $90 \div 5 = 18$
(c) $18 + 32 = 50$
10° Celsius = 50° Fahrenheit

To convert °F to °C
(a) Subtract 32 then
(b) Multiply by 5 then
(c) Divide by 9

Example: to convert 104°F to °C
(a) $104 - 32 = 72$
(b) $72 \times 5 = 360$
(c) $360 \div 9 = 40$
104° Fahrenheit = 40°Celsius

2 Basic chemistry

All foods are either pure chemical compounds or mixtures of chemical compounds. Therefore, in order to understand something of the nature of food substances and the way in which they behave, it is necessary to have a fundamental knowledge of chemistry. Substances, also termed matter, can exist in three states: solid, liquid and gaseous. Chemistry is the study of the composition and behaviour of matter.

Atoms and elements

All substances that exist, either living or non-living, are made up of atoms. Atoms themselves are made up of smaller particles, the three main ones being the **proton**, the **neutron** and the **electron**. The nucleus of an atom consists of protons and neutrons. The proton has a positive electrical charge and the neutron has no charge. The electron orbits the nucleus and has a negative electrical charge, which is equal but opposite to the charge on the proton.

The simplest type of atom is the hydrogen atom. Its nucleus consists of a single proton and it has one electron orbiting the nucleus (see Figure 2.1). The carbon atom, on the other hand, has six protons and six neutrons in the nucleus and six electrons orbiting the nucleus. There are two electrons in the first orbit and four in the second orbit. Simple representations of a hydrogen atom and a carbon atom are shown in Figure 2.1.

It will be noticed that, in each case, the number of protons is equal to the number of electrons. Since the charges on the proton and electron are equal but opposite, the atom is electrically neutral.

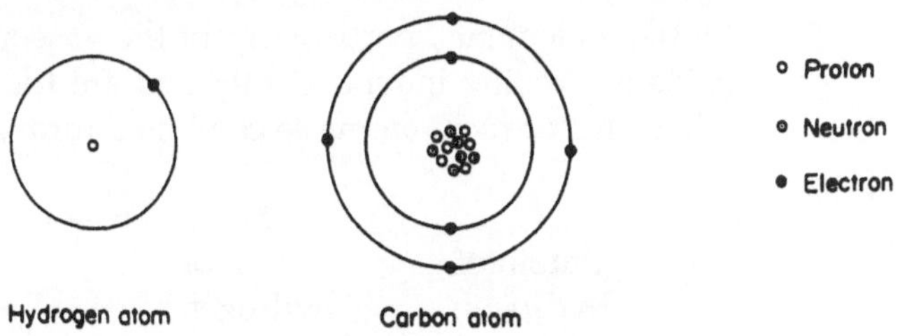

Figure 2.1 *Diagrammatic representation of a hydrogen atom and a carbon atom.*

So far, 105 different types of atoms have been discovered. This means that matter is made up of 105 fundamental substances called elements. Each element has its own type of atom; the hydrogen atom, for example, is different from the carbon atom.

An element is a simple substance consisting of atoms of only one type. It cannot be broken down into anything simpler by any known chemical process. By including the phrase 'by any known chemical process' in this definition, allowance is made for the fact that, since the discovery of radioactivity, certain elements, e.g. uranium, have been shown to undergo a *physical* process of decay producing other substances, i.e. other elements.

An atom may be defined as the smallest particle of an element which can exist and still show the properties of that element.

Of the 105 elements, 92 occur naturally in the Earth's crust or its atmosphere. The remainder have been made artificially by the use of nuclear processes.

Elements can be divided into two groups, according to their chemical behaviour. They are either metals or non-metals.

Each element has a chemical symbol, i.e. one or two letters which represent one atom of the element. In many cases this symbol is the first letter of the name written as a capital:

C for carbon

Since many elements start with the same letter, it is often necessary to use the first letter and another:

Ca for calcium Cl for chlorine

For some elements, the symbol is not derived from the English name but from the name in another language:

Na for sodium K for potassium

Table 2.1 gives the symbols of elements of importance in food science.

Molecules and compounds

In many elements, particularly in the gaseous state, atoms are incapable of existing independently and are found combined with each other. Two or more atoms so combined form a molecule.

H	+	H	$\longrightarrow$	H_2
1 atom of hydrogen		1 atom of hydrogen		1 molecule of hydrogen

Table 2.1 *Elements of importance in food science*

Element	*Symbol*	
Carbon	C	Non-metals. The constituents of proteins, fats and carbohydrates.
Hydrogen	H	
Oxygen	O	
Nitrogen	N	
Sulphur	S	
Phosphorus	P	
Sodium	Na	Reactive metals. Found in foods and essential for the functioning of the body.
Potassium	K	
Calcium	Ca	
Magnesium	Mg	
Chlorine	Cl	Halogens. A group of non-metals with similar chemical properties. Chlorine and iodine are essential in the diet.
Iodine	I	
Fluorine	F	
Bromine	Br	
Iron	Fe	Metals. All are essential in the diet.
Zinc	Zn	
Copper	Cu	
Cobalt	Co	
Manganese	Mn	
Aluminium	Al	Metals. Not essential in the diet.
Lead	Pb	
Tin	Sn	

A small number after the symbol H indicates the presence of two hydrogen atoms in the molecule. The number of atoms contained in each molecule is constant and is termed the atomicity. Most common gases are diatomic (one molecule contains two atoms), e.g. oxygen (O_2), nitrogen (N_2) and chlorine (Cl_2).

A molecule may be defined as the smallest portion of a substance capable of existing independently and retaining the properties of the original substance.

Atoms of different elements may also combine chemically to form molecules, e.g. one molecule of water (H_2O) consists of two atoms of hydrogen combined with one atom of oxygen. In nature elements rarely occur in the pure state. They are usually found in combination with each other as more complex substances. These substances are called compounds.

A compound is a substance containing two or more elements chemically combined.

Water is a substance formed when the elements oxygen and hydrogen combine. Sodium chloride (NaCl) or table salt is another example of a compound; it contains the elements sodium and chlorine. It can be seen that a molecule is the smallest particle of a compound that can exist.

The formation of molecules

Some elements are very reactive and readily form compounds; others are unreactive or stable. The electrons of an atom are arranged in orbits or **shells**. The reactivity of an atom depends on the number of electrons in the outer shell and these are called the valency electrons. Each shell can only contain a certain number of electrons. The first or innermost shell can contain two electrons but no more. The second shell is capable of holding eight electrons. The third can also hold eight, though atoms of some elements can hold eighteen, ten being in a subshell.

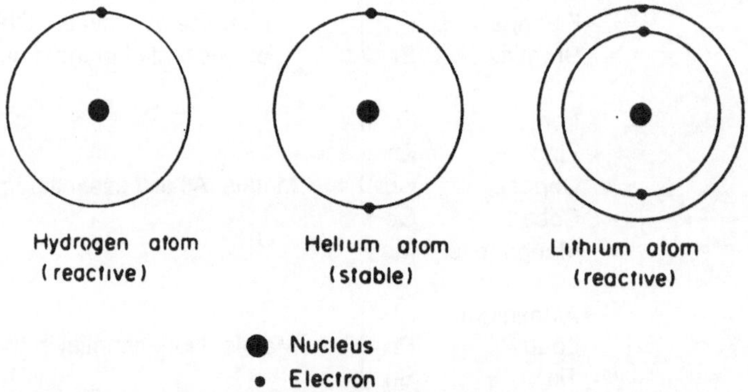

Figure 2.2 *Atoms of the three lightest elements.*

Table 2.2 *Electron arrangements in inert gases and halogens*

Inert gases	*Electron shells*			*Halogens*	*Electron shells*				
	1st	*2nd*	*3rd*		*1st*	*2nd*	*3rd*	*4th*	*5th*
Helium	2			Fluorine	2	7			
Neon	2	8		Chlorine	2	8	7		
Argon	2	8	8	Bromine	2	8	18	7	
				Iodine	2	8	18	18	7

Each shell is filled in turn starting with the innermost shell and moving outwards. If the outer shell is 'full up' with electrons then that atom will be stable and unreactive. If a shell is not 'full up' then the atom is said to be reactive, because it will tend to combine with other atoms to obtain full shells.

Looking at the three lightest elements (shown in Figure 2.2) it can be seen that hydrogen has one electron only and it therefore needs one more electron to become stable. Helium has two electrons; this is a stable number (first shell) and therefore helium is unreactive. Lithium has two electrons in the first shell and one electron in the second shell. It needs to lose one electron to become stable. Lithium is a very reactive metal.

Elements with the same number of electrons in the outer shell of their atoms have similar chemical properties since they will react in a similar way with other elements. The inert gases are a group of elements which all have outer shells which are 'full up'. The halogens are a group of elements which all have seven electrons in the outer shell (see Table 2.2).

Elements combine in one of two ways to form compounds.

1 Ionic compounds

Ionic bonding involves the transfer of electrons. Atoms containing one, two or three electrons in the outer shell, i.e. metallic elements, may lose electrons in order to obtain a stable structure. These electrons are donated to atoms of non-metallic elements containing six or seven electrons in the outer shell, thus filling these shells.

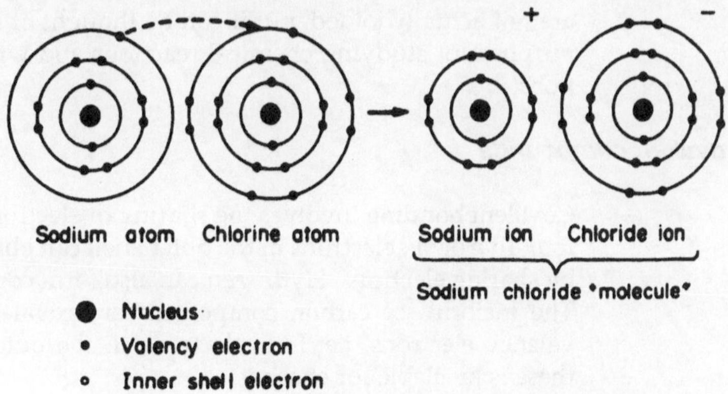

Figure 2.3 *Formation of a sodium chloride 'molecule'.*

For example, during the formation of sodium chloride each sodium atom loses an electron and this is transferred to the outer shell of a chlorine atom (see Figure 2.3). Since the sodium atom has lost an electron it will have an overall positive charge. A charged atom is called an **ion.** Similarly the chlorine atom becomes a chloride ion.

The positively and negatively charged ions attract each other and are held together by this electrostatic force forming a 'molecule' of sodium chloride. The structure of sodium chloride is three-dimensional but can be represented in two dimensions as illustrated in Figure 2.4.

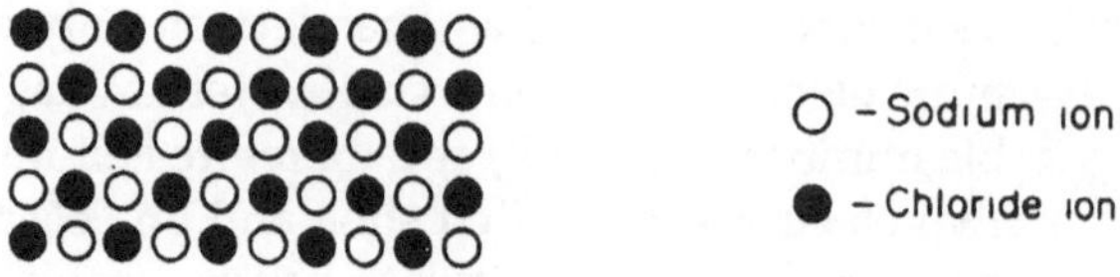

Figure 2.4 *The structure of sodium chloride.*

An ion is represented by the symbol for an element together with a sign indicating the number and nature of the charges it carries:

Na^+ represents a sodium ion
Cl^- represents a chloride ion

An atom which loses two electrons, e.g. calcium, forms ions with two positive charges:

Ca^{2+} represents a calcium ion

A 'molecule' of sodium chloride contains one sodium and one chloride ion and can be represented as Na^+Cl^-. It is more usual to write Na^+Cl^- simply as NaCl. NaCl is not strictly a molecule, since the ions are not actually joined, but it can be thought of as a molecule for the purposes of studying chemical reactions and writing chemical equations.

2 *Covalent compounds*

Covalent bonding involves the sharing of electrons. Atoms containing four, five or six electrons in the outer shell can obtain a stable structure by sharing electrons. Hydrogen can also form compounds in this way. The majority of carbon compounds are covalent. Carbon has four valency electrons, i.e. four electrons in the outer shell, and each of these is available for sharing.

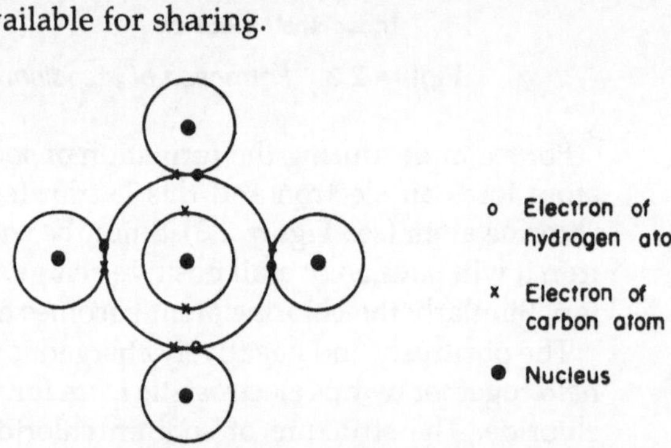

Figure 2.5 A methane molecule.

In the formation of a molecule of methane one carbon atom combines with four hydrogen atoms as shown in Figure 2.5. It can be seen that the carbon atom will now have a stable number of eight electrons in its outer shell and each hydrogen nucleus will have two electrons orbiting it. This is a stable number for hydrogen since the first shell can only hold two electrons.

Mixtures

A substance may be composed of two or more elements or compounds which are physically mixed together but are not chemically combined. This type of substance is called a mixture. It is important to distinguish between compounds and mixtures. When compounds are formed a **chemical change** takes place. If substances are only mixed together it is a **physical change.** Changes of state, e.g. from solid to liquid, are also physical changes. In a physical change no new substances are produced but a chemical reaction always produces new substances.

A compound is a substance which has a fixed composition. For example, water always contains twice as many hydrogen atoms as oxygen atoms. A mixture, on the other hand, has no fixed composition. A mixture of hydrogen and oxygen could contain 50% hydrogen and 50% oxygen, or 90% hydrogen and 10% oxygen or any other proportions. A further difference between compounds and mixtures is that a mixture will always show the same properties as the elements or compounds from which it is made. A compound does not show the properties of its constituent elements. For example, the compound sodium chloride (common salt) is made of the elements sodium and chlorine. Sodium is a dangerous, reactive metal and chlorine is a poisonous gas but the compound sodium chloride is neither dangerous nor poisonous.

A compound can only be separated into its constituent elements by chemical means whereas a mixture can be separated by physical means. For example, a mixture of salt and water can be separated into its components (salt and water) by a physical process of distillation. The formation of a compound is accompanied by a significant energy change. For example, in the burning of coal, when carbon combines with oxygen to form carbon dioxide, a large amount of heat is produced.

Table 2.3 summarises the main differences between compounds and mixtures.

Salt is a compound of the elements sodium and chlorine, whereas a salt solution is a mixture of the two compounds salt and water. Air is a mixture of the elements oxygen and nitrogen and the compound carbon dioxide. Milk, flour and most other foods are complex mixtures of many substances.

Table 2.3 *The main differences between compounds and mixtures*

Compounds	*Mixtures*
Have a definite composition	No fixed composition
Do not show properties of constituent elements	Show properties of constituent elements and compounds
Can only be separated into their constituent elements by chemical means	Can be separated into their constituents by physical means
Examples:	Examples:
Water	Air
Salt	Salt solution
Carbon dioxide	Flour
	Milk

Chemical formulae and equations

Molecular formulae

Chemical compounds may be represented by molecular formulae, which show the number of atoms of each type of element present in one molecule.

H_2O represents one molecule of water containing two atoms of hydrogen and one atom of oxygen.

NaCl represents one molecule of sodium chloride containing one atom of sodium and one atom of chlorine.

CH_4 represents one molecule of methane containing one atom of carbon and four atoms of hydrogen.

The small number after the symbol indicates how many atoms of that element are present in the molecule. A large number in front of the molecule indicates the number of molecules present, e.g. $2H_2O$ represents two molecules of water.

Equations

All chemical reactions can be represented by using molecular formulae and writing a **chemical equation.** An equation shows the rearrangement of atoms which takes place during a chemical reaction. In a chemical reaction matter is neither created nor destroyed and therefore the same number of atoms of each element must remain after the reaction has taken place.

The following is an example of a chemical equation:

$2H_2$	+	O_2	$\longrightarrow$	$2H_2O$
two molecules of hydrogen (four atoms of hydrogen)		one molecule of oxygen (two atoms of oxygen)		two molecules of water (four atoms of hydrogen and two atoms of oxygen)

Sometimes in a reaction a group of atoms remain joined together and tend to behave as a single ion. These groups of atoms are called **radicals.** They are incapable of an independent existence and always combine with other ions.

Table 2.4 shows some of the common radicals.

Table 2.4 *Some common radicals and their symbols*

Radical	*Symbol*
Ammonium	NH_4^+
Hydrogen carbonate	HCO_3^-
Carbonate	CO_3^{2-}
Hydroxide	OH^-
Nitrate	NO_3^-
Nitrite	NO_2^-
Phosphate	PO_4^{3-}
Sulphate	SO_4^{2-}
Sulphite	SO_3^{2-}

In order to write a chemical formula or equation, it is necessary to know the **valency** of the elements and radicals involved. The valency of an atom or radical is a whole number indicating its combining power. It is related to the atomic structure and more precisely to the number of valency electrons. Valency is equal to the number of electrons needed to be gained or lost in order to obtain a stable number of electrons in the outer shell (2,8,8, etc.). The hydrogen atom is the simplest atom and contains one valency electron. This electron can be given to another atom or can be used to form part of a covalent bond. Valency is defined using hydrogen as a standard. **Valency is the number of hydrogen atoms which will combine with or replace an atom or radical.**

One atom of oxygen (which has six valency electrons and requires two more to become stable) combines with two atoms of hydrogen to form water. Therefore, the valency of oxygen is two.

Table 2.5 shows the valencies of common elements and radicals.

Hydrogen is capable of showing both metallic and non-metallic behaviour, when it takes part in chemical reactions. Some elements, e.g. copper and iron, exhibit more than one valency. In compounds, the valency is indicated by a Roman numeral placed in brackets after the name of the element, e.g. copper(I) oxide and copper(II) oxide.

Table 2.5 *Valencies of common elements and radicals*

Valency	*Elements*		*Radicals*
	Metals	*Non-metals*	
1	Hydrogen (H) Copper (Cu) Potassium (K) Sodium (Na)	Chlorine (Cl) Hydrogen (H) Iodine (I)	Ammonium (NH_4) Hydrogen carbonate (HCO_3) Hydroxide (OH) Nitrate (NO_3) Nitrite (NO_2)
2	Calcium (Ca) Copper (Cu) Iron (Fe) Magnesium (Mg) Zinc (Zn)	Oxygen (O) Sulphur (S)	Carbonate (CO_3) Sulphate (SO_4) Sulphite (SO_3)
3	Aluminium (Al) Iron (Fe)	Nitrogen (N)	Phosphate (PO_4)
4		Carbon (C)	

The valency of atoms and radicals may be represented by drawing the atoms and radicals with hooks. If the valency is one, the atom or radical is drawn with one hook; if the valency is two, it is drawn with two hooks, etc. When atoms and radicals combine, all the hooks must link up. For example, when magnesium combines with oxygen:

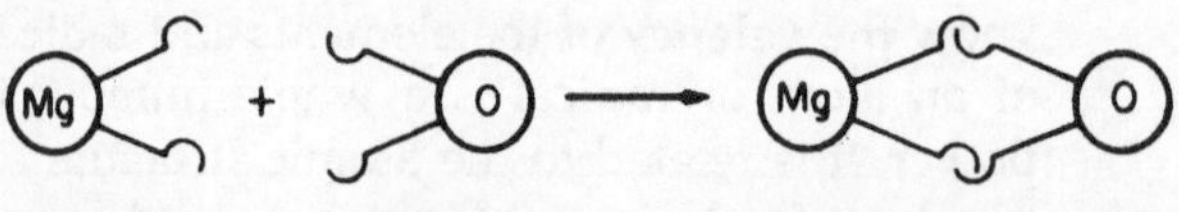

Magnesium (valency 2)   Oxygen (valency 2)   Magnesium oxide MgO

When aluminium ions combine with sulphate radicals:

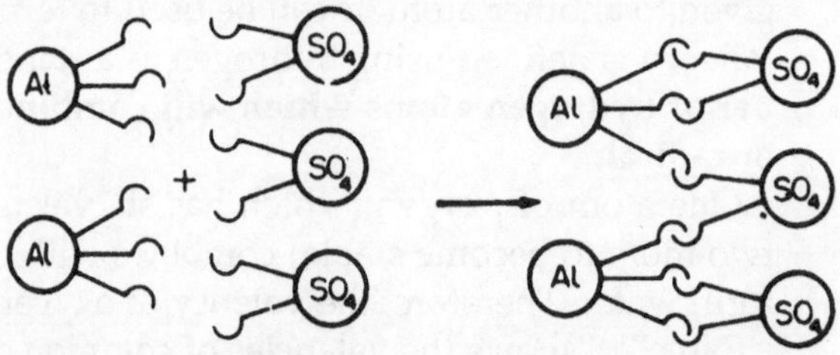

Aluminium (valency 3)   Sulphate (valency 2)   Aluminium sulphate $Al_2 (SO_4)_3$

Three sulphate ions are present in the aluminium sulphate molecule and this is represented by using brackets with a small '3' outside.

Having determined the formulae of the starting materials and products in a chemical reaction, an equation can be written. For example:

$NaHCO_3$	$\longrightarrow$	Na_2CO_3	+	CO_2	+	H_2O
sodium hydrogen carbonate		sodium carbonate		carbon dioxide		water

This equation is not correct, since it is not balanced. There are not the same number of atoms of each element on each side of the equation. There are two sodium atoms on the right-hand side and only one on the left-hand side. There must, therefore, be two molecules of sodium hydrogen carbonate taking part in this reaction. It can now be seen that the equation will balance:

$$2NaHCO_3 \longrightarrow Na_2CO_3 + CO_2 + H_2O$$

A more complicated reaction is the oxidation of glucose. Glucose, when oxidized, produces carbon dioxide and water.

$C_6H_{12}O_6$	+	O_2	$\longrightarrow$	CO_2	+	H_2O
glucose		oxygen		carbon dioxide		water

To balance this equation it must be written:

$$C_6H_{12}O_6 + 6O_2 \longrightarrow 6CO_2 + 6H_2O$$

Acids, alkalis and salts

Nearly all foods contain water and the nutrients are dispersed in this water. Therefore, in the study of food science it is necessary to understand something of the nature of water and the way in which it behaves. Nearly all the water is in the form of molecules but a small number of molecules are ionized.

H_2O	$\rightleftharpoons$	H^+	+	OH^-
water molecule		hydrogen ion		hydroxyl ion

In pure water the number of hydrogen ions is equal to the number of hydroxyl ions, therefore pure water is neutral, i.e. neither acidic nor alkaline.

When substances are dissolved in water, the ratio of hydrogen to hydroxyl ions may be altered. If the number of hydrogen ions is greater than the number of hydroxyl ions, the solution is said to be acidic. If it is the reverse, the solution is alkaline.

pH

pH is a measure of the acidity or alkalinity of a solution. It is a term derived from the concentration of hydrogen ions in the solution.

$$pH = \log_{10} \frac{1}{[H^+]} \quad \text{where } [H^+] = \text{hydrogen ion concentration}$$

If the concentration of hydrogen ions (i.e. acidity) increases, the pH decreases.

The pH scale extends from 0 to 14, 7 being neutral.

$$0 \quad \longleftarrow \quad 7 \quad \longrightarrow \quad 14$$

increasing acidity ← 7 (neutral) → increasing alkalinity

Alterations in pH of solutions are important and can have dramatic effects, e.g. egg white coagulates when the solution is made very acidic or very alkaline. The growth of micro-organisms can be controlled by reducing the pH of food. For example, the pickling of foods in vinegar, which contains acetic acid, is a method of preventing microbial food spoilage.

When foods are pickled, they may change colour, because the vegetable dyes responsible for colour are altered by changes of pH. Red cabbage is red when pickled but purple when fresh and blue if placed in alkali. Vegetable dyes may be used as indicators of pH, e.g. litmus is red in acids and blue in alkalis. Universal indicator is a mixture of several indicators and shows the degree of acidity or alkalinity of a solution.

Acids

Acids are substances which dissolve in water, producing hydrogen ions. For example:

$$\underset{\text{hydrochloric acid}}{HCl} \longrightarrow \underset{\text{hydrogen ion}}{H^+} + \underset{\text{chloride ion}}{Cl^-}$$

Hydrochloric acid is a strong acid, since it ionizes completely. Weak acids are those which ionize partially in dilute solution, e.g. acetic acid.

CH_3COOH	$\rightleftharpoons$ CH_3COO^-	+	H^+
acetic acid	acetate ion		hydrogen ion

The terms 'strong' and 'weak' should not be confused with concentration. Concentrated solutions of some weak acids, e.g. acetic acid, are dangerous and should be handled with care.

Properties of acids

1 The pH of acids is in the range 0 to 7. Acids will turn blue litmus paper red.
2 Acids have a sour taste, e.g. citric acid is responsible for the sour taste of lemon juice.
3 Concentrated solutions of strong acids are corrosive and may damage skin and clothing.
4 Acids react with carbonates or hydrogen carbonates producing carbon dioxide. This is the basis of the action of baking powders (see page 24).

Inorganic acids

Hydrochloric acid	HCl
Sulphuric acid	H_2SO_4
Nitric acid	HNO_3

These are strong acids and are useful as laboratory reagents. Hydrochloric acid is one of the constituents of gastric juice. It is secreted by the stomach wall and assists the action of the enzyme pepsin (see Chapter 11).

Organic acids

These are weak acids and many are found in foods. Some of the more important ones are shown in Table 2.6. The formulae of some of these acids are given in Chapter 3.

Alkalis

Alkalis are substances which dissolve in water, producing hydroxyl ions. Alkalis are usually oxides or hydroxides of metals, e.g. sodium hydroxide.

$NaOH$	$\longrightarrow$	Na^+	+	OH^-
sodium hydroxide		sodium ion		hydroxyl ion

Table 2.6 *Some acids found in foods*

Common name of acid	*Chemical name*	*Found in/used in*
Acetic	Ethanoic acid	Vinegar
Ascorbic (Vitamin C)		Fresh fruits and vegetables
Benzoic		Preservative. Added to fruit drinks
Citric	Hydroxypropane 1,2,3 tricarboxylic acid	Citrus fruits
Lactic	2-hydroxypropanoic acid	Sour milk, yoghurt
Malic	2-hydroxybutanedioic acid	Apples, cherries
Oxalic	Ethanedioic acid	Spinach, rhubarb. Poisonous in large quantities
Tartaric	2,3-dihydroxybutanedioic acid	Grapes. Used in baking powders

Properties of alkalis

1 The pH of an alkali is in the range 7 to 14. Alkaline solutions turn red litmus paper blue.

2 Alkalis have a bitter taste. Very few foods are alkaline.

3 Solutions of alkalis have a soapy feel. A solution of soap in water is alkaline.

4 Concentrated solutions of alkalis are corrosive.

Some common alkalis are shown in Table 2.7.

Table 2.7 *Some common alkalis*

Alkali	*Common name*	*Formula*	*Uses*
Ammonium hydroxide		NH_4OH	Cleaning agents, e.g. non-scratch bath cleaners
Calcium hydroxide	Slaked lime	$Ca(OH)_2$	Water softener. Commercial extraction of gelatin from bones and skin
Potassium hydroxide	Caustic potash	KOH	Manufacture of toilet soap
Sodium hydroxide	Caustic soda	NaOH	Manufacture of soap and soap powder. Grease remover

Neutralization

Neutralization is the reaction between an acid and an alkali producing a salt and water only.

$$\text{Acid} + \text{Alkali} \longrightarrow \text{Salt} + \text{Water}$$

For example:

HCl	+	NaOH	$\longrightarrow$	NaCl	+	H_2O
hydrochloric acid		sodium hydroxide		sodium chloride (a salt)		water

The hydrogen ions produced by the acid combine with the hydroxyl ions produced by the alkali and form water.

$$H^+ + OH^- \longrightarrow H_2O$$

Vinegar can be used for rinsing woollen garments after they have been washed in soap. This neutralizes the alkaline soap solution, which can damage wool.

Salts

Salts are ionic compounds, which can be produced by neutralization or by the reaction between a metal and an acid.

$$\text{Metal} + \text{Acid} \longrightarrow \text{Salt} + \text{Hydrogen}$$

For example:

Zn	+	H_2SO_4	$\longrightarrow$	$ZnSO_4$	+	H_2
zinc		sulphuric acid		zinc sulphate		hydrogen

If an acid which contains more than one hydrogen ion is not completely neutralized, an acid salt is produced. For example:

H_2SO_4	+	NaOH	$\longrightarrow$	$NaHSO_4$	+	H_2O
sulphuric acid		sodium hydroxide		sodium hydrogen sulphate (sodium bisulphate)		water

Sodium hydrogen sulphate is an acid salt, since it still contains a replaceable hydrogen atom.

Properties of salts

1 Salts have a high melting point and can be obtained as crystalline solids.

2 Salts in solution in water usually have a pH of 7, i.e. they are neutral. This is not always the case. If the salt is formed from a strong

alkali and a weak acid, the solution will be alkaline. Sodium carbonate is formed from sodium hydroxide, a strong alkali and carbonic acid, a weak acid, and therefore sodium carbonate is alkaline in solution.

3 The solubility of salts varies. Many, but not all, salts are soluble in water. In general, salts of sodium and potassium are soluble and calcium salts are insoluble.

Table 2.8 lists some salts, together with their formulae and uses.

Table 2.8 *Some salts of importance in food science*

Salts of inorganic acids	*Formula*	*Use*
Ammonium carbonate 'Vol'	$(NH_4)_2CO_3$	Raising agent
Calcium carbonate 'chalk'	$CaCO_3$	Flour additive (increases calcium content)
Potassium chloride	KCl	Salt substitute for low sodium diets
Potassium iodide	KI	Iodine constituent of 'iodized' salt
Potassium nitrate 'saltpetre'	KNO_3	Meat preservative
Sodium carbonate 'washing soda'	Na_2CO_3	Water softener
Sodium chloride 'salt'	NaCl	Flavouring agent and preservative
Sodium hydrogen carbonate 'baking soda'	$NaHCO_3$	Raising agent
Sodium hypochlorite	NaOCl	Bleach and disinfectant
Sodium metabisulphite 'Campden tablets'	$Na_2S_2O_5$	Fruit and vegetable preservative
Sodium nitrate 'Chile saltpetre'	$NaNO_3$	Meat preservative
Sodium sulphite	Na_2SO_3	Fruit and vegetable preservative
Salts of organic acids		*Use*
Monosodium glutamate 'MSG'		Flavour enhancer
Potassium hydrogen tartrate 'cream of tartar'		Baking powder

Chemical aeration

Baking powders

Baking powders are mixtures of substances which produce carbon dioxide when water is added and they are heated. The carbon dioxide gas causes baked goods to rise.

The most usual type of baking powder contains sodium hydrogen carbonate (bicarbonate of soda) and an acid ingredient. On the addition of water the acid reacts with the hydrogen carbonate, producing a salt, water and carbon dioxide.

$NaHCO_3$	+	HX	$\longrightarrow$	NaX	+	H_2O	+	CO_2
sodium hydrogen carbonate		acid		salt		water		carbon dioxide

One of the most usual acid ingredients is potassium hydrogen tartrate (cream of tartar). This is an acid salt of tartaric acid, since it still retains some replaceable hydrogen.

Sodium hydrogen carbonate	+	Potassium hydrogen tartrate	$\longrightarrow$	Sodium potassium tartrate	+	Water	+	Carbon dioxide

Other acid ingredients which are used include tartaric acid, acid calcium phosphate (ACP) and acid sodium pyrophosphate (ASP).

Tartaric acid, cream of tartar and ACP are used in quick-acting baking powders, in which most of the carbon dioxide is produced when water is added. ASP is used in slow-acting baking powders, which produce most of their carbon dioxide during baking. Most commercial baking powders contain both slow-acting and quick-acting ingredients. They also contain a filler, usually corn starch, which helps to keep the ingredients dry and prevents them reacting with each other before baking.

The acid ingredients may be supplied by a food. The best example of this is the use of sour milk, containing lactic acid, in the making of soda bread. Vinegar or lemon juice may also be used to provide acids.

Hydrogen carbonates or carbonates can be used on their own without an acid ingredient; they release carbon dioxide on heating. If sodium hydrogen carbonate is used alone, sodium carbonate, carbon dioxide and water are produced.

$2NaHCO_3$	$\longrightarrow$	Na_2CO_3	+	H_2O	+	CO_2
sodium hydrogen carbonate		sodium carbonate		water		carbon dioxide

Sodium carbonate is present in the baked product as an alkaline residue, which is yellow in colour and slightly bitter in taste. In a dark, strongly flavoured product, such as gingerbread, this does not matter.

Ammonium hydrogen carbonate and ammonium carbonate are

used commercially in the production of some biscuits. They do not leave an alkaline residue. Ammonia is released as a vapour during baking.

NH_4HCO_3	$\longrightarrow$	NH_3	+	H_2O	+	CO_2
ammonium hydrogen carbonate		ammonia		water		carbon dioxide

$(NH_4)_2CO_3$	$\longrightarrow$	$2NH_3$	+	H_2O	+	CO_2
ammonium carbonate		ammonia		water		carbon dioxide

Oxidation and reduction

Oxidation is a reaction in which an element or compound combines with oxygen. For example, when iron rusts, the metal combines with oxygen forming the oxide.

$4Fe$	+	$3O_2$	$\longrightarrow$	$2Fe_2O_3$
iron		oxygen		iron(III) oxide (rust)

When methane is oxidized, the hydrogen is removed and is combined with oxygen, forming water.

CH_4	+	$2O_2$	$\longrightarrow$	CO_2	+	H_2O
methane		oxygen		carbon dioxide		water

The term 'oxidation' can be extended to include the displacement of hydrogen in reactions in which there is no oxygen present. Hydrogen sulphide can be oxidized by chlorine, which combines with the hydrogen, forming hydrochloric acid.

H_2S	+	Cl_2	$\longrightarrow$	$2HCl$	+	S
hydrogen sulphide		chlorine		hydrochloric acid		sulphur

Examples of oxidation processes:

1 *Combustion*, in which substances combine with oxygen, forming oxides. Heat and light are produced during the reaction, e.g. the burning of coal in air.

C	+	O_2	$\longrightarrow$	CO_2
carbon in coal		oxygen in air		carbon dioxide

2 *Aerobic respiration is* the liberation of energy from food by reaction with oxygen, e.g. the oxidation of glucose.

$C_6H_{12}O_6$	+	$6O_2$	$\longrightarrow$	$6CO_2$	+	$6H_2O$
glucose		oxygen		carbon dioxide		water

3 *Bleaching* involves the addition of oxygen to a coloured compound, converting it into a colourless compound, e.g. chlorine dioxide is used to bleach flour.
4 *Rusting is* a slow process, in which oxygen combines with iron in the presence of water, forming rust (iron(III) oxide).
5 *Rancidity* in fats is partly due to the addition of oxygen to fatty acids and the production of peroxides, which are responsible for 'off' flavours.
6 *Enzymic browning* occurs when oxygen from the air reacts with substances in food, in the presence of enzymes, forming brown compounds, e.g. the browning of freshly cut apples.
7 *Tarnishing* of metals is the slow addition of oxygen to the surface layer of a metal, forming a dull oxide layer. Aluminium is one of the metals which tarnish in this way.

$4Al$	+	$3O_2$	$\longrightarrow$	$2Al_2O_3$
aluminium		oxygen		aluminium oxide

8 *Action of disinfectants.* Chlorine, which is used as a disinfectant, i.e. it kills bacteria, combines with water forming hypochlorous acid.

Cl_2	+	H_2O	$\longrightarrow$	HCl	+	$HOCl$
chlorine		water		hydrochloric acid		hypochlorous acid

The hypochlorous acid kills bacteria by oxidation and is converted to hydrochloric acid.

An **oxidizing agent** is a substance which brings about oxidation. For example, chlorine and chlorine dioxide are oxidizing agents.
Oxidation of foods can be prevented by the use of antioxidants, substances which are oxidized in preference to the food, e.g. butylated hydroxytoluene (BHT) is added to fats to prevent rancidity. Vitamin E, often found in fats and oils, is a naturally occurring antioxidant.

Reduction is the reverse of oxidation, i.e. it is the addition of hydrogen or removal of oxygen. There are fewer common examples of reduction since hydrogen is not present in the air.

1 *Photosynthesis is* a process which occurs in green plants. Glucose is formed from carbon dioxide and water, and oxygen is produced.

$$\underset{\text{carbon dioxide}}{6CO_2} + \underset{\text{water}}{6H_2O} \longrightarrow \underset{\text{glucose}}{C_6H_{12}O_6} + \underset{\text{oxygen}}{6O_2}$$

It can be seen that this is the reverse of aerobic respiration.

2 *Hydrogenation of oils.* The addition of hydrogen to an oil hardens the oil and converts it into a fat. This process is used in the manufacture of margarine (see page 75).

3 *The cleaning of silver.* Hydrogen, produced by a reaction involving sodium carbonate and aluminium, removes sulphide tarnish from silver.

$$\underset{\text{silver sulphide (tarnish)}}{Ag_2S} + \underset{\text{hydrogen}}{H_2} \longrightarrow \underset{\text{silver}}{2Ag} + \underset{\text{hydrogen sulphide}}{H_2S}$$

A **reducing agent** is a substance which brings about reduction, e.g. hydrogen.

3 Organic chemistry

All the components of food, with the exception of water and the mineral salts, are organic compounds. Therefore, a knowledge of organic chemistry is essential in the study of food science and nutrition.

Organic chemistry is the study of covalent carbon compounds. All forms of life are based on these organic carbon compounds. When the term organic chemistry was first introduced, it was thought that these compounds were found only in living organisms and that they could not be produced synthetically. This is now known to be incorrect and a wide variety of organic compounds are produced commercially. Nowadays, it is possible to synthesize vitamins, some sugars and fats, and some simple proteins. Many synthetic organic compounds are an important part of our life; these include plastics, such as polythene and polystyrene, and man-made fibres, such as nylon and polyester.

Carbon is unique among the elements in that it is capable of forming thousands of different compounds. The reason for this is that carbon atoms join together very easily and, therefore, a large number of different molecules can be obtained. These molecules are sometimes very large and complex. Carbon atoms, as well as forming bonds with other carbon atoms, also form bonds with atoms of other elements. The elements which most often combine with carbon to form organic compounds are hydrogen, oxygen and nitrogen. Sulphur, phosphorus and the halogens (fluorine, chlorine, bromine and iodine) may also be present in organic compounds.

Carbon has a valency of four, since the four electrons in the outer shell readily form covalent bonds. The covalent bonds can be represented by lines. When a carbon atom is present in a molecule the atom and bonds can be represented as follows:

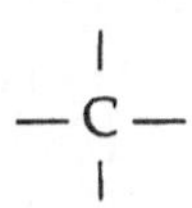

Carbon atoms may be joined by single, double or triple bonds. In a single bond, one pair of electrons is shared between the two carbon atoms. Two pairs of shared electrons form a double bond and three pairs a triple bond. The conventional representations of single, double and triple bonds are shown in Figure 3.1.

Table 3.1 shows the valency of some of the other elements which are found in organic compounds.

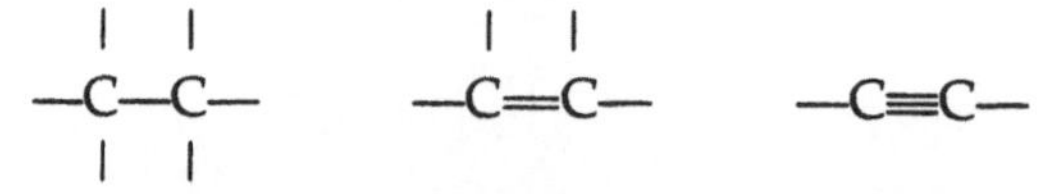

Figure 3.1 *Bonds between carbon atoms.*

The simplest organic compounds are the hydrocarbons which contain carbon and hydrogen only. There are basically two types of organic compound: aliphatic and aromatic. The structures of these can be illustrated by considering simple hydrocarbon structures.

Table 3.1 *Valency of some of the elements (other than carbon) commonly found in organic compounds*

Elements	*Valency*	*Representation*
Hydrogen	1	H—
Oxygen	2	—O—
Nitrogen	3	—N— (with a third bond below)
Sulphur	2	—S—
Phosphorus	3	—P— (with a third bond below)
Fluorine	1	F—
Chlorine	1	Cl
Bromine	1	Br—
Iodine	1	I—

1 Aliphatic compounds

These compounds contain chains of carbon atoms. The length of the chain ranges from two to several thousand carbon atoms. The chains may be either straight or branched.

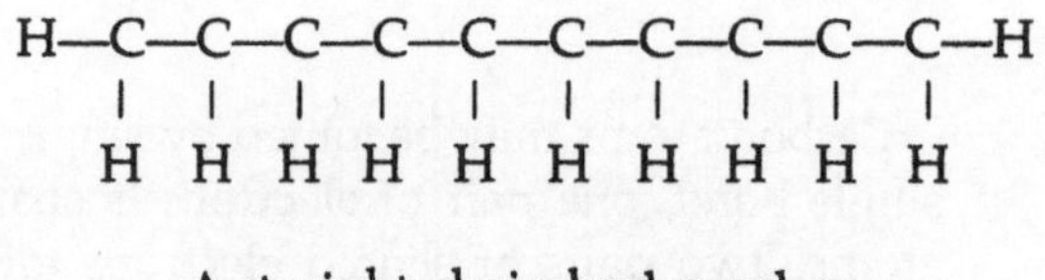

A straight-chain hydrocarbon

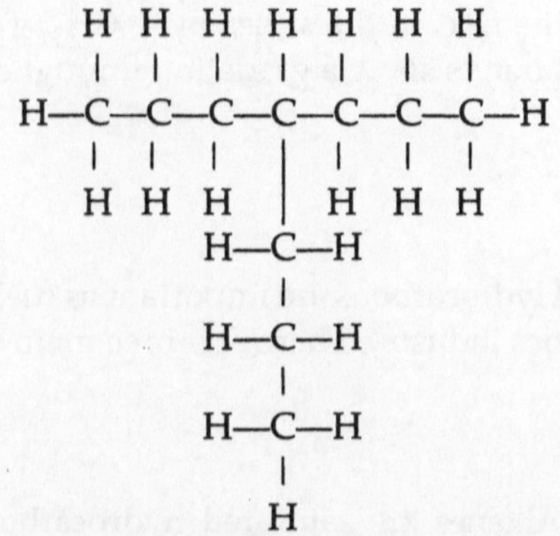

A branched-chain hydrocarbon

2 *Aromatic compounds*

Aromatic compounds, as their name suggests, often have a distinctive smell. In addition to forming chains, carbon atoms form ring structures. The most stable of these is the six-membered benzene ring, which is the basis of aromatic compounds.

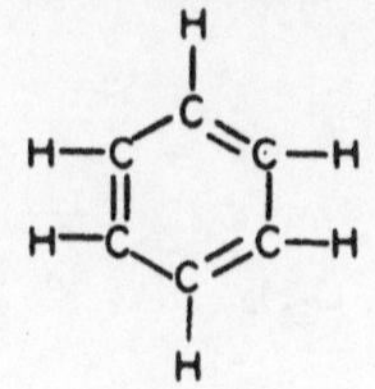

Benzene

The carbon and hydrogen atoms may be omitted, and the formula of benzene may be conveniently written as:

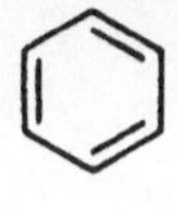

Homologous series

There are several million organic compounds and therefore it is almost impossible to study each compound individually. It is more convenient to place the compounds in groups and to study the properties of these groups. Organic compounds are therefore classified into groups known as homologous series. A homologous series is a group of compounds which have similar structures and therefore similar chemical properties. All members of the group can be represented by the same general formula. The molecular formula of a compound differs from the next in the series by —CH_2. The physical properties of the compounds show a gradation throughout the series.

Hydrocarbons

Hydrocarbons are important as fuels and as raw materials for the plastics industry. There are three main types of aliphatic hydrocarbons.

1 Alkanes

Alkanes are saturated hydrocarbons, i.e. all the bonds between the carbon atoms are single bonds. The structures and formulae of the simplest members of this series are shown in Table 3.2.

Table 3.2 *The simpler alkanes*

Name	*Molecular formula*	*Structural formula*	
Methane	CH_4	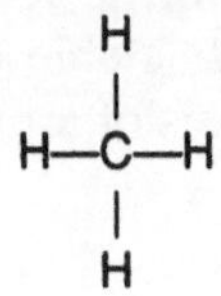	or CH_4
Ethane	C_2H_6	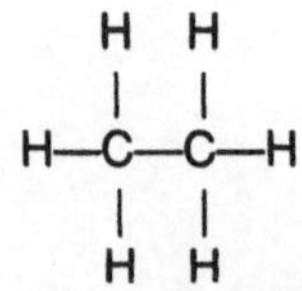	or CH_3CH_3
Propane	C_3H_8	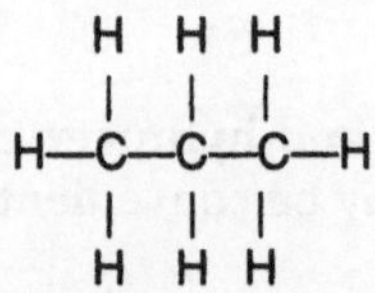	or $CH_3CH_2CH_3$
n-Butane	C_4H_{10}	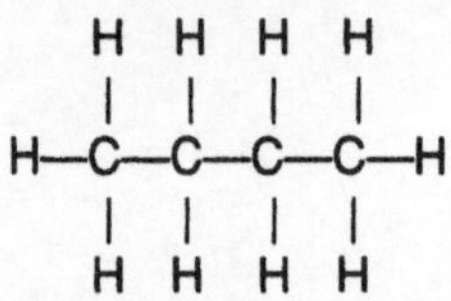	or $CH_3CH_2CH_2CH_3$
iso-Butane	C_4H_{10}	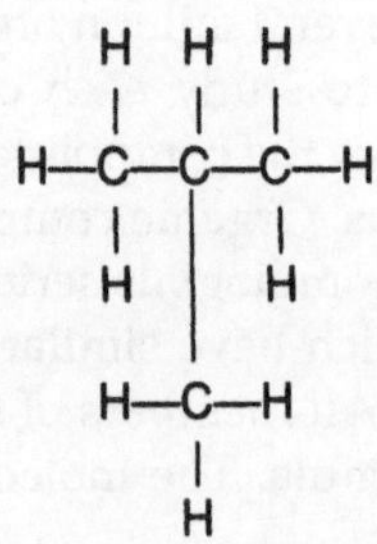	or $CH_3CHCH_3CH_3$

The main use of alkanes is as fuels. They all undergo combustion, i.e. are oxidized by burning in air to produce heat energy. One of the most important members of the series is methane. Over 90% of the gas in 'natural gas' is methane.

When methane is burned in a plentiful supply of air the products are carbon dioxide and water. The complete combustion of methane is shown by the following equation:

CH_4	+	$2O_2$	$\longrightarrow$	CO_2	+	$2H_2O$
methane		oxygen		carbon dioxide		water

If combustion is incomplete carbon monoxide may be formed. Carbon monoxide is poisonous and therefore it is essential to have an adequate air supply for gas water heaters and other gas equipment.

Propane and butane are used in gas cylinders for portable camping stoves and for industry.

Crude oil is a mixture of hydrocarbons. After the oil is refined a variety of products, including petrol, paraffin, diesel oil and lubricating oils, is produced.

Formulae

It can be seen from Table 3.2 that there are three ways of writing the formulae of organic compounds.

The **molecular formula** shows the total number of atoms of each element present in one molecule of the compound. It does not, however, give any indication as to how the atoms are joined to each other. Several or many organic compounds may exist with the same molecular formula. For instance, the formula C_4H_{10} may equally well refer to n-butane and iso-butane. Similarly, the formula $C_2H_4O_2$ may apply to both acetic acid and methyl formate. The **structural formula** indicates the arrangement of atoms within the molecule. This may be written as a *graphic formula*, using lines to represent the bonds between atoms, or as a *condensed structural formula* in which most of the lines are omitted and the way in which the atoms are joined is shown by writing their symbols in conventional groups. The graphic and condensed structural formulae of n-butane and iso-butane are shown in Table 3.2. The structural formulae of acetic acid and methyl formate are shown in Table 3.3.

Isomerism

Isomerism is the occurrence of two or more compounds with the same molecular formula but different structural formulae. There are two isomers of butane. The two isomers contain the same number of atoms of each element but the atoms are joined to each other in a different manner. Normal butane (abbreviated to n-butane) is an isomer of butane in which the chain of carbon atoms is unbranched. Iso-butane is a branched chain isomer. As the number of carbon atoms per molecule increases the number of possible isomers also increases. Pentane, the next alkane in the series after butane, has three isomers.

Table 3.3 *Structures of acetic acid and methyl formate*

Compound	*Molecular formula*	*Structural formulae*	
		Graphic	*Condensed*
Acetic acid (ethanoic acid)	$C_2H_4O_2$	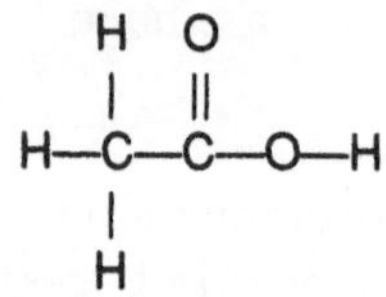	CH_3COOH
Methyl formate (methyl methanoate)	$C_2H_4O_2$	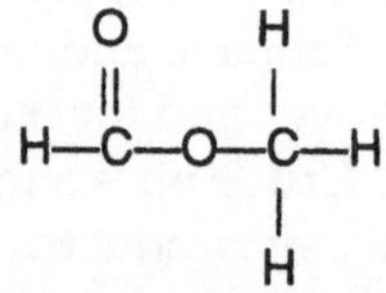	$HCOOCH_3$

Acetic acid and methyl formate are isomers since they have the same molecular formula, $C_2H_4O_2$.

2 Alkenes

Alkenes are unsaturated hydrocarbons, i.e. they contain carbon–carbon double bonds. The first two members of the series are ethene (ethylene) and propene (propylene), see Table 3.4.

Table 3.4 *The simpler alkenes*

Name	*Molecular formula*	*Structural formula*
Ethene (ethylene)	C_2H_4	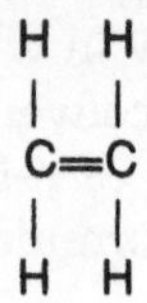 or $CH_2 = CH_2$
Propene (propylene)	C_3H_6	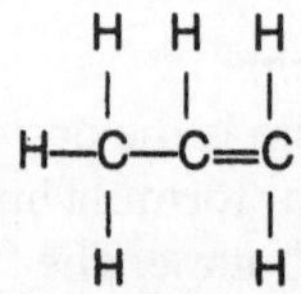 or $CH_3CH = CH_2$

All unsaturated compounds are reactive and will combine with hydrogen or other elements to form saturated compounds. A molecule containing one double bond will react with two atoms, i.e. one molecule, of hydrogen. For example, ethene combines with two atoms of hydrogen to form ethane.

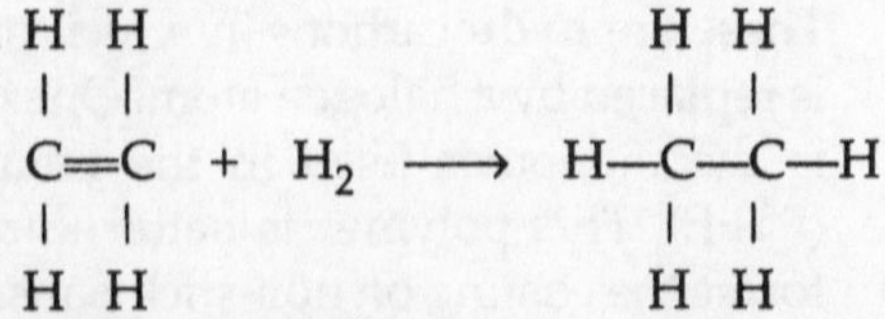

ethene hydrogen ethane

This type of reaction is called an **addition reaction.**

Polymerization

Polymerization is a chemical reaction in which small molecules, known as **monomers,** combine to form long chains, known as **polymers.** Molecules such as ethene and propene, which contain double bonds, undergo **addition polymerization.** In the formation of the polymer the double bonds are broken.

The following equation shows the formation of the plastic material polyethene (polyethylene), commonly known as polythene, from ethene:

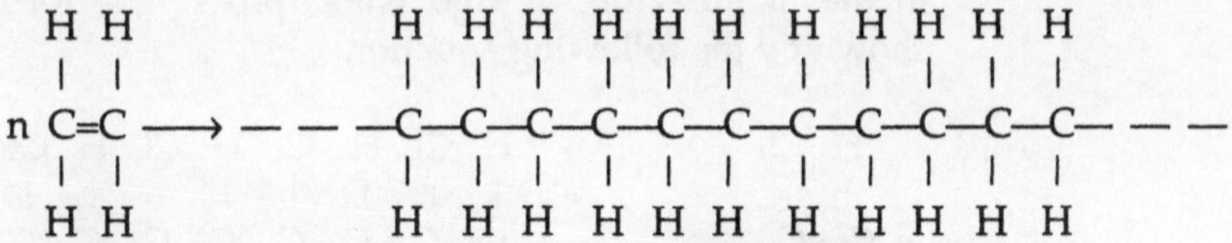

ethene (monomer) polyethene (polymer)

n = a large number

Propene polymerizes in a similar way to form polypropene (polypropylene).

3 Alkynes

Alkynes are a series of unsaturated hydrocarbons containing a carbon–carbon triple bond. The first member of the series is ethyne (acetylene); its structure is shown in Table 3.5.

Table 3.5 *The simplest alkyne*

Name	*Molecular formula*	*Structural formula*
Ethyne (Acetylene)	C_2H_2	H—C≡C—H or HC≡CH

Alkynes also undergo addition reactions and ethyne is used as a starting material in the production of many organic compounds.

Halogen derivatives of hydrocarbons

There are several important halogen derivatives of hydrocarbons. These are hydrocarbons in which one or more of the hydrogen atoms is replaced by a halogen atom. One of these is tetrafluoroethene, which is the monomer used in the manufacture of polytetrafluoroethene (PTFE). This polymer is better known by its trade name Teflon and forms the coating on non-stick pans. The following equation shows the polymerization of tetrafluoroethene:

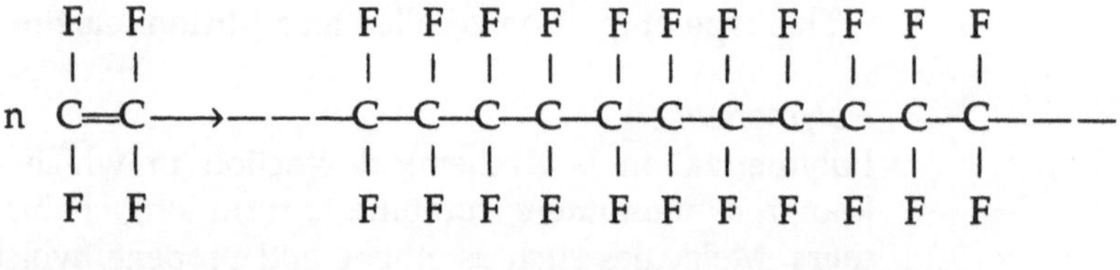

tetrafluoroethene polytetrafluoroethene (PTFE)

Chloroethene (vinyl chloride) is the monomer used in the manufacture of polychloroethene (polyvinyl chloride or PVC). PVC has many uses as a plastic. It is used as packaging film in the food industry and in the manufacture of cold water pipes. The formation of PVC is shown by the following equation:

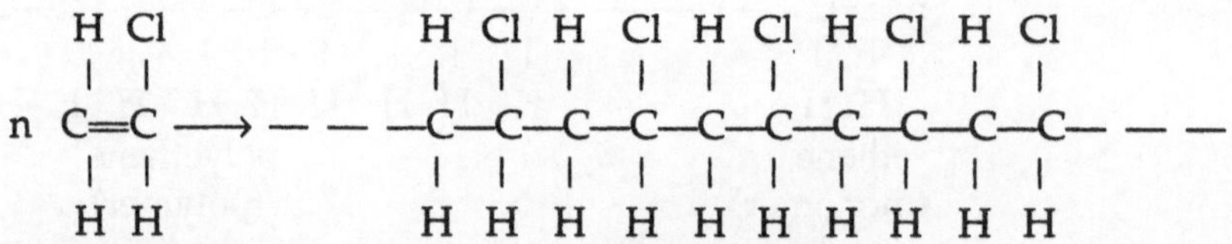

chloroethene (vinyl chloride) polychloroethene (polyvinyl chloride, PVC)

Functional groups

Many organic compounds have structures in which one of the hydrogen atoms in a hydrocarbon molecule is replaced by a functional group. A functional group is a group of atoms which, to a large extent, determines the chemical properties of the compound. Compounds containing the same functional group are members of the same homologous series.

Names of simpler organic compounds consist of two parts. The first part indicates the number of carbon atoms present in the molecule. This is shown in Table 3.6.

Table 3.6 *Naming of organic compounds according to the number of carbon atoms*

Name of compound	*Number of carbon atoms*
Meth-	1
Eth-	2
Prop-	3
But-	4
Pent-	5
Hex-	6
Hept-	7
Oct-	8
Non-	9
Dec-	10

The last part of the name of an organic compound indicates the functional group. Table 3.7 lists the names and formulae of functional groups of importance in this book.

Table 3.7 *Functional groups and their formulae*

Name of compound	*Functional group*	*Formula*	*Name of homologous series*
-ane		—H	alkanes
-anol	hydroxyl	—OH	alcohols
-anoic acid	carboxyl	—COOH	carboxylic acids
-anal	aldehyde	—CHO	aldehydes
-anone	carbonyl	$>$CO	ketones
-amine	amino	$—NH_2$	amines

Ethanol is derived from ethane and is composed of a hydrocarbon stem containing two carbon atoms (C_2H_5—) and a hydroxyl group (—OH). The formula of ethanol is C_2H_5OH. Acetic acid (ethanoic acid) contains two carbon atoms and has the formula CH_3COOH.

Naming organic compounds

Many organic compounds have two names: a systematic name and a trivial name. The systematic names have been derived under the IUPAC system (IUPAC stands for International Union of Pure and Applied Chemistry). Under this system the names used are based on the structure of the compounds. Using this system it is possible to write the structural formula of any compound from its name. The only disadvantage of the system is that for complicated molecules the name becomes very cumbersome; in such cases it is more sensible to use the trivial or common name. For example, 'glucose' is to be preferred to '2,3,4,5,6-pentahydroxyhexanal'. The trivial name is the common name by which the compound was originally known. Wherever possible systematic names have been used in this book but, for the sake of convenience, trivial names have sometimes been preferred, either because the systematic name is too long or because the trivial name is more meaningful. Where alternative names are given, the preferred name has been used in the main text and the alternative has been given in parentheses.

The Iupac system

The procedure for naming a compound, given its structural formula, is as follows:

1 Look for the longest unbranched chain in the molecule and select the systematic name for this skeleton.

2 Number the carbon atoms in this skeleton 1, 2, 3, etc., starting at a functional group if there is one present.

3 Look for the side groups attached to the main chain and the numbers of the carbon atoms to which they are attached.

4 The name then consists of the name of the longest unbranched chain, prefixed by the names of the side groups preceded by the numbers of the carbon atoms to which they are attached.

Alcohols

Alcohols are a homologous series of compounds in which one of the hydrogen atoms of a hydrocarbon molecule is replaced by a hydroxyl (—OH) group. The simplest members of the series are methanol and ethanol (see Table 3.8).

Table 3.8 *The simplest alcohols*

Name	*Structural formula*	
Methanol	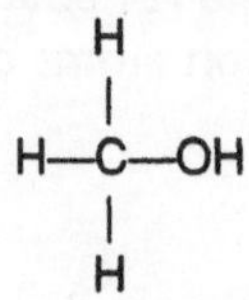	or CH_3OH
Ethanol	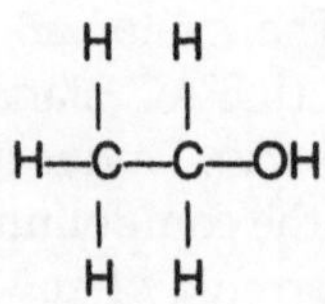	or C_2H_5OH

Methanol, also called methyl alcohol, is found in methylated spirits and badly distilled liquor. It is harmful and may cause blindness if taken in sufficient quantity. Ethanol, also called ethyl alcohol, is the alcohol found in beers, wines and spirits. It is produced by a fermentation process whereby yeast enzymes break down sugars forming ethanol and carbon dioxide (see page 218).

Methanol and ethanol are monohydric alcohols, i.e. each molecule contains one hydroxyl group. Some compounds contain more than one hydroxyl group per molecule. The most important of these is glycerol (propanetriol), which is a constituent of fats and oils. It is a trihydric alcohol, i.e. each molecule contains three hydroxyl groups.

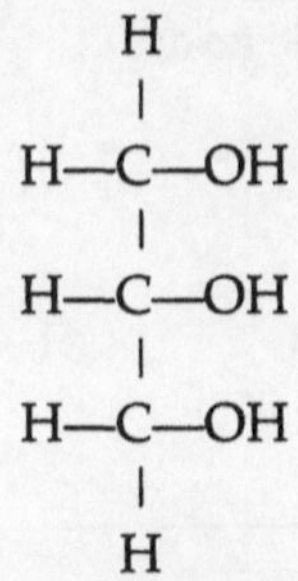

glycerol
(propanetriol)

Glycerol, also known as glycerine, is used as a softening and moistening agent in confectionery. It prevents hardening of Royal icing during storage. Sorbitol, a sugar substitute used in diabetic foods, is also an alcohol.

Carboxylic acids

Carboxylic acids, also known as organic acids, contain one or more carboxyl (—COOH) groups. These compounds are weak acids; the molecules partially dissociate to produce hydrogen ions. Organic acids resemble inorganic acids in that they are capable of forming salts.

Monocarboxylic acids contain one —COOH group. The simplest members of the series are shown in Table 3.9.

Monocarboxylic acids from butyric acid upwards combine with glycerol to form fats, and are known as fatty acids.

Vinegar is a dilute solution of acetic acid (ethanoic acid). In the presence of air certain bacteria convert ethanol into acetic acid. This process is used in the commercial production of vinegar. Propionic acid (propanoic acid) and its calcium and sodium salts are widely used as preservatives in flour confectionery. The salts are also used to impregnate wrapping materials to preserve fruits and vegetables.

Table 3.9 *The simplest monocarboxylic acids*

Name	*Structural formula*	
Acetic acid (ethanoic acid)	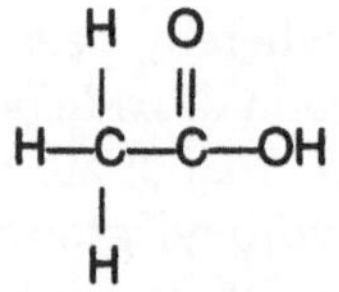	or CH_3COOH
Propionic acid (propanoic acid)	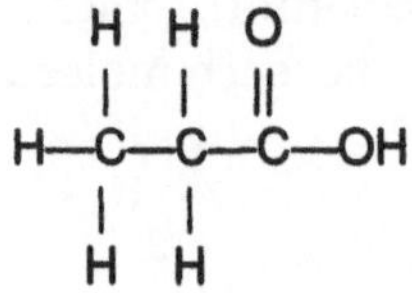	or CH_3CH_2COOH
Butyric acid (butanoic acid)	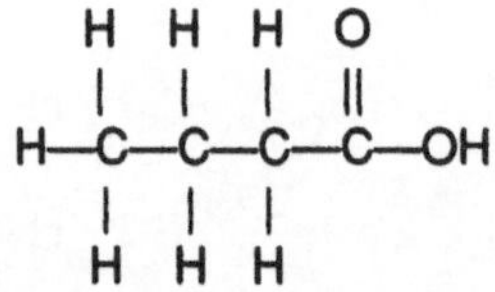	or $CH_3CH_2CH_2COOH$

Some organic acids contain more than one functional group. Lactic acid (2-hydroxypropanoic acid) contains both a carboxyl group and a hydroxyl group and has the following structure:

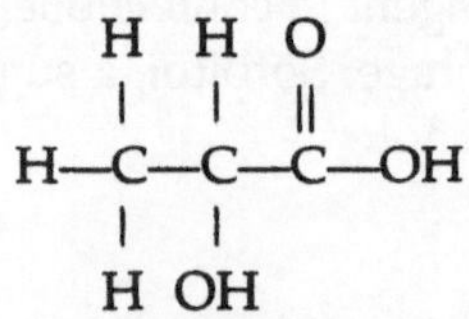

lactic acid
(2-hydroxypropanoic acid)

Lactic acid is found in muscle tissue. It is also formed, during the souring of milk, by the action of certain bacteria on lactose, the sugar in milk. There are two optical isomers of lactic acid. **Optical isomerism** occurs when a compound has an asymmetric carbon atom, i.e. a carbon atom with four different groups attached to it. The four groups in the lactic acid molecule are $—CH_3$, —H, —COOH and —OH. The isomers cannot be shown in two dimensions and it is necessary to imagine the three-dimensional structure of the molecule. The four covalent bonds of the carbon atom are arranged in space so that they are directed towards the corners of a tetrahedron. If the molecule has four different groups attached to the central carbon atom, two different structures or isomers are possible. The isomers are mirror images of one another, as shown below.

The main difference between the isomers is that they rotate the plane of polarized light in different directions. Light consists of waves vibrating in all directions, at right angles to the direction of the beam. Polarized light consists of waves vibrating in one direction or plane only.

Unpolarized light　　　　Polarized light

If a beam of polarized light is passed through a solution of one isomer, it is rotated to the right and this isomer is known as the dextro- (or d-) form of the compound. A solution of the other isomer will rotate the light to the left and is, therefore, called the laevo- (or l) form of the compound. Substances which show this type of isomerism are described as optically active compounds.

An instrument known as a polarimeter can be used to measure concentrations of optically active substances in solution by measuring the degree of rotation of polarized light.

Pyruvic acid (2-oxopropanoic acid) also contains two functional groups. It contains a carboxyl group and a carbonyl group (>C=O) and has the following structure:

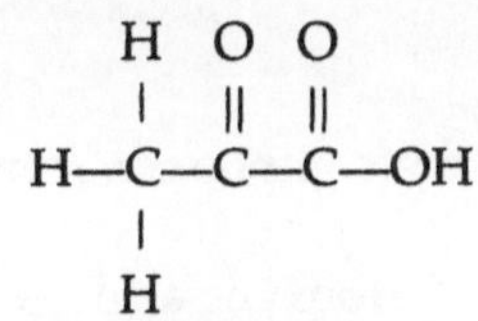

pyruvic acid
(2-oxopropanoic acid)

Pyruvic acid is formed in the body as a step in the breakdown of glucose to produce energy (see page 144).

Tartaric acid (2,3-dihydroxybutanedioic acid) is a dicarboxylic acid, i.e. each molecule contains two carboxyl groups. In addition there are two hydroxyl groups in each molecule. It has two asymmetric carbon atoms and is optically active.

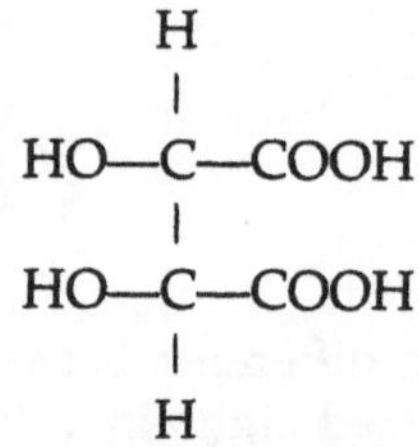

tartaric acid
(2,3-dihydroxybutanedioic acid)

It is found in fruits, especially in grapes, and is obtained commercially as a by-product in the production of wines.

Citric acid (2-hydroxypropane tricarboxylic acid) is a tricarboxylic acid, i.e. each molecule contains three carboxyl groups. In addition there is a hydroxyl group attached to the central carbon atom.

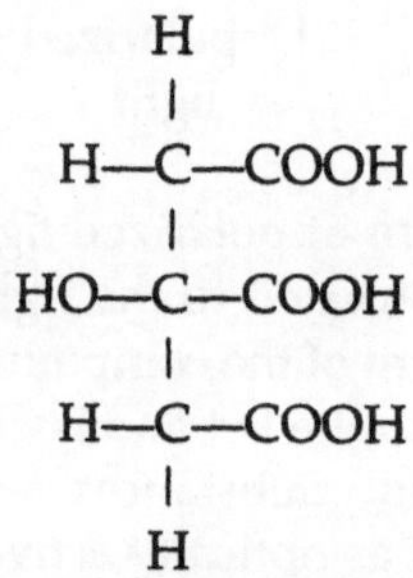

citric acid
(2-hydroxypropane tricarboxylic acid)

It occurs in citrus fruits and is widely used in the food industry for flavouring fruit drinks and other fruit products.

Esters

Esters are compounds formed when carboxylic acids react with alcohols.

Carboxylic acid + Alcohol ⟶ Ester + Water

For example:

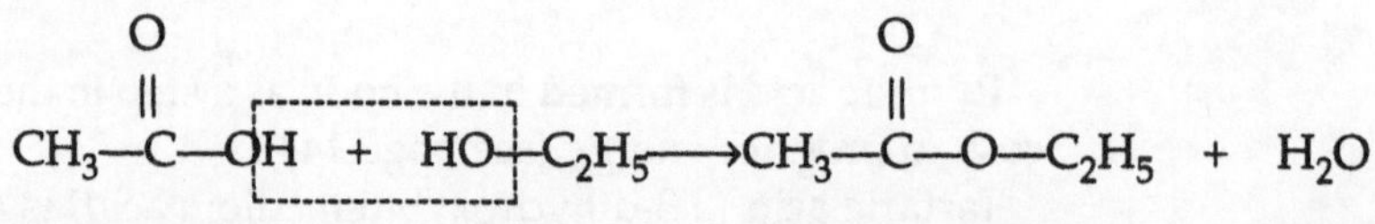

Acetic acid (ethanoic acid) | Ethanol | Ethyl acetate (ethyl ethanoate) | Water

A large variety of esters are found in food, especially in fruits. They are responsible for some of the characteristic flavours and odours of foods and are particularly important in wines, where they contribute to the bouquet. Esters can be produced synthetically and are used in the production of artificial flavours. For example, ethyl lactate (ethyl hydroxypropanoate) is used in synthetic grape flavouring and amyl acetate (pentyl ethanoate) is responsible for the characteristic flavour of pear drops.

Fats and oils are esters of fatty acids and glycerol (see Chapter 6).

Aldehydes

Aldehydes are a homologous series of compounds in which one of the hydrogen atoms of a hydrocarbon molecule is replaced by an aldehyde (—CHO) group. The names and structural formulae of some aldehydes are shown in Table 3.10.

Formaldehyde (methanal) is used in the manufacture of plastics, such as Melamine, and as a disinfectant. Aldehydes contribute to the flavour of foods. Acetaldehyde (ethanal), for example, is partly responsible for the characteristic flavour of yoghurt. Many aldehydes are used in the production of synthetic flavours. For example, benzaldehyde is used in artificial almond essences.

Table 3.10 *Some of the simpler aldehydes*

Name	*Structural formula*	
Formaldehyde (methanal)	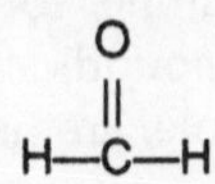	or HCHO
Acetaldehyde (ethanal)	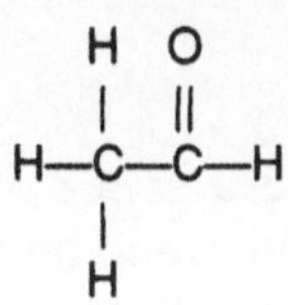	or CH_3CHO
Benzaldehyde	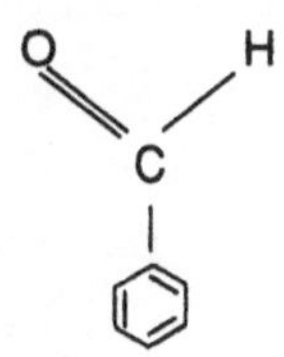	or C_6H_5CHO

Ketones

Ketones are a homologous series of compounds containing a carbonyl (>CO) group. The simplest member of the series is acetone (propanone) which has the following structure:

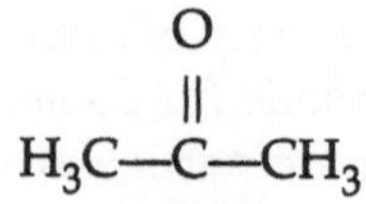

acetone
(propanone)

Many organic compounds dissolve in acetone and therefore acetone is used as a solvent in many industries.

Amines

Amines are a series of compounds in which a hydrogen atom of a hydrocarbon molecule is replaced by an amino (—NH_2) group. The simplest member of the series, methylamine (methamine), has the following structure:

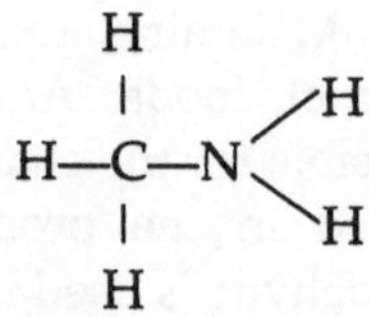

methylamine
(methamine)

Amines are produced during the spoilage and decay of protein foods. Trimethylamine, for example, has the characteristic odour of rotting fish. Compounds called diamines, which contain two amino groups per molecule, are used in the manufacture of nylon.

Amino acids

Amino acids are a series of compounds containing two functional groups, an amino group and a carboxylic acid group, attached to the same carbon atom. The simplest amino acid, glycine, has the following structure:

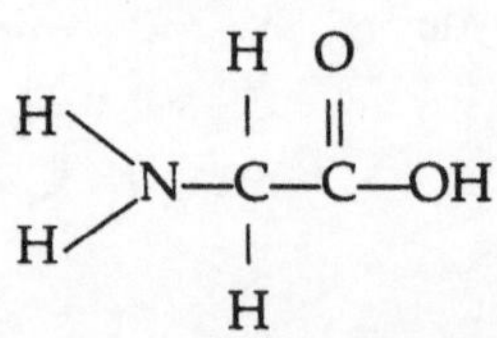

glycine

Amino acids are the monomers from which the polymers, proteins are made. The formation of proteins is an example of **condensation polymerization.** In this type of polymerization, when the monomers join together, a small molecule, usually water, is produced. Unlike addition polymerization it does not involve the breaking of double bonds.

4 Food dispersions

Nearly all foods contain water. The nutrients present in these foods are dispersed in water. Solids, liquids and gases may be dispersed in water to form either solutions or colloids.

Solutions

If sugar is placed in water it dissolves and produces a solution. A solution is homogeneous, i.e. the composition is uniform throughout.

A solution is made up of two components: the **solute,** which is the substance dissolved, e.g. sugar in the above example, and the **solvent,** the liquid in which the solute is dissolved, e.g. water in the above example. Solutions are not necessarily composed of a solid dissolved in a liquid. Soda water is a solution of a gas (carbon dioxide) dissolved in a liquid (water). Vinegar is a solution of one liquid (acetic acid) dissolved in a second liquid (water).

Dissolved substances cause an increase in the boiling-point and a depression of the freezing-point of solutions. The effect of a solute on the boiling-point and freezing-point of a solution is directly proportional to its concentration. Sugar solutions, used in confectionery, have boiling-points well above 100°C, the boiling-point of water. Salt is used to lower the freezing-point of water and to prevent ice forming on roads in winter.

Solutions are formed by inorganic compounds, in which the particles or ions have an affinity for water. If the particles of a compound have a greater attraction for each other than they have for water, the compound will be insoluble.

Mineral elements found in foods, such as sodium and chlorine, are usually present as ions and form true solutions. Small organic molecules, such as sugars, which have an affinity for water, also form true solutions. Vitamins, depending on their structure, may be either dissolved in the water or in the fat present in foods.

Solubility

The solubility of a substance is the extent to which the substance will dissolve in a given solvent. It is usually expressed as g solute per 100 ml solvent. The solubility of most substances increases with an increase in temperature.

A **saturated solution** is one in which no more solute will dissolve in the solvent at a given temperature.

Under certain conditions a **supersaturated solution** may be formed. A super saturated solution contains more dissolved solute than a saturated solution. (It can be obtained by cooling a saturated solution.) Supersaturated solutions are unstable and the excess dissolved solvent will readily revert to the solid form by the formation of crystals.

Crystallization

Under normal circumstances, when a saturated solution is cooled, particles of the solute will be deposited from the solution. The particles of the solid solute assume a characteristic geometrical shape and are known as crystals. Crystals may be a variety of different shapes. For example, crystals of salt (sodium chloride) are cubic. Crystallization is a useful method of purifying solids. It is used to purify many crystalline substances in the food industry, such as sugar, salt and citric acid.

Sugar boiling and crystallization

Pure water boils at 100°C (212°F). A solution of sugar in water boils at a temperature above 100°C. As the solution boils, water is evaporated from the surface of the solution and the sugar concentration will therefore increase. Different concentrations of sugar solutions are used for different purposes. Some examples are given in Table 4.1.

Table 4.1 *Boiling points of sugar solutions used in catering*

Boiling point °C	*Name*	*Use*
115	Soft ball	Making of marzipan and fondant
121	Hard ball	Making of nougat, petit fours, etc.
138	Soft crack	Making of Italienne meringue
143	Pulled sugar	Making of ornaments for decoration
154	Hard crack	Dipping of fruit and marzipan for petit fours. To make spun sugar for decoration
177	Caramel	Used for flavouring and colouring

When sugar solutions are cooled, the size of the sugar crystals which are formed depends on the rate of cooling. Slow cooling produces large crystals, which tend to give confectionery a gritty texture.

Therefore a variety of techniques are used to reduce crystal size or to avoid the formation of crystals.

Sugar products can be divided into two types:

1 **Crystalline,** e.g. fondant, soft toffee, fudge. These are boiled at lower temperatures and, therefore, have a higher water content.

In the manufacture of these products crystallization has been partly inhibited in order to result in the production of many microcrystals. This is brought about by the following:

(a) beating. For example, in the manufacture of fondant, a saturated sugar solution is cooled from 115°C to 40°C and is beaten steadily throughout. Care is needed, since a sugar or dust particle can trigger premature crystallization and the production of large crystals;
(b) inversion, the breakdown of sucrose to produce glucose and fructose (see page 63). For example, in the manufacture of fondant, an acid (cream of tartar) may be added to produce a mixture of glucose and fructose, which crystallizes more slowly;
(c) adding glucose;
(d) adding fat. For example, in the manufacture of toffee, cream or butter is added and acts by inhibiting crystal growth.

2 **Non-crystalline,** e.g. boiled sweets, butterscotch, spun sugar. If sugar is heated to 150°C–160°C in an acidic solution, i.e. with vinegar or lemon juice, inversion occurs. The resulting syrup is cooled quickly without agitation and it solidifies without crystallising, forming a glass-like solid, which has a hard, amorphous texture. The degree of inversion must be controlled or else the product will be too hygroscopic, i.e. will absorb water and become sticky on exposure to the atmosphere.

Diffusion

If there is a higher concentration of dissolved solute in one part of a solution, diffusion will take place, i.e. solute particles will move from a region of high solute concentration to a region of low solute concentration. This is due to the particles being in constant motion. Therefore if a solution is left to stand the particles will eventually become thoroughly mixed and the concentration will be equal throughout. Diffusion also takes place in mixtures of gases.

Osmosis

Filter paper is a permeable membrane since true solutions will pass through it. There are, however, some membranes which are only semi-permeable. Water molecules are small enough to pass through or 'permeate' the fine pores of these membranes but the larger solute molecules are not.

If a semi-permeable membrane forms a barrier between two solutions of unequal concentration, diffusion cannot take place, since the membrane forms a barrier preventing the free passage of solute molecules. Instead, water passes through the semi permeable membrane from the dilute to the more concentrated solution, and the solutions tend to become equal in concentration. This process is called osmosis and is shown diagrammatically in Figure 4.1.

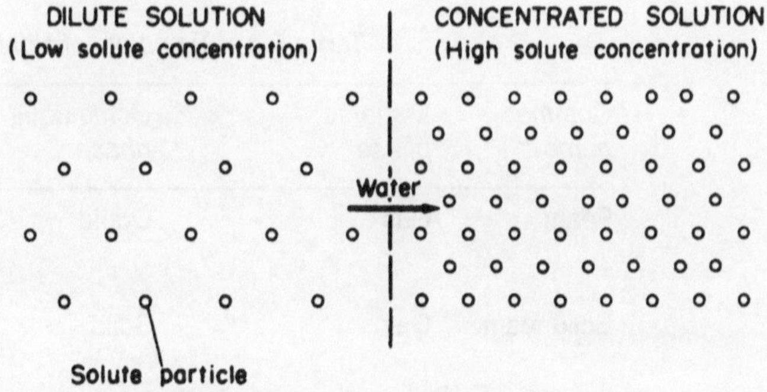

Figure 4.1 *Diagram illustrating osmosis.*

The force or pressure set up by the movement of the water is called **osmotic pressure.** The rate at which osmosis takes place depends on the difference between the concentrations of the two solutions.

The membranes of both plant and animal cells are semi-permeable. The root hairs of plants take in water by osmosis, since the dissolved mineral salts inside the cells of the root hairs exert an osmotic pressure. Osmosis plays a part in the regulation of the water content of the body tissues of animals. There are many examples of osmosis in food preparation and processing. If sugar is placed on a half grapefruit it will be noticed that, after a time, juice comes out of the grapefruit and dissolves the sugar. The sugar exerts an osmotic pressure. Both salt and sugar are used as food preservatives because of their osmotic effect on the microorganisms responsible for spoilage (see page 231).

Colloids

If a substance such as albumin, the protein in egg white, is mixed with water it does not dissolve but forms a colloidal dispersion. This dispersion is not a solution and is not homogeneous, since the molecules of protein do not dissolve. The molecules are dispersed throughout the water producing a heterogeneous or two-phase system. The substance which is dispersed in known as the **disperse phase** and it is suspended in the **continuous phase.** In the above example protein is the disperse phase and water the continuous phase. The particles of the disperse phase of a colloid are usually between 1 and 100 nm in diameter. They are intermediate in size between the small particles of a true solution and the larger, visible particles of a suspension. After a period of time the particles in a suspension settle out as a sediment, due to the effect of gravity.

There are various types of colloidal system depending on the physical state (solid, liquid or gas) of the two phases. Some of the colloidal systems found in foods are listed in Table 4.2.

Table 4.2 *Types of colloidal system*

Common name	*Disperse phase*	*Continuous phase*	*Examples*
Foam	Gas	Liquid	Beaten egg white Whipped cream 'Head' on beer
Solid foam	Gas	Solid	Bread Cake Meringue
Emulsion	Liquid	Liquid	Milk Cream Mayonnaise
Gel	Liquid	Solid	Jelly Baked egg custard
Sol	Solid	Liquid	Egg white

Aerosols, which are also colloidal systems, consist of solids or liquids dispersed in a gas. There are no food examples of aerosols.

Colloids are formed by large organic molecules or by aggregates of smaller organic molecules. Some inorganic materials may also form colloids if they are of a suitable particle size. In foods, proteins, polysaccharides, such as starch, and fats are often present in the form of colloids.

Most colloidal dispersions are fairly stable but the two phases may separate out over a long period of time. The rate of separation is accelerated by an increase in temperature or by mechanical agitation. Many colloids separate out on freezing; this causes problems when foods containing emulsions of fat and water are frozen.

Colloids in which the continuous phase is a liquid are important in food science, since many foods contain water and/or oil. These liquid-based colloids can be broadly categorized into two groups:

1 **Lyophilic colloids,** in which there is an attraction between the colloidal particles (the disperse phase) and the liquid of the continuous phase, e.g. sols and gels. If the continuous phase is water, these colloids are said to be hydrophilic.

2 **Lyophobic colloids,** in which there is no attraction between the particles of the disperse phase and the continuous phase, e.g. emulsions. If the continuous phase is water, these colloids are said to be hydrophobic.

Sols and gels

In the study of foods we are often concerned with colloidal systems in which the continuous phase is water. Water molecules possess the ability to form bonds, known as **hydrogen bonds,** either with other water molecules or with molecules of other substances. Water molecules consist of two hydrogen atoms joined by covalent bonds to an oxygen atom. The pairs of electrons which make up the covalent bonds are not shared equally but are attracted more strongly by the oxygen atom. The oxygen atom has a very slight negative charge, represented by the symbol δ–. The hydrogen atoms consist of an unshielded proton, since there are no electrons other than the one shared with the oxygen atom. Therefore, there will be a very slight positive charge, δ+, on both of the hydrogen atoms. Water molecules, therefore, have regions of localized charge and are attracted to one another by hydrogen bonds which are weak cohesive forces arising from electrostatic attraction (see Figure 4.2).

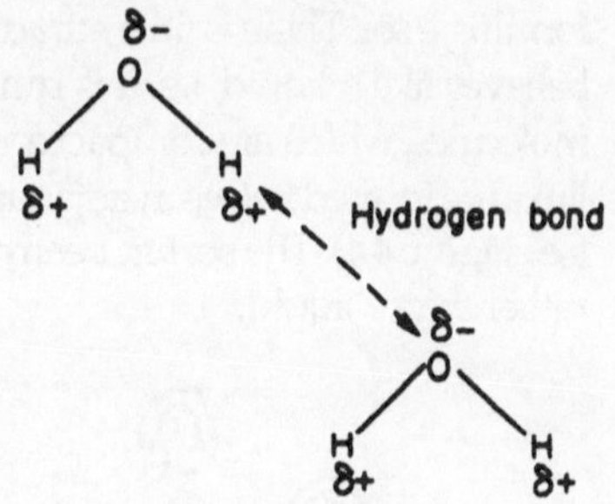

Figure 4.2 *Diagram showing hydrogen bonding between water molecules.*

The proteins and starch in foods may be present in the form of sols or gels. Proteins consist of amino acids joined by peptide links (see page 87). Each amino acid has a side chain which is basically a hydrocarbon chain but which may contain an amino group or a carboxylic acid group. Hydrogen bonding may take place either between the water molecules and the peptide links (as shown in Figure 4.3) or between the water molecules and the amino and carboxyl groups on the side chain.

Because of the attraction between parts of the protein chain and the water, the protein can be readily dispersed in the form of a colloid.

Starch consists of long chains of glucose units and contains many hydroxyl groups which can form hydrogen bonds with water molecules. Therefore starch can form colloids.

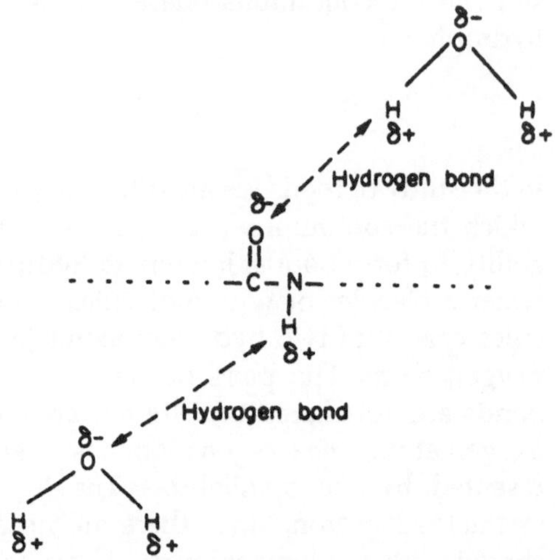

Figure 4.3 *Diagram showing hydrogen bonding between water molecules and atoms in a peptide link.*

When a jelly is made, gelatin (a protein) is dispersed in water and heated forming a sol. There is little attraction between the protein molecules and the sol behaves like a liquid, i.e. it is runny and can easily be poured. On cooling, the molecules, which are compact and coiled in the sol, begin to unwind and cross-links are formed between adjacent molecules and a mesh or network is formed (see Figure 4.4). The sol has been converted to a gel and the gel resembles a solid rather than a liquid.

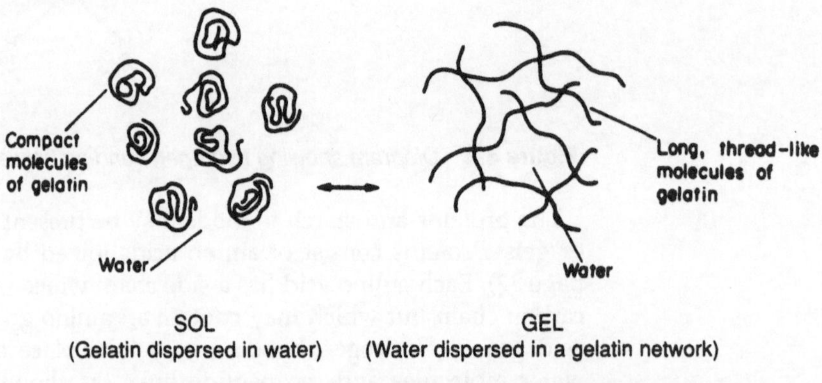

Figure 4.4 *Diagram showing the formation of a gel.*

Sometimes gel formation can be reversed. For example, if a jelly is heated it liquefies and forms a sol.

Corn starch (cornflour) and arrowroot are used as thickening agents, since they are both capable of forming sols and gels.

Syneresis is the shrinkage of a gel and the subsequent loss of liquid. This process may take place if a jelly is left to stand for a long time. A pool of liquid surrounding the base of the jelly indicates that syneresis has taken place. Scrambled egg is a gel and if it is overcooked syneresis may occur.

Emulsions

There are two main types of emulsions found in foods:

1 *Oil-in-water* emulsions, where the disperse phase consists of droplets of oil dispersed in the continuous phase, which is mainly water.

2 *Water-in-oil* emulsions, where the disperse phase consists of droplets of water dispersed in the continuous phase, which is mainly oil.

The structures of these two types of dispersions are shown diagrammatically in Figure 4.5.

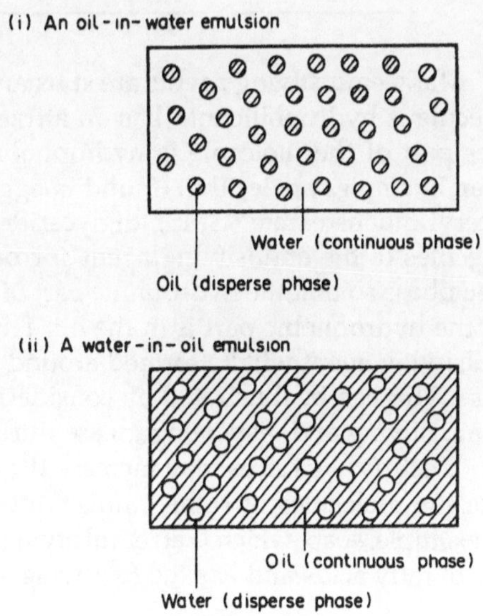

Figure 4.5 *Types of emulsions.*

Table 4.3 lists some examples of emulsions occurring in foods.

If water and oil are shaken up together and left for a short time the two liquids will separate, with the oil forming a layer on top of the water. Two such liquids which will not normally mix are said to be immiscible. In an emulsion two immiscible liquids are held in a stable colloidal state by means of a third substance, present in small quantities, known as an **emulsifying agent or emulsifier.** The mechanisms by which emulsifying agents assist in the formation of stable emulsions are complex and incompletely understood. However, the following types of action, which can occur either alone or in combination, have been investigated and have been shown to be important.

Table 4.3 *Emulsions found in foods*

Type of emulsion	*Food*
Oil-in-water	Milk Cream Mayonnaise Salad cream Gravy Cream soups Ice cream
Water-in-oil	Butter Margarine Egg yolk

1 Many emulsifying agents are substances in which one part of the molecule is hydrophilic and has an attraction for water, whereas the other part of the molecule is hydrophobic and has little affinity for water. Examples are lecithin (found in egg yolk), monoglycerides, e.g. glyceryl monostearate (GMS), diglycerides and most detergents. The molecules of the emulsifying agent surround the droplets of the disperse phase so that the hydrophilic part of the molecule is in the water and the hydrophobic part is in the oil. Thus a coating of molecules of emulsifying agent will be formed around the particles of the disperse phase. This can be illustrated by considering the action of a detergent in emulsifying and dispersing grease during washing (see Figure 4.6).

2 Electrostatic forces may increase the stability of some emulsions, since the molecules of some emulsifying agents are readily ionized. For example, soap, which is an emulsifying agent consists of the sodium salts of fatty acids and has the following structure:

$$\mathrm{R{-}\overset{\displaystyle O}{\overset{\|}{C}}{-}O^{-}Na^{+}}$$

(R is a hydrocarbon chain)

When grease is dispersed during washing, the sodium ions separate from the fatty acid chain and are dispersed throughout the water. The

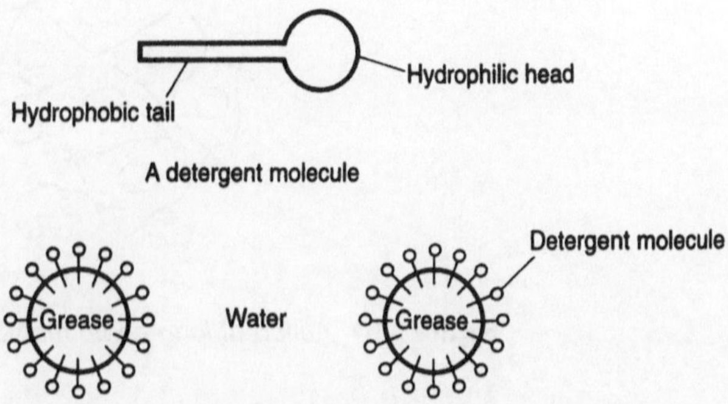

Figure 4.6 Diagram showing the action of a detergent (an emulsifying agent).

coating which remains around the droplets of grease consists of the fatty acid ions and has a negative charge. Since like charges repel each other, this coating will keep the droplets apart and prevent them from coalescing (see Figure 4.7).

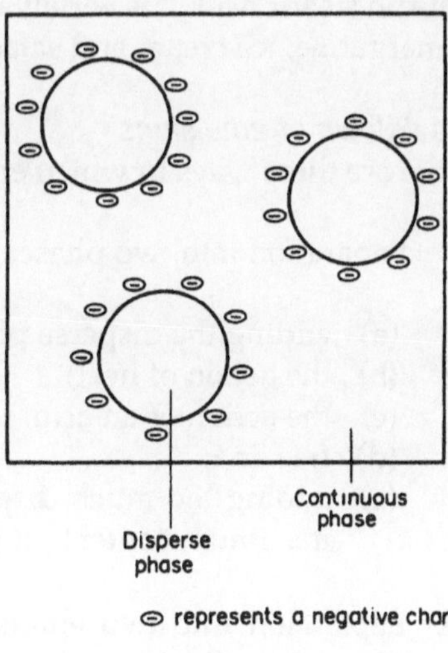

Figure 4.7 *Diagram showing coating of electrostatic charge around particles of the disperse phase.*

3 Stabilizers help to maintain an emulsion once it has been formed. Stabilizers are long chain molecules, e.g. proteins and starches, which form a network within the continuous phase which separates the droplets of the disperse phase and prevents coalescence (see Figure 4.8).

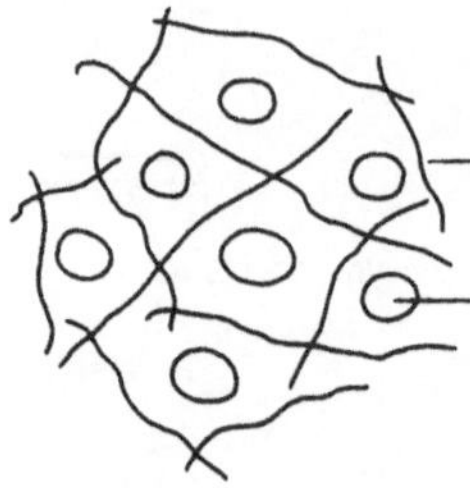

Figure 4.8 *Action of long chain molecules in preventing coalescence.*

Stabilizers also increase the stability of the emulsion by increasing the viscosity of the continuous phase. Stabilizers used commercially include proteins, such as gelatin, and carbohydrates, such as pectin, sodium alginate and a variety of gums.

Emulsifying agents, both natural and artificial, are widely used in food preparation. Lecithin is an important naturally occurring emulsifying agent. It is present in egg yolk and many vegetable oils. Commercially it is extracted from soya bean oil. The most important of the artificial emulsifiers is glyceryl monostearate, which is an ester of glycerol and stearic acid. It is widely used in the manufacture of foods such as margarine, ice cream and salad cream.

Breakdown of emulsions

There are three ways in which emulsions may break down.

1 Separation into two phases. This may be caused by:

(a) adding the disperse phase too quickly during preparation;
(b) the action of heat;
(c) the action of an acid, i.e. lowering the pH;
(d) freezing;
(e) adding too much disperse phase during preparation. (The maximum content of the disperse phase is about 74%.)

2 Separation into two emulsified layers, e.g. the formation of a cream layer in milk.

3 Phase inversion. The disperse phase becomes the continuous phase and vice versa. This occurs during the formation of butter from cream and is caused by mechanical agitation.

Foams

A foam consists of very small bubbles of a gas, usually air, dispersed in a liquid. It is the action of substances dissolved in the liquid which stabilizes the foam, since the dissolved substances decrease the surface tension of the liquid and prevent the molecules of the liquid from massing together (see page 262).

Egg white foams

Egg white foams are stabilized in two ways:

1 The protein in egg white, albumin, is a thick, viscous solution. When the egg white is beaten and bubbles of air are incorporated, the albumin drains more slowly out of the bubble walls than a thin liquid would. All of the proteins present in egg white probably act in a similar way. They are large molecules, which get in the way of each other and of the water that surrounds them and therefore contribute to the high viscosity.

2 The various proteins present in egg white confer a mechanical stability on the bubble walls. When egg white is beaten and air is incorporated, one part of the protein molecule is attracted to the water through hydrogen bonds, while other parts of the molecule will align themselves so that they are in contact with the pocket of air, since they have no attraction for the water. This action causes the molecules, which are normally compact, to unfold. Once unfolded, the protein molecules bond with each other forming a network, which holds the water in place while shielding it from the pockets of air.

Added ingredients affect the stability of egg white foams. Fat, even in small amounts, e.g. a little egg yolk, interferes with foam formation and reduces the volume by as much as two-thirds. Acid, on the other hand, improves stability. Many meringue recipes include a small amount of acid in the form of cream of tartar. Salt increases whipping time and reduces foam stability. Sugar has a mixed effect. It delays foaming and reduces maximum volume but helps to prevent drainage and collapse during cooking. It is, therefore, normally folded into egg white after whipping but before baking.

If an egg white foam is heated, the protein coagulates and a meringue, a solid foam, is formed. Bread is a further example of a solid foam.

Ice cream

Ice cream is a complex substance being both an emulsion and a foam. It has four phases:

1 Fat globules. Milk fat is used in dairy ice cream, whereas vegetable fat is used in non-dairy ice cream.

2 Air cells. In order to impart a creamy texture these should be small (less than 0.1 mm diameter).

3 Ice crystals. These consist of pure water. They should be small and well dispersed, otherwise the product will have a gritty texture.

4 Liquid containing dissolved sugar, suspended milk proteins, stabilizers, flavours, colours, etc. The stabilizers, such as alginates or gelatin, give the ice cream body and prevent rapid melting.

5 Carbohydrates

Carbohydrates are a group of nutrients important in the diet as a source of energy. They contain the elements carbon, hydrogen and oxygen and are produced in plants by the process of **photosynthesis**, which may be represented by the following equation:

$$6CO_2 + 6H_2O \xrightarrow{\text{chlorophyll}} C_6H_{12}O_6 + 6O_2$$

$6CO_2$	+	$6H_2O$	$\xrightarrow{\text{chlorophyll}}$	$C_6H_{12}O_6$	+	$6O_2$
carbon dioxide (from the air)		water (from the soil)	sunlight (solar energy)	glucose ↓ other carbohydrates		oxygen (released into the air)

Chlorophyll is a green pigment which absorbs energy from sunlight and enables plants to build up carbohydrates from carbon dioxide and water.

There are various different carbohydrates but they may be divided into three main groups according to the size of their molecules:

increasing size of molecule ↓		
	MONOSACCHARIDES	SUGARS
	DISACCHARIDES	SUGARS
	POLYSACCHARIDES	NON-SUGARS, e.g. starch

Sugars

1 *Monosaccharides*

The monosaccharide sugars commonly found in food contain six carbon atoms and have the general formula $C_6H_{12}O_6$. The three most important members of this group are:

(A) Glucose (Dextrose)

The structure of a molecule of glucose is shown in Figure 5.1. In the conventional representation the carbon atoms in the ring are omitted.

Glucose is found in varying amounts in fruits and vegetables. Large amounts are found in fruits such as grapes and smaller quantities in vegetables such as young peas and carrots. It is also found in the blood of animals.

Glucose syrup or commercial glucose is not pure glucose but a mixture of glucose, other carbohydrates and water (see page 65).

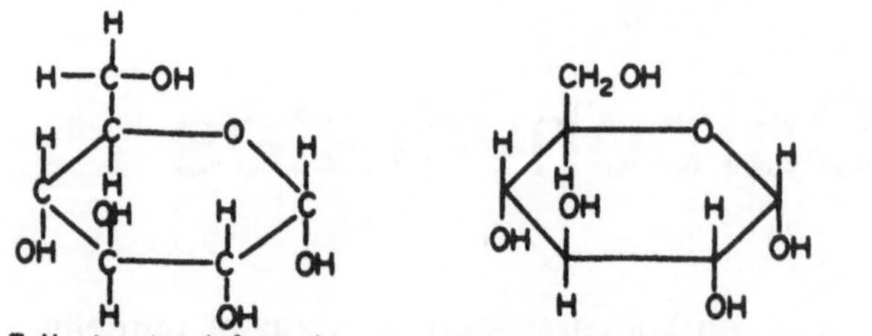

Figure 5.1 *Structure of glucose.*

(B) Fructose (Laevulose)

This is chemically similar to glucose except that the arrangement of the atoms within the molecule is slightly different. Fructose is found, together with glucose, in many fruits and in honey.

(C) Galactose

This is also chemically similar to glucose. It does not exist as such in foods but is produced when lactose, a disaccharide, is broken down during digestion.

2 Disaccharides

These sugars have the general formula $C_{12}H_{22}O_{11}$. They are formed when two monosaccharide molecules combine with the elimination of a water molecule.

$C_6H_{12}O_6$	+	$C_6H_{12}O_6$	$\longrightarrow$	$C_{12}H_{22}O_{11}$	+	H_2O
monosaccharide		monosaccharide		disaccharide		water

This is an example of a **condensation reaction**, i.e. a reaction in which two small molecules combine to form one larger molecule with the elimination of a small molecule, usually water, from between them.

(A) Sucrose

This is ordinary household 'sugar' and is produced in plants by the condensation of glucose and fructose. The structure of sucrose is shown in Figure 5.2.

Sucrose is found in many fruits and vegetables, some of which, e.g. sugar cane and sugar beet, contain relatively large quantities. It is from cane and beet that sugar is extracted commercially.

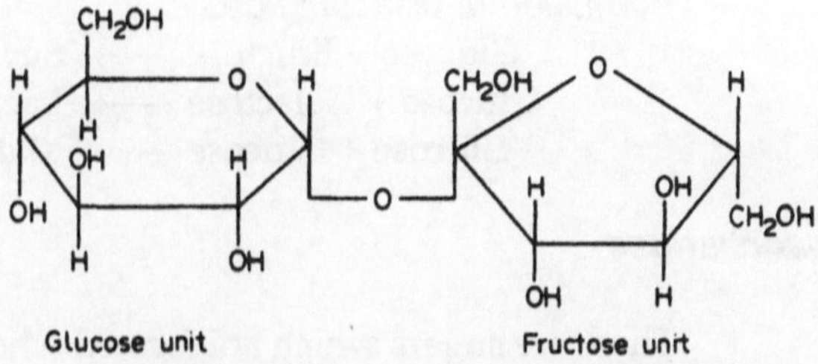

Figure 5.2 *Structure of sucrose.*

Production and refining of sugar

Both sugar cane and sugar beet contain about 15% sucrose. Sugar cane is grown in tropical countries. The sugar is extracted by crushing the canes and spraying them with water so that the sucrose diffuses into the water. Impurities in the solution are removed by treatment with lime and carbon dioxide, followed by evaporation. Raw sugar is then separated from the molasses by centrifugal spinning. This raw sugar, which contains about 96% sucrose, is exported to sugar-consuming countries such as Britain to be refined. The refining process involves centrifuging and washing to remove any remaining molasses. This is followed by treatment with lime and carbon dioxide to remove other impurities, treatment with charcoal to decolorize the solution and vacuum evaporation to crystallize the sucrose. At this stage the mixture consists of sugar crystals suspended in syrup. The syrup is removed by spinning in centrifugal separators and the damp sugar is dried in a current of hot air.

Sugar beet, which is produced in countries with a temperate climate such as Britain, is processed to white sugar as one continuous process. The beets are sliced and steeped in hot water to extract the sucrose. The solution is purified with lime and carbon dioxide. This is followed by evaporation and crystallization. The sugar crystals are centrifugally separated from the remaining syrup and molasses, and finally dried.

Molasses, the main by-product of sugar production, is used as an ingredient by food manufacturers and animal food producers. It can also be fermented and made into rum.

(B) Lactose

This sugar is formed by the condensation of glucose and galactose. It is found only in milk, where it is the sole carbohydrate.

(C) Maltose

A molecule of maltose is formed by the condensation of two glucose molecules. During the germination or sprouting of barley, starch is broken down into maltose. Malt, a vital ingredient in brewing, is produced by this process.

Formation of disaccharides

Glucose + Fructose ⟶ Sucrose + Water
Glucose + Galactose ⟶ Lactose + Water
Glucose + Glucose ⟶ Maltose + Water

3 Oligosaccharides

These are sugars which are formed when more than two monosaccharide molecules combine. They are normally present in foods in only small amounts. Examples of oligosaccharides include:

raffinose, a trisaccharide (3 monosaccharide units)
stachyose, a tetrasaccharide (4 monosaccharide units)

Properties of sugars

1 Appearance and solubility
All sugars are white, crystalline compounds which are soluble in water.

2 Sweetness
All sugars are sweet but they do not all have the same degree of sweetness. The sweetness of different sugars may be compared, using a point scale in which the sweetness of sucrose is taken as 100. Table 5.1 shows the relative sweetness of various sugars.

Table 5.1 *The relative sweetness of various sugars*

Sugar	*Relative sweetness*
Fructose	170
*Invert sugar	130
Sucrose	100
Glucose	75
Maltose	30
Galactose	30
Lactose	15

*A mixture of glucose and fructose (see below).

3 Hydrolysis
Disaccharides undergo a process of hydrolysis to form monosaccharides. Hydrolysis is the chemical breakdown of a molecule, by combination with water, producing smaller molecules. This process may be represented by the following equation:

AB	+	H_2O	$\longrightarrow$	*AOH*	+	*BH*
large molecule		water		small molecule		small molecule

For example:

$C_{12}H_{22}O_{11}$	+	H_2O	$\longrightarrow$	$2C_6H_{12}O_6$
1 molecule of disaccharide		water		2 molecules of monosaccharide

Sucrose + Water $\longrightarrow$ Glucose + Fructose
Lactose + Water $\longrightarrow$ Glucose + Galactose
Maltose + Water $\longrightarrow$ Glucose + Glucose

It can be seen that these are the reverse of the condensation reactions by which disaccharides are formed.

The hydrolysis of sucrose is also known as the **inversion of sucrose** and the product, a mixture of glucose and fructose, is called 'invert sugar'. Inversion may be brought about either by heating sucrose with an acid or by adding the enzyme invertase. Invert sugar is used in the production of jam, boiled sweets and some other sugar confections. A small quantity of invert sugar, added to a hot sucrose solution will help reduce the likelihood of crystallization when the solution is cooled.

4 *Effect of heat*

When sugars are heated they caramelize. Although caramelization occurs most readily in the absence of water, sugar solutions (syrups) will caramelize if heated strongly enough. Caramel is a sweet, brown substance and is a mixture of carbohydrate-like compounds.

5 *Reducing properties*

All the monosaccharides and disaccharides mentioned, with the exception of sucrose, act as reducing agents (see page 28) and are therefore known as **reducing sugars**. The ability of these sugars to reduce oxidizing agents forms the basis of several tests for glucose and other reducing sugars. For example, these sugars reduce the copper(II) ions of Fehling's solution to copper(I) ions on boiling, producing an orange precipitate. Sucrose is a non-reducing sugar and therefore does not reduce Fehling's solution.

Polysaccharides

Polysaccharides are condensation polymers of monosaccharides and are made up of many monosaccharide molecules joined together, with the elimination of one water molecule at each link. They have the general formula $(C_6H_{10}O_5)n$, where 'n' represents a large number.

1 Starch

Starch is the major food reserve of plants. It is a mixture of two different polysaccharides:

(a) *Amylose*. The amylose molecule consists of between 50 and 500 glucose units joined in a straight chain.

(b) *Amylopectin*. This molecule consists of up to 100,000 glucose units joined in a branched-chain structure.

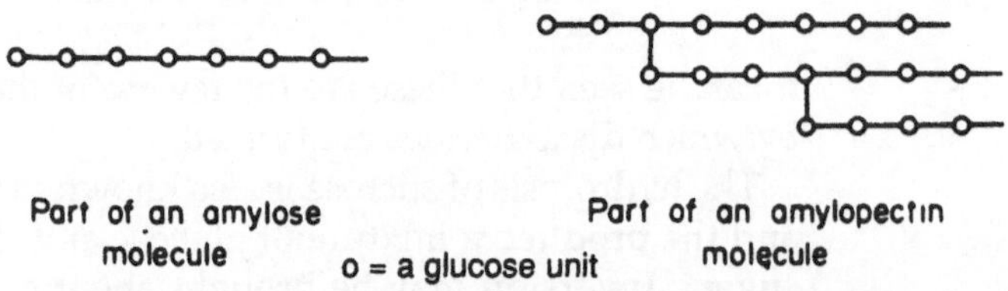

Figure 5.3 *Structure of amylose and amylopectin.*

The starch in many plants, including wheat, rice, corn and potato, consists of approximately 80% amylopectin and 20% amylose. Microscopic examination shows that the starch in plant cells occurs as small grains or **granules**. The outer layer of each granule consists of closely packed starch molecules which are impervious to cold water. The different plant sources of starch are characterized by the shape of the granules and by the distribution of granule sizes. Typical potato and corn starch granules are shown in Figure 5.4.

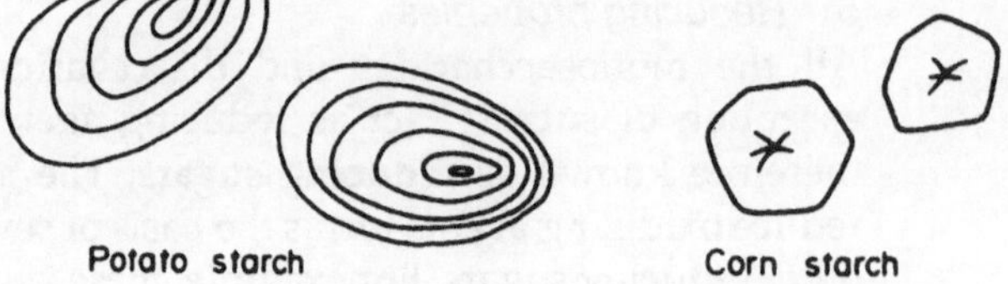

Figure 5.4 *Typical starch granules.*

Properties of starch

1 Appearance and solubility

Starch is a white, non-crystalline powder which is insoluble in cold water.

2 *Sweetness*

Unlike monosaccharides and disaccharides, starch and other polysaccharides do not have a sweet taste.

3 *Hydrolysis*

Hydrolysis of starch may be brought about by the action of an acid or an enzyme. If starch is heated with an acid it is broken down into successively smaller molecules, the final product being glucose.

$$\underset{\text{starch}}{(C_6H_{10}O_5)n} \quad + \quad \underset{\text{water}}{nH_2O} \quad \longrightarrow \quad \underset{\text{glucose}}{nC_6H_{12}O_6}$$

There are various stages in this reaction. The large starch molecules are first broken down into shorter chains of glucose units known as dextrins. The dextrins are further broken down into maltose (two glucose units) and, finally, the maltose is broken down into glucose.

$$\text{starch} \longrightarrow \text{dextrins} \longrightarrow \text{maltose} \longrightarrow \text{glucose}$$

Hydrolysis of starch may also be brought about by enzymic action. During digestion the enzyme amylase breaks down starch into maltose. Amylase is also present in flour and germinating grain where it is also known as diastase. It is important in breadmaking and brewing since it produces a sugar (maltose) which yeast enzymes are able to break down further to produce carbon dioxide and alcohol. For a more detailed description of the action of enzymes in digestion and breadmaking, see Chapter 11.

Commercial glucose syrups (liquid glucose) are produced by hydrolysing corn (maize) starch with hydrochloric acid and/or the enzyme amylase. Hydrolysis is not complete and the syrups are a mixture of glucose, maltose and longer chains of glucose units. The extent of hydrolysis of a glucose syrup is measured in terms of its dextrose equivalent (DE). A high DE syrup contains more dextrose (glucose) and is therefore sweeter than a low DE syrup.

4 *Effect of heat*

(a) **Gelatinization** (with water). If a suspension of starch in water is heated, the water penetrates the outer layers of the granules and the granules begin to swell. This occurs as the temperature rises from 60°C to 80°C. The granules may swell until the volume is as much as five times the original. As the size of the granules increases the mixture becomes viscous. At about 80°C the starch granules break up and the contents become dispersed throughout the water. The long-chain molecules begin to unfold and the starch/water mixture becomes more viscous, i.e. thickens, forming a sol (see page 51). On cooling, if the proportion of starch to water is sufficiently great, the starch molecules form a network with the water enclosed in its meshes so producing a gel. The entire process is known as the gelatinization of starch and is very important in cooking. For example, it is responsible for the thickening of sauces, soups and gravies by the addition of flour or cornflower. It is also important in the baking of bread and other flour goods where it contributes to the desired crumb structure and texture of the product.

The strength of a starch gel depends on a variety of factors including:

(i) the proportions of starch and water present. The more starch the stronger the gel;
(ii) the proportion of amylose in the starch. Amylose aids gelling because the molecules are spiral-shaped and form a network in which water is trapped. High amylose starches are used, therefore, where a rigid gel is needed. Amylopectin molecules are larger than amylose but are more compact and, therefore, do hot hold water as well. High amylopectin starches (i.e. waxy starches) gel only at high concentration;
(iii) the presence of sugar. Sugar competes with the starch for water and therefore reduces gel strength;
(iv) the presence of acid. Acid hydrolyses starch and reduces gel strength forming a viscous paste. This occurs, for example, in lemon pie filling.

Although amylose-containing starches gel best, they are less stable than high amylopectin starches. The amylose molecules tend to unwind and the gel becomes opaque and like a pulpy sponge. This change is called **retrogradation** and occurs particularly when foods are frozen and then thawed. High amylopectin starches, e.g. waxy corn starch, should be used when preparing foods for a freeze/thaw process. Alternatively, chemically-modified starches are widely used in frozen manufactured foods as they do not retrograde easily.

Pregelatinized starches are used in some manufactured foods. These are cooked in water, i.e. gelatinized, and then dried. They are used, for example, in instant dessert mixes.

(b) **Dextrinization** (dry heat). Many foods containing starch also contain small amounts of dextrins. On heating, dextrins polymerize to form brown-coloured compounds called pyrodextrins. Pyrodextrins contribute to the brown colour of many cooked foods including toast and bread crust.

2 Cellulose

Cellulose is another polysaccharide consisting of long chains of glucose units. It acts as a structural material in plants, being found in cell walls where it gives rigidity. The basic structure of cellulose is similar to that of starch but the glucose units are linked in a different way. Man does not possess enzymes capable of breaking this type of linkage and therefore is unable to use cellulose as a food. However, cellulose is important for providing fibre (NSP) in the diet. Dietary fibre is necessary for the efficient passage of food through the alimentary canal and the regular emptying of the bowel (see page 71). Cows, and other ruminant animals, are able to break down and utilize cellulose for energy due to the presence of cellulose-digesting bacteria in the rumen (the first of the four stomachs of the cow). This explains why cows can utilize grass as food, whereas man cannot.

3 Glycogen

This is a carbohydrate found only in animals. It can be thought of as the carbohydrate reserve in animals in the same way as starch is the carbohydrate reserve in plants. Animals store glycogen in the muscles and liver, and when required it is converted into glucose which is then broken down to provide energy. Glycogen, like amylopectin, is composed of branched chains of glucose units.

4 Pectin

Pectin is a complex mixture of polysaccharides found in many fruits and some root vegetables. Apples and the peel of citrus fruits are particularly rich in pectin. Its main importance is as a gelling agent, especially in jam making. Sugar is needed for gel formation, about 65% giving best results. This is about the amount normally present in jam. pH also affects gel strength, the optimum for gel formation being pH 3.0–3.5. In jams made from fruit with a low pectin content, such as strawberries, the addition of an acid, e.g. lemon juice, lowers pH and aids setting. Pectin is broken down in fruit as the fruit ripens. Jam will not gel satisfactorily if made from overripe fruit.

In some instances the presence of pectin may be undesirable; for example, in wines, pectin produces an unacceptable haze. Unwanted pectin can be removed by the addition of pectolytic enzymes.

5 Gums, alginates and agar

Gums such as tragacanth, arabic and guar are produced by plants and are used in food manufacturing as thickeners, stabilizers and gelling agents in a wide range of foods including ice cream, salad dressings and fruit pie fillings. Certain seaweed extracts are used in a similar manner. These include carageenan (Irish moss), alginates, e.g. sodium alginate, and agar (or agar-agar). Agar is also used in the preparation of microbiological media.

Functions of carbohydrates in the body

Available carbohydrates (starch and sugars) are digested and absorbed into the bloodstream. Starch and disaccharides are hydrolysed by digestive enzymes and are therefore absorbed as monosaccharides. In the liver, fructose and galactose are converted into glucose. Carbohydrates are used in the body in the following ways.

1 *Energy*

Glucose is oxidized in the cells. It is broken down in a series of reactions and energy is released when this takes place (see Chapter 10).

1 g of carbohydrate provides 17 kJ (4 kcal)

2 *Storage*

Glucose in excess of energy requirements can be:

(a) converted into glycogen and stored in the liver and muscles as a readily available source of energy;
(b) converted into fat and stored all over the body in the fatty cells of the adipose tissue.

An average adult has about 400 g of stored glycogen and about 12 kg of stored fat. However, an excessive energy intake over a period of time leads to larger fat stores and obesity.

3 *Dietary fibre*

Unavailable carbohydrates (i.e. those not broken down by digestive enzymes) give bulk to the faeces (see page 71).

Sources of carbohydrate in the diet

1 *Cereals and cereal foods*

All cereals contain a high percentage of starch. Wheat is the most important cereal in Britain. However, rice, maize (corn), oats, rye and barley are also included in the diet. Many foods made from cereals, such as bread, cakes, pastry, pasta and breakfast cereals, also contain considerable quantities of starch.

Cereal foods account for 47% of the total carbohydrate content of the average British diet.

2 *Refined sugar (sucrose)*

Sugar is eaten in large quantities, both in the form of table sugar and in manufactured foods, such as biscuits, sweets, chocolates, ice cream, jams, cakes and soft drinks.

Sugar, preserves and confectionery account for 14% of the total carbohydrate content of the average British diet.

3 *Vegetables*

Vegetables contain starch and sugars in varying amounts. The most important vegetable supplying carbohydrate in the diet is the potato. Pulse vegetables also contain a significant amount of carbohydrate but root and green vegetables contain smaller quantities.

Vegetables account for 14% of the total carbohydrate content of the average British diet.

4 *Fruits*

As fruit ripens starch is turned into sugars. Most fruits contain between 5% and 10% sugars, the sweeter fruits (e.g. grapes) containing the most. Bananas are the only common fruit which contain starch as well as sugar when ripe.

Fruit accounts for 6% of the total carbohydrate content of the average British diet.

5 *Milk*

Milk contains the sugar lactose. Foods such as cheese and butter which are made from milk usually do not contain carbohydrate, though soft cheeses such as cottage cheese contain small amounts.

Milk and related foods account for 8% of the total carbohydrate content of the average British diet.

The available carbohydrate content of some of these foods is shown in Table 5.2.

Carbohydrates and health

1 *Sugars and starch*

The main energy-giving foods in the diet are those which contain considerable amounts of sugar, starch or fat. Generally speaking, foods rich in sugar or fat are more expensive than starchy foods. Most countries have a staple food which is a cheap, starchy cereal food. In countries which still have a low standard of living and a poor diet, up to 90% of the energy content of the diet may be provided by one of the staple foods. In most affluent countries the cheap, starch staple is less important, but more sugars and fats are eaten. In Britain, sugars provide 18% of the total energy in the diet and fats about 40%.

Table 5.2 *Carbohydrate content of some foods*

Food	*% Carbohydrate*	*% Sugars*	*% Starch*
Sugar	100	100	0
Frosties	94	42	52
Rice	86	0	86
Cornflakes	86	8	78
White flour	78	1.5	76
Honey	76	76	0
Biscuits, semi-sweet	75	22	53
Spaghetti	74	3.3	71
Jam	69	69	0
Chocolate, milk	59	57	2.9
White bread	49	2.6	47
Potatoes	17	0.6	17
Apple	12	12	0
Peas	11	4.3	7.0
Carrots	7.9	7.6	0.3
Milk	4.8	4.8	0
Cabbage	4.1	4.0	0.1

Sugars can be divided into two types according to the way in which they are found in foods:

(a) **Intrinsic sugars**. These are sugars which are naturally present and are built into the cellular structure of food, e.g. glucose and fructose found in the cells of fruit and vegetables. When these intrinsic sugars are eaten as part of the cellular structure of food, as with fruit, there is no evidence of any adverse effects on health.

(b) **Extrinsic sugars**. These are not incorporated in cells. They may be from natural, unprocessed foods such as lactose in milk and fructose in honey or more frequently from refined or processed foods such as table sugar, fruit juices and manufactured foods with added sugar or glucose syrup.

The term **'non-milk extrinsic sugars (NMES)'** is used to describe the sugars other than lactose which are not within the cellular structure of food. NMES consist largely of sucrose and are associated with tooth decay. Tooth decay (dental caries) is caused by acids produced by oral bacteria which break down sugars in the plaque on teeth. There is a link between the incidence of tooth decay and a high NMES intake, or more acurately a frequent NMES intake. Present NMES consumption is nearly 70 g per person per day but less than one-third of this is sold as packet sugar. The remainder comes from manufactured foods such as cakes, biscuits, ice creams and other desserts, sweets and soft drinks.

As well as contributing to tooth decay, sugar-containing foods being very palatable are often eaten in excess and are, therefore, a contributory factor in the development of obesity. Sugar is said to provide 'empty calories'. In other words, it is a source of energy but contains no other essential nutrients, such as vitamins and minerals.

Since there are health risks associated with diets containing a lot of sugar and fat, it is recommended that more starchy foods (cereals, bread, potatoes, etc.) should be eaten to provide the necessary energy in the diet. Most starchy foods also provide other important nutrients. For example, bread is a good source of protein, calcium, iron, B vitamins and fibre, and potatoes contain vitamin C and B vitamins.

Current nutritional guidelines recommend a reduction in sugar intake to 20 kg per person per year (about 55 g per day) or approximately 10% of dietary energy, while at the same time increasing the intake of starch and intrinsic sugars in fruit so that total intake of carbohydrates increases to 50% of dietary energy. This allows for a reduction in fat intake.

2 Non-starch polysaccharides (dietary fibre)

Non-starch polysaccharides (NSP) are found in the cell walls of plants where they give structural support. They include insoluble cellulose (insoluble fibre) and soluble pectins, hemicellulose and gums (soluble fibre). Non-starch polysaccharides are resistant to breakdown by enzymes in the small intestine and they pass unchanged into the large intestine (bowel). The more familiar term 'dietary fibre' also includes the non-carbohydrate material lignin, the woody substance found, for example, in old vegetables but this is excluded from 'non-starch polysaccharide'.

The outer layers of cereal grains (the bran or husk) are a rich source of NSP. In wheat, maize and rice the NSP is mainly insoluble whereas in oats, rye and barley a large proportion is soluble. Vegetables contain approximately equal amounts of soluble and insoluble NSP.

Insoluble NSP acts by binding water in the intestines. This increases the bulk of the material passing through the large intestine and stimulates movements of the intestinal wall (peristalsis) thus giving bulk to the faeces and aiding the voiding of faeces. Some NSP is broken down in the large intestine by the action of bacteria normally found there. The carbon dioxide and methane gases produced as a result of this are the cause of flatulence or 'wind'.

Research has shown that the average UK diet contains insufficient NSP. In Western, industrialized countries much of the carbohydrate consumed is in a highly refined form such as sugar, white flour and white bread. In these countries there is a relatively high incidence of diseases of the alimentary tract such as diverticular disease (small bulges in the wall of the large intestine), cancer of the colon and haemorrhoids (piles). These conditions are associated with constipation and the slow transit of food through the alimentary canal. In some rural communities in Africa these diseases are virtually unknown. The diet in these areas contains many coarser unrefined foods and is, therefore, much higher in NSP and the transit time of food through the alimentary canal is much shorter.

There is evidence that some soluble forms of NSP (e.g. from beans and oats) reduce blood cholesterol levels (both total and LDL cholesterol) and so reduce the risk of coronary heart disease (see page 85). It has been suggested that high fibre diets slow the rate of sugar absorption and reduce the risk of developing diabetes.

At present the average intake of NSP in the UK is 12 g per day with about half of this provided by cereals and the remainder mainly from vegetables. The 1994 COMA report recommends an increase in the intake of NSP by adults from 12 g to 18 g per day. People should therefore be encouraged to eat more wholegrain cereal products (wholemeal bread, wholegrain breakfast cereals, brown rice, etc.) and to increase the amount of fruit and vegetables in the diet. However, the NSP present in cereals, especially wheat, contains phytates (see page 127) which can form complexes with minerals, such as calcium and iron, making them unavailable to the body. This could present a problem to people with a diet unusually high in NSP (especially from unprocessed wheat bran) and low in minerals. Table 5.3 shows the NSP content of a variety of foods.

Table 5.3 *NSP (fibre) content of some foods*

Food	*g NSP per 100 g food*
All Bran	24.5
Weetabix	9.7
Peanuts	6.2
Wholemeal bread	5.8
Peas	4.7
Baked beans	3.7
Carrots	2.4
Cabbage	2.4
Digestive biscuits	2.2
Raisins	2.0
Brown rice	1.9
Apples	1.8
White bread	1.5
Potatoes	1.3
Bananas	1.1
Cornflakes	0.9
White rice	0.4

6 Fats and oils (lipids)

Fats and oils, also known as **lipids,** are like carbohydrates in that they contain the elements carbon, hydrogen and oxygen. They are esters of glycerol and fatty acids (see Chapter 3). Glycerol is a trihydric alcohol, i.e. it has three —OH groups. The general formula of a fatty acid (alkanoic acid) is RCOOH where R represents a hydrocarbon chain. Each —OH group of the glycerol reacts with the —COOH of a fatty acid to form a molecule of fat or oil. This is an example of a condensation reaction (see page 60).

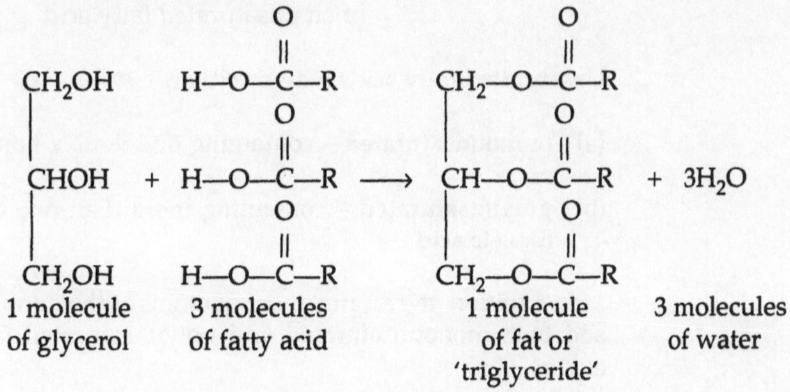

Fats and oils are mixtures of **triglycerides.** A triglyceride consists of one molecule of glycerol combined with three fatty acid molecules, as shown in the above equation. Diglycerides consist of glycerol combined with two molecules of fatty acid, and in monoglycerides only one fatty acid molecule is present. Diglycerides and monoglycerides are used as emulsifiers (see page 54).

The simplest type of triglyceride is one in which all three fatty acids are the same. However, triglycerides usually contain two or three different fatty acids and are known as mixed triglycerides. Naturally occurring fats and oils are mixtures of different mixed triglycerides and therefore may contain a number of different fatty acids. There are about 40 different fatty acids found in foods.

There are basically two types:

1 **Saturated fatty acids** in which the hydrocarbon chain is saturated with hydrogen

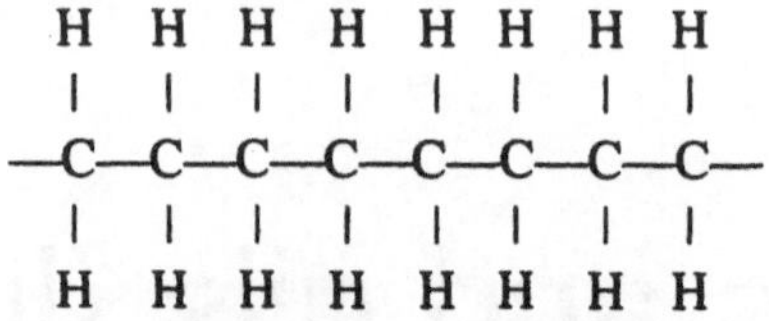

part of the hydrocarbon chain
of a saturated fatty acid

2 **Unsaturated fatty acids** in which the hydrocarbon chain is not saturated with hydrogen and therefore has one or more double bonds.

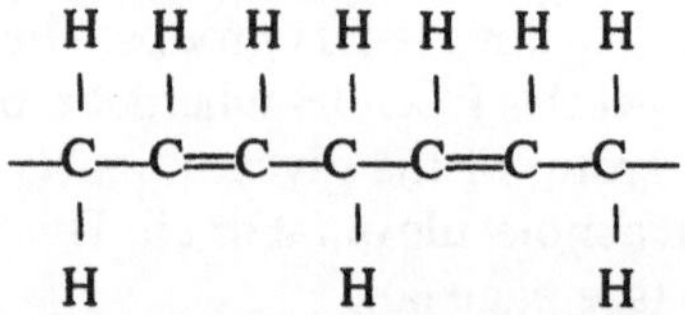

part of the hydrocarbon chain
of an unsaturated fatty acid

Unsaturated fatty acids may be either:

(a) **monounsaturated** – containing one double bond, e.g. oleic acid; or

(b) **polyunsaturated** – containing more than one double bond, e.g. linoleic acid.

In addition, the arrangement of atoms at the double bond may vary and both monounsaturated and polyunsaturated fatty acids can be either:

(a) cis fatty acids – with the two hydrogen atoms on the same side of the double bond;
or

(b) trans fatty acids – with the hydrogen atoms on geometrically opposite sides of the double bond.

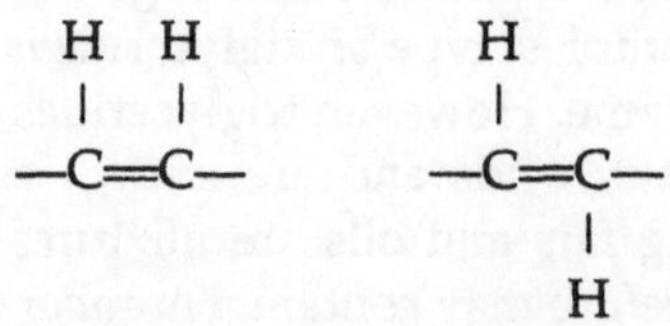

cis trans

Some of the more important fatty acids are listed in Table 6.1.

Fats and oils have the same general chemical structure. In common use the word 'fat' is used to refer to mixtures of triglycerides which are solid at normal air temperature, whereas the word 'oil' refers to those which are liquid at the same temperature. The difference between a fat and an oil may be explained by the presence of different fatty acids. Fats contain a large proportion of saturated fatty acids distributed among the triglycerides, and oils a large proportion of unsaturated fatty acids. The presence of unsaturated fatty acids lowers the slip point, i.e. the temperature at which the fat or oil starts to melt. In general, fats are obtained from animal sources and oils from vegetable sources. Both fats and oils contain small amounts of non-triglyceride; in particular, fatty acid complexes containing phosphate, called phospholipids.

Table 6.1 *Some common fatty acids*

Type	*Name*	*Formula*	*Number of double bonds*	*Occurrence*
Saturated	Butyric acid	C_3H_7COOH	0	Milk fat and butter
	Palmitic acid	$C_{13}H_{31}COOH$	0	Occur widely, particularly in solid fats
	Stearic acid	$C_{17}H_{35}COOH$	0	
Monounsaturated	Oleic acid	$C_{17}H_{33}COOH$	1	Occur in fats and oils
Polyunsaturated	Linoleic acid	$C_{17}H_{31}COOH$	2	
	Linolenic acid	$C_{17}H_{29}COOH$	3	Found mainly in vegetable and fish oils

The degree of unsaturation, i.e. the number of double bonds, of a fat or oil may be measured in terms of its **iodine value.** A molecule of iodine (I_2) will react with each double bond, and thus unsaturated oils have higher iodine values than saturated fats.

Vegetable oils should not be confused with either mineral oils or essential oils. Mineral oils are obtained from crude oil and are mixtures of hydrocarbons (see page 32). Essential oils are found in plants but are not triglycerides. They are volatile organic compounds, i.e. they evaporate easily, and are responsible for the flavour of many spices and other foods. Eugenol, for example, is responsible for the flavour of cloves.

In countries where bread is the staple food there is a greater demand for spreadable fats than for liquid oils. Since vegetable oils are more readily available than animal fats much of the vegetable oil produced in the world is converted into fat by a process of **hydrogenation.** Hydrogenation is the addition of hydrogen across a double bond. Thus an unsaturated fatty acid is turned into a saturated fatty acid. In this way vegetable oils can be used in the manufacture of margarine, other spreadable fats and cooking fats.

Properties of fats and oils

1 Solubility

Fats and oils are insoluble in water. However, in the presence of a suitable substance known as an emulsifying agent, it is possible to form a stable mixture of fat and water. This mixture is termed an emulsion. The emulsion may be a fat-in-water emulsion, e.g. milk, or a water-in-fat emulsion, e.g. butter. Emulsions are explained in more detail in Chapter 4.

Fats and oils are soluble in organic solvents such as petrol, ether and carbon tetrachloride. Solvents of this type can be used to remove grease stains from clothing.

2 Effect of heat

As fats are heated there are three temperatures at which noticeable changes take place.

(A) Melting point

Fats melt when heated. Since fats are mixtures of triglycerides they do not have a distinct melting point but melt over a range of temperature. The temperature at which melting starts is called the slip point. Most fats melt at a temperature between 30°C and 40°C. The melting point for oils is below normal air temperature. The more double bonds the lower the melting point.

(B) Smoke point

When a fat or oil is heated to a certain temperature it starts to decompose, producing a blue haze or smoke and a characteristic acrid smell. Most fats and oils start to smoke at a temperature around 200°C. The smoke point for lard is 185°C and for corn oil is 232°C. In general, vegetable oils have a higher smoke point than animal fats. Decomposition of the triglycerides produces small quantities of glycerol and fatty acids. The glycerol decomposes further producing a compound called acrolein. This decomposition is irreversible and, when using a fat or oil for deep frying, the frying temperature should be kept below the smoke point. Smoke point is a useful measure when assessing the suitability of a fat or oil for frying purposes. Repeated heating of a fat or oil or the presence of burnt food particles will reduce the smoke point. Repeated heating will also produce oxidative and hydrolytic changes in the fat and result in the accumulation of substances giving undesirable flavours to the foods cooked in the fat.

(C) Flash point

When a fat is heated to a high enough temperature, the vapours given off will spontaneously ignite. This temperature is known as the flash point. For corn oil the flash point is 360°C. Water should **never** be used on a fat fire. It will only spread the fire because the fat will float on the water. The heat should be turned off and the oxygen supply cut off by covering the container of burning fat with a lid or blanket.

3 Plasticity

Substances which possess the property of plasticity will change their shape, when pressure is applied to them, but will remain in their final shape when the pressure is removed. They do not return to their original shape. Fats are plastic at certain temperatures, i.e. they are soft and can be spread. The plasticity of a fat is due to the fact that fats are mixtures of triglycerides and that each triglyceride has its own melting point; this means that at a given temperature some of the fat will be liquid and some will be in the form of a crystalline solid. Fats containing smaller crystals, which are produced by rapid cooling of the fat during manufacture, will be more plastic.

The range of temperature over which a fat shows plastic behaviour is known as the plastic range of the fat. A mixture of triglycerides with a large range of melting points will form a fat with a wide plastic range. This type of fat is better for certain purposes; for example, for creaming and spreading. Margarines are manufactured to have a wide plastic range and will therefore spread straight from the refrigerator. Most animal fats have a narrow plastic range and are hard and difficult to spread.

4 Rancidity

Rancidity is the term used to describe the spoilage of fats and oils. There are basically two types.

(A) Oxidative rancidity

This occurs as a result of the reaction between unsaturated triglycerides and oxygen from the air. Oxygen molecules join across the double bond of the triglyceride molecule and a variety of compounds are formed including aldehydes and ketones, which give rise to an unpleasant rancid taste. The reaction is accelerated by heat, light and traces of metals, such as copper and iron.

(B) Hydrolytic rancidity

Enzymes known as lipases hydrolyse fats, breaking them down into glycerol and fatty acids.

$$\text{Fat} + \text{Water} \xrightarrow{\text{lipase}} \text{Glycerol} + \text{Fatty acids}$$

Lipases may occur naturally in fats and oils, but they can be inactivated by heat treatment. They may also be produed by micro-organisms present in fatty foods. The free fatty acids, especially the short-chain ones, which are produced by this reaction can give fats an unpleasant taste and smell. For example, the unpleasant taste of rancid butter is mainly due to the fatty acid butyric (butanoic) acid.

Rancidity can be reduced by storing fats and oils in a cool, dark place in a non-metal container and by keeping fats well wrapped. Antioxidants, such as BHT (butylated hydroxytoluene), are added commercially to many fats and fatty foods to reduce oxidative rancidity. Vegetable oils contain natural antioxidants such as vitamin E, though this is destroyed by heat treatment.

5 Saponification

Triglycerides react with alkalis forming a soap and glycerol. This process is known as saponification. Sodium hydroxide (caustic soda) is the alkali most commonly used in soap manufacture but potassium hydroxide (caustic potash) may also be used. The reaction may be represented by the following equation:

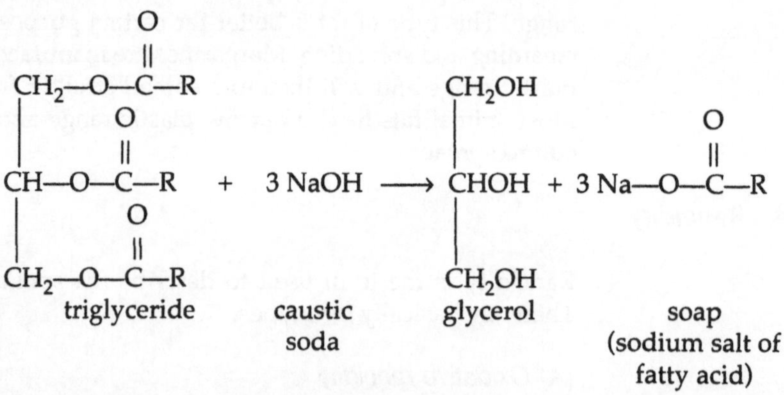

R represents a hydrocarbon chain which varies in structure depending on the nature of the fatty acids contained in the fat used. Soap is a mixture of sodium salts of different fatty acids.

Some uses of fats and oils in food preparation

1 Frying

Frying is a rapid method of cooking because high temperatures, usually about 180°C, are employed and heat transfer from the fat or oil to the food is rapid. Fats with a high smoke-point are best for frying. It is important to keep fats free from water. Fried food has a characteristic colour and flavour found very acceptable by most people.

2 Shortening effect

Fats have a shortening effect in baked goods, i.e. they make products, such as cakes and biscuits, more crumbly and palatable. They surround the starch granules and protein molecules and thus break up the structure. Fat also prevents contact between the protein in the flour and water in the dough and so restricts the formation of gluten (see "Bread" section in Chapter 14). The gluten that does form is in short lengths and not long elastic strands. Pure fats (rather than emulsions such as butter and margarine which contain water) are the best shortening agents and plastic fats are best as they coat the flour particles readily.

3 Creaming and aerating effect

When making rich cakes, fat and sugar are beaten or creamed together. This process incorporates small air bubbles into the mixture, forming a foam and so lightening the product. The addition of an emulsifying agent to the fat used for creaming helps to disperse the air bubbles.

The production of oils and fats

1 Vegetable oils

About 70% of all oils and fats produced in the world are of vegetable origin. Oils are obtained from nuts and seeds of plants such as corn (maize), groundnut (peanut), soya bean, olive, sunflower, cottonseed, palm, coconut and rapeseed. The composition of these oils varies considerably. Soya, sunflower and corn oils are particularly high in polyunsaturated fatty acids (PUFA), olive oil and rapeseed oil in monounsaturates and coconut and palm oils are higher in saturates (see Figure 6.1). Rapeseed is now grown in some quantity in Europe. Bright yellow fields of rape in flower in early summer are a common sight in Britain. The original varieties used contained erucic acid, a fatty acid which has been associated with heart disease. However, present varieties contain little or no erucic acid.

Oils are extracted from the nuts or seeds by crushing and by the use of solvent extraction, which involves dissolving the oil in an organic solvent with a low boiling point and then removing the solvent by evaporation. The oils at this stage are impure and have to be refined. Neutralization with sodium hydroxide removes the free fatty acids. The soap formed by this process is present as an insoluble solid and can be easily removed. The oil is then bleached with Fuller's earth, which absorbs the coloured matter. Finally, the oil is deodorized by heating under vacuum and injecting steam. This process removes the volatile substances responsible for odour.

2 Margarine

Margarine is an emulsion of water in fat. The fat phase is a blend of refined vegetable oils, a portion of which has been hardened by hydrogenation to produce the desired plasticity in the final product. Fish oils and animal fats may also be incorporated in the blend. The hydrogenation is carried out by heating the oil in large sealed vessels under pressure. Hydrogen is bubbled into the oil, and finely divided nickel, which is subsequently removed by filtration, is required as a catalyst. The oil blend is mixed with the water phase, which is skimmed milk, soured under controlled conditions to give the desired flavour to the product. Artificial colouring, salt and vitamins A and D are then added. In Britain these vitamins must be added by law. This law is necessary because margarine often replaces butter in the diet and butter is an important source of vitamins A and D. The emulsion is formed in a machine called a votator, in which mixing and cooling occur together, and a fat of the desired consistency is produced.

Hard margarines are more hydrogenated, i.e. saturated, than soft tub margarines. Sunflower margarines are high in PUFA.

3 Spreads and low fat spreads

These are not margarines as they contain less than 80% fat, the legal minimum for margarine. However, they are made in a similar way. Many, e.g. Flora, contain about 70% fat but low fat spreads have a much lower fat content (about 40%) and very low fat spreads only about 25% fat or less. The low fat spreads have a much higher water content than margarine and, therefore, are not suitable for cooking.

4 Cooking fats and shortenings

These were first produced in the USA as a substitute for lard. They are pure fat products rather than emulsions. The fat is a blend of vegetable and fish oils and animal fats. The oils are partially hydrogenated. The fat blend is cooled to give the desired consistency and air is usually incorporated into the product to improve the texture.

Some fats have an emulsifying agent added. These fats, known as high ratio fats, are specifically designed for high ratio cakes, i.e. cakes made from a batter with a high moisture content.

5 Lard

Lard is fat extracted from pigs. The extraction is carried out by heating or 'rendering'. Lard is almost 100% pure fat.

6 Butter

Butter is made by churning pasteurized cream. During churning the cream becomes more viscous and finally a mass of solid butter is produced. The liquid by-product, known as buttermilk, is removed and the butter is mixed to give the desired consistency. Salt and colouring matter may be added at this stage, although some butter is sold unsalted.

The churning or agitation process reverses the emulsion. Cream is an emulsion of fat globules dispersed in a water phase. During churning the fat globules aggregate and form a solid phase which is interspersed by small water droplets. Butter is therefore a water-in-fat emulsion.

7 Suet

Suet is the fat from around the kidneys of animals such as the ox. Nowadays it is usually sold in the form of shredded suet.

The composition of some of these fats is shown in Figure 6.1.

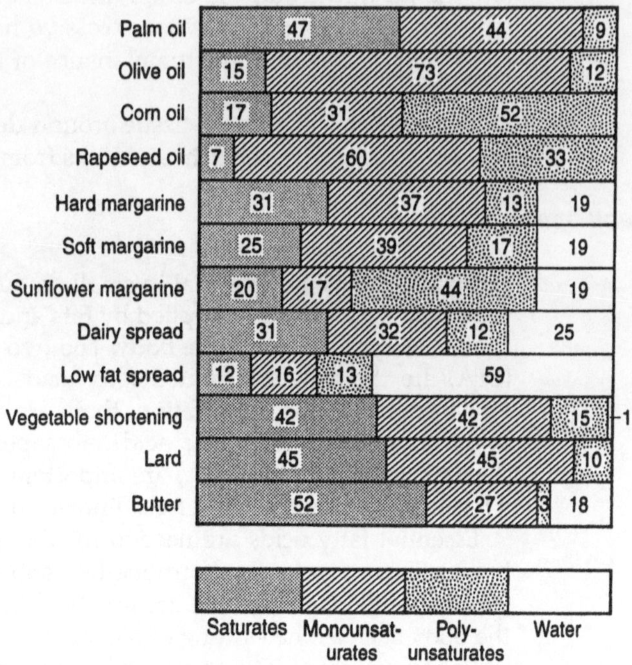

Figure 6.1 *Percentage composition of various fats and oils.*

Functions of fats in the diet

1 *Energy*

Fat is broken down in the body by a process of oxidation and energy is released. A description of this process is given in Chapter 10.

1 g of fat provides 37 kJ (9 kcal)

Fat has more than twice the calorific value of carbohydrates and is therefore a more concentrated source of energy. For people whose energy requirements are high it is useful to include a reasonable quantity of fat in the diet, as it reduces the bulk of food which must be eaten.

2 *Formation of adipose tissue*

Excess fat, which is not immediately required for energy, is stored in the adipose tissue where it has three functions:

(a) fat stored in this way constitutes an energy reserve;
(b) the fat in the adipose tissue under the skin forms an insulating layer and helps to prevent excessive heat loss from the body. It therefore assists in the maintenance of a constant body temperature;
(c) fat is stored in adipose tissue around delicate organs, such as the kidneys, and protects these organs from physical damage.

3 *Essential fatty acids*

Some fatty acids are essential in small amounts for the functioning of the body. They must be supplied by fats and oils in the diet since they cannot be synthesized in the body. The two main essential fatty acids (EFA) are the polyunsaturated fatty acids (PUFA) linoleic acid and alpha linolenic acid. In addition, there are several longer chain fatty acids of which arachidonic acid, eicosapentaenoic acid (EPA) and docosahexaenoic acid (DHA) are important, but these can be made to a limited extent in the body from linoleic and alpha linolenic acids.

Essential fatty acids are needed for the maintenance of cell membranes. They also make hormone-like substances called eicosanoids (prostaglandins, etc.) which are involved in a number of functions in the body such as the clotting of blood.

Polyunsaturated fatty acids can be divided into two main groups or series, according to the positions of the double bonds. The two main series of PUFA are called the n-3 and n-6 series and these are derived from alpha linolenic and linoleic acids, respectively. The n-3 (or omega-3) series includes the long chain fatty acids EPA and DHA. The n-6 (or omega-6) series includes gamma linolenic acid (GLA) and arachidonic acid as well as linoleic acid. We obtain the n-3 PUFA mainly from oily fish and the n-6 PUFA from seed oils (vegetable oils) and polyunsaturated margarines. There is evidence that eating more of the long chain n-3 PUFA reduces the risk of death from heart attacks by decreasing the tendency of the blood to clot. It is recommended in the 1994 COMA report that consumption of long chain n-3 PUFA should be increased from 0.1 g per day to 0.2 g. This could be achieved by eating more oily fish such as mackerel, herring, pilchards, sardines, trout and salmon.

4 *Fat-soluble vitamins*

Certain fats included in the diet help to ensure an adequate intake of the fat-soluble vitamins A, D and E. However, in countries where fat intake is low, these vitamins can be obtained in other ways.

Sources of fat in the diet

Fats and oils are obtained from both animals and plants. They are formed from carbohydrate and represent a concentrated store of energy.

1 *Meat and fish*

All meat contains fat, though the percentage of fat varies from animal to animal and from one part of an animal to another. Meat provides 25% of the total fat content of the average British diet. Oily or fatty fish, such as herring and sardines, contain up to 20% oil but they contribute only 2% to the total intake because they are eaten infrequently.

2 *Butter and margarine*

These are important sources of fat in the British diet. Butter contributes 6% and margarine 11% of the total fat content of the average diet.

3 *Spreadable fats, cooking fats and oils*

Spreadable fats (spreads) are now used extensively in place of butter and margarine for spreading on bread. Vegetable oils and cooking fats are used in the preparation of a large number of goods, such as fried foods and pastry products. Together these account for 15% of the fat content of the average British diet.

4 Milk, cream and cheese

Milk contains between 3% and 4% fat; some products made from milk, such as cream and cheese, contain much larger amounts. Milk and cream account for 11% of the total fat content of the average British diet, and cheese contributes a further 6%.

5 Baked goods

Fat is used in the manufacture of cakes, pastry, biscuits and bread. These foods provide 11% of the total fat content of the average British diet.

6 Eggs

Eggs contain fat in an emulsified form in the yolk. They contribute 2% to the total fat content of the average British diet.

Many other foods contain a considerable amount of fat. These include ice cream, chocolates and some sweets, nuts and salad dressings.

Vegetables and fruits contain insignificant amounts of fat. Notable exceptions are the soya bean which contains 19% fat and the avocado pear which is 20% fat.

Table 6.2 shows the fat content of a variety of foods.

Table 6.2 *Fat content of some foods*

Food	*% Fat*
Cooking oils	100
Lard	99
Butter	82
Margarine	81
Spread, e.g. Flora	70
Peanuts, roasted	49
Cream, double	48
Low fat spread	41
Cheese, Cheddar	34
Chocolate, milk	30
Beef, average	24
Cream, single	21
Herring	14
Eggs	11
Chicken	4.3
Milk, full cream	3.8
Milk, semi-skimmed	1.7
Cod	0.7

Fats and health

A small amount of fat (about 2% of total energy intake) is necessary in the diet in order to supply the essential fatty acids (EFA). However, in the UK we tend to eat a lot more fat than we need. On average fat intake provides 40% of total energy.

There is much concern about the link between a high fat intake and the incidence of coronary heart disease (CHD) and stroke. Cardiovascular diseases (CHD and stroke) are the major causes of death in Britain. Coronary heart disease is caused by narrowing of the arteries of the heart due to the build-up of fatty deposits in the lining of the arteries (atherosclerosis). The presence of a blood clot in these arteries can lead to a blockage which cuts off the supply of blood to part of the heart and to a subsequent heart attack (coronary thrombosis). Stroke is the sudden loss of brain function most usually due to a blood clot in an artery supplying the brain.

It has been shown that there is an increased risk of death from CHD if a person has a high level of cholesterol (a fat-like substance) in their blood. Cholesterol is carried in the blood by specific proteins which direct its metabolism. The two main lipid-protein complexes (lipoproteins) are low density lipoproteins (LDL) and high density lipoproteins (HDL). Coronary heart disease is linked mainly with LDL which carries 70% of the blood cholesterol. A high level of LDL cholesterol in the blood (especially if it is oxidized) can lead to deposits in the arteries (plaques) which cause narrowing. HDL cholesterol, on the other hand, is beneficial as it transports cholesterol from places where there is too much to the liver where it is disposed of. A high intake of saturated fatty acids increases both LDL cholesterol and total cholesterol in the blood. Increasing the intake of dietary n-6 polyunsaturated fatty acids (PUFA) decreases both total and LDL cholesterol.

The n-3 PUFA such as DHA and EPA in fish oils may reduce the risk of heart attacks by inhibiting the formation of blood clots or reducing blood pressure.

Lower rates of CHD are found in countries such as Greece where the people have a 'Mediterranean diet'. This diet is low in saturates and total fat but high in monounsaturated fatty acids, largely from olive oil. It also includes high intakes of fruit and vegetables. Monounsaturates do not lower the 'protective' HDL cholesterol.

At the present time, fat in the UK diet provides about 40% of total food energy with saturates providing 16% of energy. The 1994 COMA report recommends reducing total fat intake to 35% of energy and that from saturated fats from 16% to 10%. It also recommends increasing the n-3 PUFA (mainly from oily fish) from about 0.1 g per day to 0.2 g per day, but not to increase the intake of n-6 PUFA. Over the last 10 years the n-6 PUFA (mainly from polyunsaturated margarines and spreads) have often been used as substitutes for saturated animal fats but the monounsaturates (olive oil, etc.) could also be used. Trans fatty acids (mainly from hydrogenated margarines and shortenings and products made from them such as cakes and biscuits) also probably raise blood cholesterol levels and the COMA report recommends that ways of reducing their intake should be considered.

We should, therefore, be looking for practical ways of reducing the intake of total fat, particularly saturated and trans fatty acids while increasing our intake of n-3 PUFA. This may be achieved without drastically altering the diet, for example by:

1 Eating less red meat but more chicken and fish (both white and oily).

2 Eating oily fish (mackerel, salmon, trout, sardines, pilchards, etc.) once a week.

3 Replacing butter and hard margarines by soft margarines or low fat spreads.

4 Using reduced fat products such as skimmed or semi-skimmed milk, low fat yoghurt and fromage frais.

5 Grilling, boiling, steaming or microwaving foods rather than frying them.

6 Using liquid oils (e.g. olive, corn) for cooking rather than lard or hardened cooking fats.

7 Reducing the intake of manufactured biscuits, cakes and desserts.

7 Proteins

Proteins are a very important group of nutrients. They are found in the cytoplasm of all living cells, both animal and plant. Proteins are organic substances and they resemble fats and carbohydrates in that they contain the elements carbon, hydrogen and oxygen. However, all proteins also contain nitrogen and most contain sulphur and some contain phosphorus. Proteins show a greater variety and complexity of structure than either fats or carbohydrates. Plants are able to synthesize protein from inorganic materials. Carbon dioxide from the air and water from the soil provide the carbon, hydrogen and oxygen necessary for protein synthesis. Nitrogen is obtained from the soil in the form of inorganic compounds, usually nitrates and nitrites. Some plants, such as the legumes, are able to utilize nitrogen from the air, with the aid of bacteria. Animals, unlike plants, cannot synthesize protein from inorganic compounds, therefore protein is an essential nutrient in the diet of all animals.

The structure of proteins

Protein molecules are extremely large and consist of long chains of amino acids chemically combined. About 20 different amino acids occur in the proteins found in foods (see Table 7.1). Each amino acid molecule contains at least one amino group (—NH_2) and at least one acidic group (—COOH). Therefore, amino acids show both basic and acidic properties and are said to be **amphoteric.** It is incorrect to think that because they are described as acids they all have a pH below 7.

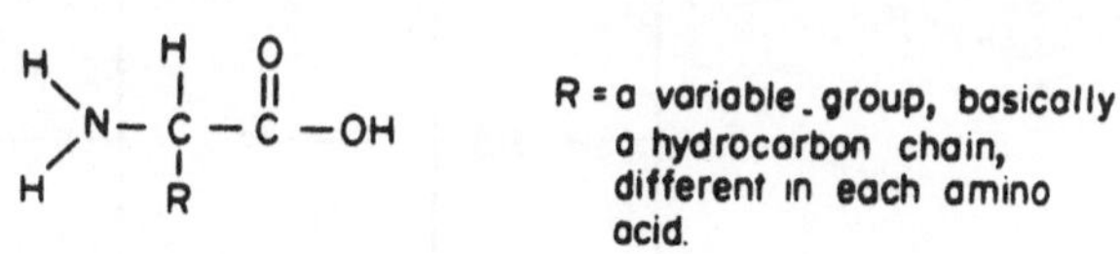

Generalized formula of an amino acid

A typical protein molecule contains about 500 amino acids, joined together by **peptide links.** A peptide link is formed when the amino

($—NH_2$) group of one amino acid reacts with the acidic (—COOH) group of an adjacent amino acid. A molecule of water is eliminated during the formation of the peptide link (see Figure 7.1). This type of reaction is an example of condensation polymerization. Two amino acids joined together form a **dipeptide,** with the —CONH— atoms forming the peptide link. Longer chains of amino acids are called **polypeptides. A protein molecule** consists of a single polypeptide chain or a number of polypeptide chains joined by cross-linkages.

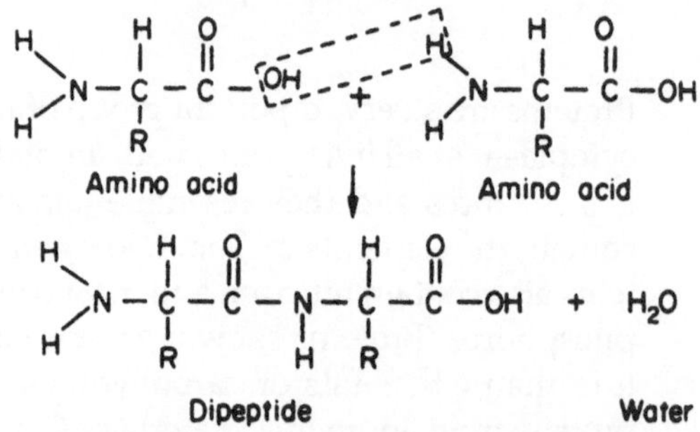

Figure 7.1 *Formation of a peptide link.*

Protein molecules have a complex nature since they can contain all 20 amino acids in any arrangement. If a polypeptide was made up of only 10 amino acid units, the possible number of amino acid arrangements would be 20^{10} or well over a billion. Since even the simplest protein contains more than 50 amino acid units, it can be seen that it is possible to have an almost infinite number of different protein molecules. The order or 'pattern' of amino acids in the protein molecule is known as the *primary* protein structure.

Cross-links may be formed between the side groups of amino acids. These links may form between different polypeptide chains or between side groups on the same polypeptide chain. One of the most important types of cross-linkage is the disulphide bridge. The amino acid cysteine contains an —SH group. When two cysteine units are adjacent, a disulphide bridge, —S—S—, may be formed by the oxidation of the —SH groups, as shown in Figure 7.2.

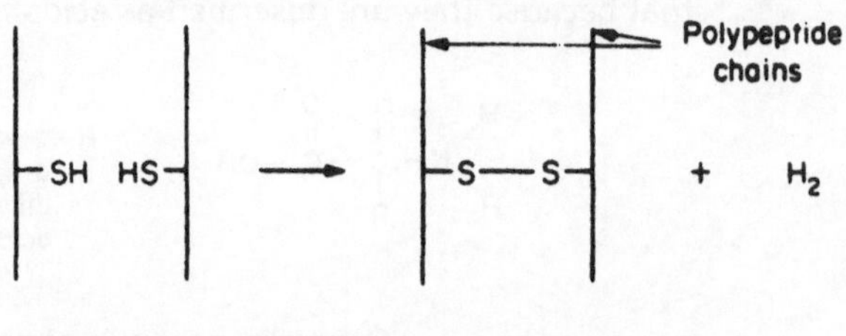

Figure 7.2 *Formation of a disulphide bridge.*

Cross-links may also be produced by the formation of hydrogen bonds. These are weak bonds arising from the tendency of hydrogen atoms, when attached to oxygen or nitrogen atoms, to share the electrons of a neighbouring oxygen atom (see page 51). Cross-linking determines the *secondary* structure of the protein, i.e. the shape and the three-dimensional configuration of the protein molecule.

Proteins vary a great deal in structure but they can be classified into two main groups, according to the shape of the molecules.

1 Globular proteins

Molecules of globular proteins are rounded in shape but are not necessarily spherical. The amino acid chain is folded and the molecule is kept in shape by cross-linkages within the amino acid chain. The structure is three-dimensional but it can be represented in two dimensions as shown in Figure 7.3.

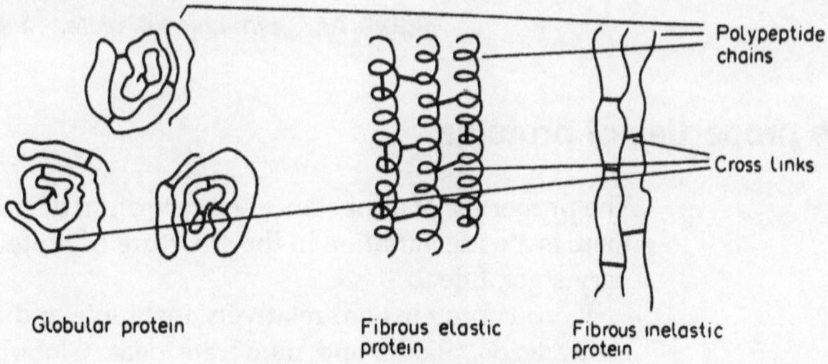

Figure 7.3 *Types of proteins.*

The molecules are not closely packed, nor is there any organized arrangement. It is easy for water molecules to penetrate the empty spaces within the protein molecules. Globular proteins are easily dispersed in either water or salt solutions to form colloids (see Chapter 4). Some examples of globular proteins found in foods are ovalbumin, found in egg white, and caseinogen, found in milk. Most of the proteins found in body cells are globular, e.g. haemoglobin and myoglobin.

2 Fibrous proteins

Molecules of fibrous proteins are straighter. They may be almost completely straight (inelastic or extended proteins) or coiled in a spiral (elastic proteins) as shown in Figure 7.3.

In fibrous proteins there is usually an organized arrangement and the molecules are closely packed together. There are cross-links between adjacent amino acid chains and it is difficult for water molecules to penetrate the structure. Therefore fibrous proteins are not usually soluble in water.

Gluten, the insoluble protein found in wheat, is an example of an elastic protein. When pulled, gluten will stretch but it tends to return to its original shape when the force is removed. This is because molecules of gluten are coiled and behave like a spring. They return to their original position due to the cross-links holding the chains together. This is shown diagrammatically in Figure 7.4. Elastin, a constituent of connective tissue which is found in meat and known as 'gristle', and keratin, the protein found in hair and wool, behave in a similar fashion. Collagen, one of the other proteins found in connective tissue, is an example of an extended protein.

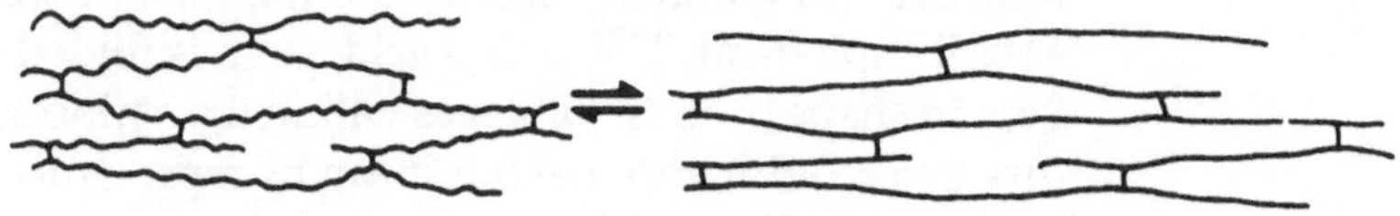

Figure 7.4 *Stretching of gluten molecules.*

The properties of proteins

The properties of a substance are determined by its structure and since there is a wide variation in the structure of proteins the properties also vary a great deal.

Fibrous proteins are relatively insoluble and are not greatly affected by acids, alkalis and moderate heat. Globular proteins form colloidal solutions and are affected by acids, alkalis and heat.

Denaturation and coagulation

Proteins undergo a process known as **denaturation** when their secondary structure is altered but their primary structure is unchanged. The molecule unfolds and changes shape but the sequence of amino acids remains the same. Denaturation is brought about by various physical and chemical means and involves the breaking of the cross-linkages which maintain the shape of the molecule. It is usually irreversible, it being impossible to regain the original structure of the molecule. As a result of denaturation the properties of the proteins alter; they become less soluble and more viscous. The unfolded molecules tend to bond with each other forming clumps. This results in the hardening or 'setting' of the protein food and is known as **coagulation.** Coagulation can be brought about by various means such as:

1 Action of heat

Many proteins coagulate when heated. For example, when an egg is cooked the proteins in the white and the yolk coagulate. Egg-white proteins coagulate first at 60°C and the yolk at approximately 66°C.

This coagulation is used extensively in the preparation of many dishes, e.g. egg custard and sponge cake. The muscle fibre proteins in meat coagulate when heated resulting in the shrinkage of meat during cooking.

Denatured proteins are more readily attacked by digestive enzymes and therefore most protein foods (e.g. eggs, meat) are more digestible when cooked.

2 Presence of acid

When milk sours, bacteria present in the milk ferment lactose, producing lactic acid. The pH of the milk is lowered and this causes the milk protein, caseinogen, to coagulate. The starter culture, used in the manufacture of some milk products, such as yoghurt and cheese, consists of lactose-fermenting bacteria. The lactic acid, produced by the bacteria, is responsible for the coagulation or 'setting' of the milk and the formation of a curd.

3 Addition of salt

Certain salts, such as sodium chloride, coagulate some proteins. If salt is added to the cooking water used for boiling eggs, the white will not escape as readily if the shell is cracked. During cheesemaking, salt is often added to the curd to increase firmness and also to suppress the growth of micro-organisms.

4 Addition of rennin

Rennin, known commercially as rennet, is an enzyme which coagulates protein. Rennet is used to make junket, which is clotted or coagulated milk. Rennin is also used, together with a bacterial starter, to form the curd in cheese manufacture (see Chapter 14).

5 Mechanical action

Mechanical action during the whisking of egg white causes a partial coagulation of the protein. The protein molecules unfold and form a reinforcing network round the air bubbles, thus stabilizing the foam. This is used in food preparation, e.g. the making of meringues and soufflés.

Maillard reaction (non-enzymic browning)

This is a browning reaction which occurs during the roasting, baking, grilling and frying of many foods. A chemical reaction takes place between the amino group of a free amino acid or a free amino group on a protein chain and the carbonyl group of a reducing sugar, e.g. glucose. Brown-coloured compounds are formed which are responsible for the attractive colour of products such as bread crust, roasted meat, fried potatoes and baked cakes and biscuits. The compounds also confer an appetizing flavour to the foods.

Although the reaction is generally considered desirable during cooking, there are two undesirable effects. Firstly, there is some loss of nutritional value of proteins. Amino acids containing an extra amino group, e.g. the essential amino acid lysine, are most likely to be involved. Secondly, the reaction can cause discoloration of foods during storage, for example the gradual browning of dried milk powder.

Functions of proteins in the body

1 Growth and maintenance

Proteins are the main constituents of the cells of the body. The membranes surrounding the cells contain protein which is also found within the cell. The number of cells in the body increases during periods of growth, therefore during childhood and adolescence protein requirements are particularly high. In addition, protein in the tissues is constantly being broken down and must be replaced from the amino acids supplied in the diet. This replacement of tissue occurs in all people at all stages of their life. An account of the process by which amino acids in body cells combine to form protein in included in Chapter 10.

Protein is necessary for the formation of enzymes, antibodies and some hormones. These substances are produced within cells and in some cases are released either into the blood-stream (antibodies and hormones) or into the intestine (digestive enzymes). For a description of enzymes see Chapter 11 and for hormones see page 154.

2 Energy

Not all of the protein supplied by food can be used for growth and repair. The amount of protein which is available for use in this way depends on the Biological Values (see page 93) of the various proteins in the diet. In addition, the diet may supply more protein than is required for growth and maintenance. Any excess protein may be used for energy. Amino acids which are not required for protein synthesis are deaminated in the liver, i.e. the nitrogen-containing parts of the amino acid molecules are removed to form urea. Urea is a waste product, which is of no value to the body, and it is carried by the blood to the kidneys, from there it is excreted in the urine. The deaminated molecules contain carbon, hydrogen and oxygen. They enter the chain of reactions in which glucose is oxidized in the cells to supply energy (see page 144).

1 g of protein provides 17 kJ (4 kcal)

Essential amino acids and protein quality

Of the 20 amino acids commonly found in proteins, eight are essential in the diet. These essential (or indispensable) amino acids must be supplied by the protein in the diet, since they cannot be synthesized in the body. Eight amino acids are essential for all people and an additional one must be supplied in the diets of rapidly growing infants. The non-essential (dispensable) amino acids can be synthesized in the body by converting one amino acid into another within the body cells. Table 7.1 indicates which of the 20 commonly occurring amino acids are essential.

Table 7.1 *Essential and non-essential amino acids*

Essential	*Non-essential*
Isoleucine	Alanine
Leucine	Arginine
Lysine	Aspargine
Methionine	Aspartic acid
Phenylalanine	Cysteine (may occur in the form of Cystine)
Threonine	Glutamic acid
Tryptophan	Glycine
Valine	Ornithine
Histidine (essential for infants)	Proline (may occur in the form of Hydroxyproline)
	Serine
	Tyrosine

Methionine and cysteine are sulphur-containing amino acids and some of the requirements of methionine can be met by cysteine or cystine.

When protein foods are eaten, the proteins are hydrolysed during digestion to produce amino acids. After absorption the amino acids are transported by the blood to the cells. In the cells the amino acids recombine and new proteins are formed. The distribution of the various essential amino acids in the food we eat is not necessarily the same as is required to synthesize protein in the cells. A protein which has a similar distribution of essential amino acids to the protein in the human body is therefore of more use, or of better quality, than one which does not supply the essential amino acids in the necessary quantities. The **Biological Value** of a protein is used as a measure of protein quality. **Biological Value (BV) is the percentage of absorbed protein which is converted into body protein.** The protein content of a food is difficult to determine by experiment. It is usual to determine the nitrogen derived from protein rather than the total protein content.

$$BV = \frac{\text{Retained nitrogen}}{\text{Absorbed nitrogen}} \times 100$$

The Biological Values of a variety of proteins are given in Table 7.2. Egg protein, which has an amino acid pattern similar to human protein, has a BV of 97. Gelatin has a BV of 0, because it is completely lacking in the essential amino acid tryptophan.

Table 7.2 *BV of proteins from a variety of sources*

Protein source	*BV %*
Egg	97
Meat	82
Fish	79
Milk	77
Soya bean	73
Rice	67
Peas	64
Peanuts	55
Corn	50
Wheat	49
Gelatin	0

Some years ago the F.A.O. (Food and Agriculture Oganization of the United Nations) published a reference standard representing a protein having a BV of 100. The amino acid pattern of this protein is shown in histogram form in Figure 7.5.

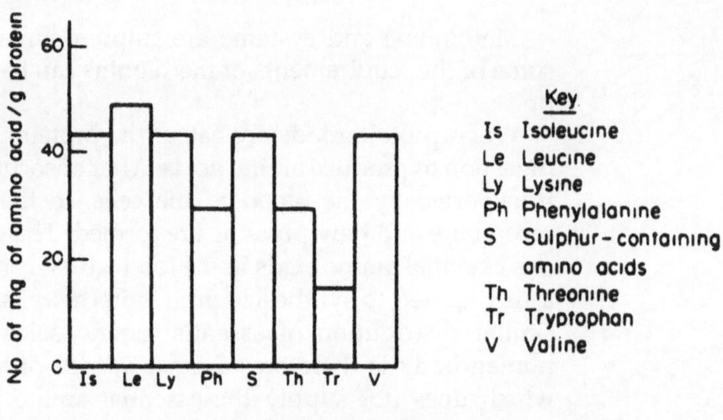

Figure 7.5 *Amino acid histogram for a perfect protein.*

Similar histograms showing the amino acid pattern of cheese protein and bread protein (see Figure 7.6) show that cheese is deficient in methionine and the other sulphur-containing amino acids and that bread has a significant deficiency of lysine, sulphur-containing amino acids and tryptophan. Sulphur-containing amino acids are limiting in cheese protein, since only 78% of the required amount is present. All other essential amino acids are present in sufficient quantity. In bread protein, lysine is the limiting amino acid; only 47% of the required amount is present.

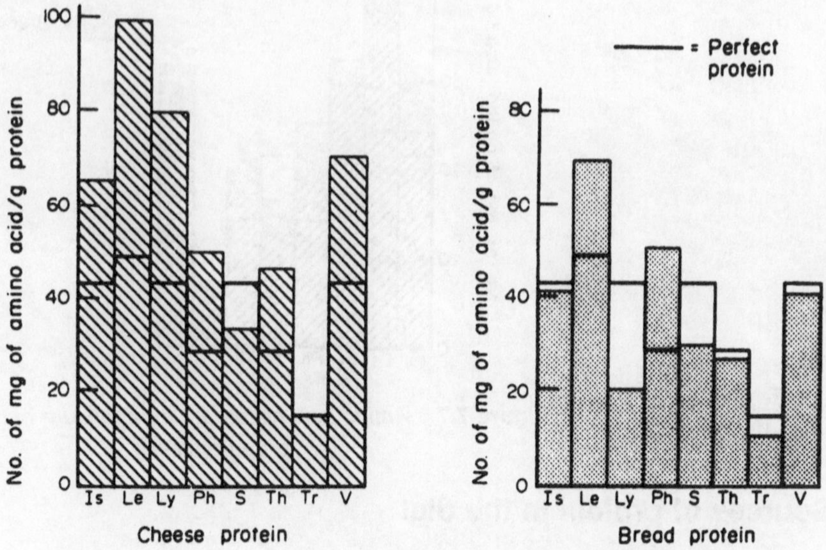

Figure 7.6 *Amino acid histograms for cheese and bread protein.*

Biological Value is a measure of protein quality when the protein concerned is the sole source of protein in the diet. However, people normally eat a mixed diet containing a variety of proteins. When two different proteins are mixed, the resulting mixture has a higher BV than the average BV of the components. One protein may have a surplus of the amino acid which is the limiting amino acid in the other protein. A good example of this complementation is bread and cheese; the lysine deficiency in the bread is made good by the excess in the cheese. This is illustrated in Figure 7.7, which shows the BV of a mixture of three parts of cheese protein to one part of bread protein.

Other examples of dishes in which the proteins complement each other include breakfast cereals and milk, baked beans on toast, pasta and cheese (e.g. macaroni cheese) and milk and rice (e.g. rice pudding).

Commercially, the BV of plant proteins can be increased by the addition of small quantities of the limiting amino acid. For example, yeast protein has a BV of 67 but the addition of 0.3% methionine (the limiting amino acid in yeast) increases the BV to 91.

When considering the value of a protein food in the diet, it is not only the BV of the protein which must be considered, but also the percentage of protein in a food and the amount of the food eaten.

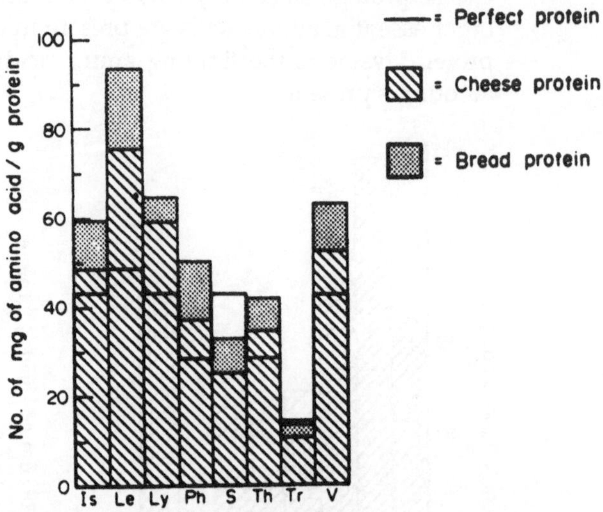

Figure 7.7 *Amino acid histogram for a mixture of cheese and bread protein.*

Sources of protein in the diet

Protein can be obtained from both animal and plant sources. In general, foods obtained from animals contain more protein than foods obtained from plants, although some vegetable materials, such as soya beans, have a high protein content. Vegetable proteins usually have a lower BV than animal proteins and in the past much emphasis was placed on this. However, in a mixed diet, this is not serious, and vegetable proteins have the advantage of being cheaper than animal proteins. In the average UK diet two-thirds of the protein comes from animal sources and one-third from plant foods.

1 *Meat and fish*

The term 'meat' usually refers to the muscle tissue of animals but it may be extended to include other parts of the animal, such as liver, kidney and sweetbreads. The contribution of all forms of meat to the protein content of the average British diet is 29%. Fish is eaten less frequently and contributes 5% of the total protein intake.

2 *Bread and cereals*

Bread contains a significant amount of protein and is one of the most important and one of the cheapest sources in the British diet. However, it is not as important as a protein source as it has been in the past since bread consumption has decreased in recent years. Nevertheless, bread and flour together account for 16% of the total protein intake. Other cereal foods, such as rice, pasta, breakfast cereals, cakes and biscuits, also contain protein and contribute a further 10%.

3 *Milk and cheese*

Milk is a valuable source of good-quality protein. Protein is present in some foods made from milk, the most important of these being cheese. Milk accounts for 17% of the protein content of the average British diet, while cheese contributes a further 6%.

4 *Eggs*

Eggs are an excellent source of high-quality protein. However, they are not eaten as much as some other protein foods, therefore their contribution to the protein content of the average British diet is only 3%.

5 *Vegetables*

The amount of protein in the cells of root and green vegetables is small, although potatoes, mainly because of the quantity in which they are eaten, do contribute 3% to the total protein content of the average British diet. Seeds of plants contain significantly more protein. Pulse vegetables such as peas and lentils contain moderate amounts of protein, though when dried, they have a much higher protein content.

6 *Nuts*

Although not an important source of protein in the average British diet, nuts are a major source of protein in the diets of many vegans and vegetarians (see page 179).

The protein content of some of these foods is shown in Table 7.3.

Protein requirements

The Department of Health (DoH) has published Reference Nutrient Intakes (RNIs) for protein. These are amounts of protein that are enough or more than enough for 97% of the population. Some of these figures are shown in Table 7.4.

The protein requirement of an individual depends mainly on their body-weight and whether or not they are growing. An adult needs approximately 0.75 g of protein per day for every kilogram of body-weight. During periods of growth proportionally more protein is required. For example, for children aged 7 to 10 years about 1 g of protein is needed per day for every kilogram of body-weight.

Table 7.3 *Protein content of some foods*

Food	*Protein %*
Soya beans, dried	36
Cheese, Cheddar	26
Peanuts, roasted	25
Lentils, dried	24
Chicken	21
Stewing beef	20
Cod and haddock	17
Brazil nuts	14
Eggs	13
White bread	8.4
Cornflakes	7.9
Broad beans	7.9
Hummus	7.6
Rice	7.3
Peas	6.9
Baked beans	5.2
Milk	3.2
Potatoes	2.1
Cabbage	1.7

Table 7.4 *Reference Nutrient Intakes (RNIs) for protein*

	Males		*Females*	
Age	*Body-weight (kg)*	*Protein (g/day)*	*Body-weight (kg)*	*Protein (g/day)*
1–3 years	12.5	14.5	12.5	14.5
4–6 years	17.8	19.7	17.8	19.7
7–10 years	28.3	28.3	28.3	28.3
11–14 years	43.0	42.1	43.8	41.2
15–18 years	64.5	55.2	55.5	45.0
19–50 years	74.0	55.5	60.0	45.0
50+ years	71.0	53.5	62.0	46.5
Pregnancy				+6
Lactation				+11

During pregnancy and lactation (breast-feeding) women need more protein in their diet to allow for the growth of the baby and adequate breast milk production.

In the UK intakes of protein are considerably higher than the RNIs. There has been some concern that there may be health risks associated with very high intakes, such as the loss of minerals from bone, though there is little firm evidence in this area.

Protein deficiency

In the less developed countries of the world, particularly in parts of Africa and the Far East, the diet is composed mainly of one staple food (a plant food) and in areas where this food is a low-protein food, such as cassava or yams, protein deficiency is common. Severe protein deficiency causes a disease known as **kwashiorkor.** This condition is caused by a diet low in protein and high in carbohydrate and is most common in young children after weaning. The disease is serious and has many symptoms. The main symptoms are wasting of the muscles, retarded growth and a distended abdomen caused by oedema (fluid in the tissues). The lack of protein also causes anaemia, since protein is necessary for the formation of red blood cells. Children in some underdeveloped countries may also be existing on diets low in energy (i.e. insufficient food). The term 'protein-energy malnutrition (PEM)' is used to cover the whole range of conditions from protein deficiency at the one extreme to energy deficiency at the other.

The treatment of PEM involves the provision of a diet adequate in energy, vitamins and minerals, containing a good quantity of easily digested protein of high biological value. Dried, skimmed milk is one of the most useful foods for the treatment of kwashiorkor. However, this is only a short-term measure and in the long term the normal diet of the people must be improved.

The technical means for increasing food production are already available. These means include the development of disease-resistant and high-yielding crops, the use of chemical fertilizers and pesticides, irrigation of infertile land and the further development of fish farming. However, the main causes of food shortage and malnutrition are economic, political and social, rather than technical. The richer, industrialized countries have the purchasing power to take more than their share, while the poorer countries do not have the money to invest in their own agriculture or to import sufficient food.

Production of animal protein is not an efficient method of obtaining protein since animals are not efficient at converting dietary protein into body protein. As little as 15% of the protein fed to an animal is actually converted into consumable protein such as meat, milk and eggs. It is therefore more economic to eat plant protein, rather than feed animals with cereals and protein concentrates and eat the animal products. One hectare of land used to graze cattle will provide enough beef to meet the protein requirement of one man for 300 days. If this hectare of land is used for the production of wheat, 3500 days' protein supply can be produced, and if it is used for the cultivation of soya beans, 8000 days' protein requirement can be supplied by the same area of land.

Another factor in food production which is now being given much consideration is the energy output: energy input ratio. The energy output is a measure of the energy value of the food obtained. The energy input is the energy required to grow crops or rear animals. Mechanical energy is necessary for ploughing, sowing and harvesting. Energy is consumed in the manufacture of fertilizers and insecticides. Animals require energy in the form of the food they eat. Intensive methods used for livestock farming necessitate the use of heat and light in animal buildings.

The energy output: energy input ratio of various foods is listed below:

Food	*Energy output: input ratio*
Wheat	2.3
Bread	1.3
Eggs	0.16
Chickens	0.13

If the ratio is less than one, more energy is used in producing the food than is obtained by its consumption. It can be seen from the figures that the production of animal foods is very energy-intensive and it is therefore preferable to concentrate on producing more vegetable foods.

Novel sources of protein

In recent years various new or 'novel' protein foods have been developed. Because they are low in saturated fat, these products can be used as a healthier alternative to meat.

1 *Textured vegetable protein (TVP)*

The protein from certain oilseeds can be used to make textured products which can be used to replace, or partly replace, meat in a wide variety of dishes. The seeds most frequently used are soya beans. Defatted soya-bean meal contains about 50% protein, but it is not suitable as a human food because it contains substances which inhibit growth. Some of these substances are heat-sensitive and are easily destroyed by cooking or roasting. Others are water-soluble and can be removed by soaking and extraction.

Soya-bean meal can be used to manufacture a product with a meat-like texture, known as textured vegetable protein (TVP). The protein is extracted by adding an alkali and fibres are formed by extruding the protein through fine nozzles or spinerettes. The fibres are combined with fat, a protein binder, colours and flavours. The product is similar to cooked meat and can be frozen, canned or dehydrated. TVP is used in catering, particularly in industrial canteens and the school meals service.

2 Single-cell protein

Micro-organisms have a high protein content and contain useful quantities of vitamins. Their rate of growth is very rapid and the rate of protein synthesis in micro-organisms has been compared favourably with the rate in animals. A 500 kg bullock produces an extra 500 g of protein per day, whereas 500 kg of yeast grown in suitable conditions can produce 50 tonnes of protein in one day. It can be seen that micro-organisms are potentially a very valuable source of protein, especially if they can be produced economically by the use of a cheap food. Many foods (or substrates) have been investigated including petroleum products, agricultural waste products and waste material from the food industry such as whey produced as a by-product of the cheesemaking industry.

Quorn is a novel protein food or meat substitute which is made from a microscopic type of fungus. It is, therefore, described as a mycoprotein. It is grown in a fermenter and 'harvested', then heat processed, flavoured and sliced or shredded. Quorn can be used instead of meat in home-cooking and is used in manufactured foods such as pies and curries. It is used extensively in vegetarian and vegan cooking.

8 Vitamins

The vitamins are a group of complex organic compounds required in small quantities by the body for the maintenance of health. They are not usually synthesized in the body and are therefore essential in the diet. They are present in foods in small amounts.

In the nineteenth century it was assumed that a diet containing carbohydrate, fat, protein and minerals was sufficient to maintain health. However, in 1888, a scientist called Lunin carried out experiments showing that mice could not survive on such a diet although they thrived on the same diet if they were also given milk. It was apparent that milk contained substances other than carbohydrates, fats, proteins and minerals, which were essential for health.

The effects of vitamin deficiencies had been recognized for centuries but the cause of these diseases was unknown. Scurvy, a disease caused by a dietary lack of vitamin C, was common among sailors on long sea voyages in the sixteenth and seventeenth centuries. In his voyage round the world from 1772 to 1775, Captain Cook demonstrated that scurvy could be prevented by the consumption of fresh fruits and vegetables.

In 1912 Hopkins published the results of his experiments on rats which showed conclusively the existence of a vitamin, or as he called it an 'accessory food factor' in milk. Since that time over 20 different vitamins have been isolated from food, identified and also synthesized in the laboratory. When the early vitamins were discovered they were named according to the letters of the alphabet. Each vitamin was also given a chemical name when its chemical composition was identified. Letters are still used for naming vitamins but they are gradually being replaced by the chemical names.

Unlike other groups of nutrients, the vitamins are not chemically similar to each other. Each vitamin has a specific chemical structure and a specific function or set of functions in the body. Many of the vitamins are involved in enzyme systems in the body (see Chapter 11).

For most people a sensible and varied diet will supply all the necessary vitamins. It is unnecessary to waste money on vitamin tablets. With few exceptions, most notably babies, young children and pregnant women, people do not require vitamin supplements.

Vitamins can be divided into two main groups.

1 *Fat-soluble vitamins*

This group includes vitamins A, D, E and K. Fat-soluble vitamins will dissolve in fats and oils but not in water. Vitamins A and D can be stored in the body, in the liver. In extreme circumstances it is possible to have an excessive intake of these vitamins leading to high levels in the body and a condition known as 'hypervitaminosis'. Quantities of vitamins A and D are measured in micrograms (μg) (see page 5).

2 *Water-soluble vitamins*

The vitamins of the B group and vitamin C will dissolve in water but not in fats. Since they are water soluble they are not stored in the body, any excess being excreted in the urine. Quantities of the three main B vitamins (thiamin, riboflavin and niacin) and vitamin C are measured in milligrams (mg).

Vitamin A (retinol)

Retinol is a pale yellow solid which dissolves in fats and oils but not in water. It is found only in animal foods, but many fruits and vegetables contain carotenes, a group of orange pigments, which can be converted into retinol in the body. The most important of these pigments is beta (β)-carotene.

Vitamin A is measured in retinol equivalents.

$$\begin{aligned} 1\ \mu g \text{ retinol equivalent} &= 1\ \mu g \text{ retinol} \\ &= 6\ \mu g\ \beta\text{-carotene} \end{aligned}$$

Only a proportion of the β-carotene present in food is converted into retinol.

Sources of retinol

Retinol is found in some fatty animal foods. Since animals and fish can store retinol in the liver, liver and fish liver oils have a high retinol content. Fish liver oils are not foods but are dietary supplements. They are so rich in vitamins A and D that they are potentially dangerous and should be taken only in the recommended doses. Retinol is also found in butter, milk, cheese, eggs and oily fish. It is not present in vegetable oils but since 1954, vitamin A has been added to margarine by law to make margarine nutritionally equivalent to butter. It is also normally added to other spreadable fats. Although liver, kidney and heart are good sources, carcase meat contains only a trace of retinol. Table 8.1 shows the retinol content of some foods.

Table 8.1 *Retinol content of some foods*

Food	*μg retinol equivalents per 100 g*
Halibut liver oil	900,000
Cod liver oil	18,000
Liver, ox	16,500
*Margarine	985
*Fat spread	940
*Butter	885
Cheese, Cheddar	365
*Eggs	190
*Milk, whole	55
Herring	45
*Milk, semi-skimmed	23

*Includes a contribution from carotene.

Sources of beta-carotene

Beta-carotene is found in yellow, orange and green fruits and vegetables. The richest source is carrots but it is also found in fruits such as mangoes, apricots and melons. In green vegetables the green pigment chlorophyll masks the carotene but the darker green the vegetable the more beta-carotene it contains. The vitamin A content of some fruits and vegetables is shown in Table 8.2.

Table 8.2 *Carotene content of some foods*

Food	*μg retinol equivalents per 100 g*
Carrots	1350
Red peppers	640
Spinach	590
Mangoes	300
Tomatoes	110
Broccoli	95
Cabbage	65
Apricots	60
Peas	50

(1 μg retinol equivalent = 6 μg β-carotene.)

In the British diet, approximately two-thirds of the vitamin A is consumed as retinol and one-third as beta-carotene. The most important sources of vitamin A are liver, carrots, milk, margarine, butter and other spreadable fats (see Table 8.3).

Table 8.3 *Contributions made by different foods to the total vitamin A content of the average British diet*

Food	*Contribution to total vitamin A intake*
Liver	32%
Carrots	13%
Milk and cream	12%
Margarine	9%
Butter	5%

Functions

1 Retinol is essential for growth and metabolism of all body cells.

2 It is also required for the formation of rhodopsin (visual purple), a complex substance formed from retinol and protein. Rhodopsin is a pigment found in the retina, a membrane at the back of the eye, and is necessary for vision in reduced light.

3 Vitamin A is also essential for the maintenance of healthy skin and surface tissues, particularly the moist mucous membranes such as the cornea at the front of the eye and the lining of the respiratory and digestive tracts.

4 Beta-carotene is thought to act as an antioxidant in body tissues removing free radicals. A high intake may give some protection against some forms of cancer (see page 123).

Deficiency

Since retinol is stored in the body it is possible to exist for a certain period of time on a diet containing little vitamin A. However, if this period is prolonged, signs of deficiency will become apparent.

1 Lack of vitamin A in the diet of children reduces the rate of growth.

2 Since without retinol the body is unable to synthesize rhodopsin, vision in reduced light is impaired, causing a condition known as **night blindness.** If the deficiency is only slight the condition is easily reversed by increasing the intake of vitamin A. The popular fallacy that 'eating carrots helps you to see in the dark' contains an element of truth since carrots contain a significant amount of vitamin A. However, since the average British diet contains sufficient vitamin A, increasing the intake above the required level will cause no improvement in eyesight.

3 Vitamin A deficiency affects the health of the skin and resistance to infection is lowered due to the poor condition of the mucous lining of the respiratory tract. In extreme cases the tear glands become

blocked and the membranes at the front of the eye become dry and inflamed. This condition is known as **xerophthalmia.** Severe and prolonged deficiency can lead to ulceration of the cornea causing blindness. Vitamin A deficiency is a common cause of blindness in developing countries where the diet is composed mainly of a staple cereal food and where fruits and vegetables containing carotene are not available. It usually develops in children after weaning when vitamin A is no longer supplied by breast milk.

Vitamin A deficiency is virtually unknown in Britain.

Excess

Very large doses of retinol are harmful. Excessive intakes are unlikely to occur with a normal diet, but there have been cases of illness when people have taken large amounts of vitamin preparations over a period of time. Hypervitaminosis A causes drowsiness, irritability, skin and bone disorders and an enlarged liver. Sometimes mothers have been unaware of the harmful effects and have given their children excessive doses of vitamin drops or fish liver oils. A relationship has been suggested between high intakes of vitamin A during pregnancy and defects of the baby. Pregnant women are, therefore, advised not to take vitamin A supplements and not to eat liver or products containing liver (e.g. pâtés, liver sausage) during their pregnancy.

Recommended intake

The Department of Health Reference Nutrient Intake (RNI) for men is **700 μg** retinol equivalents per day and for women is **600 μg** per day. Women need an extra 100 μg per day during pregnancy to meet the needs of the growing baby. During lactation when a woman needs to produce milk containing sufficient vitamin A for her baby, the RNI is 950 μg retinol equivalents per day.

Losses on cooking and storage

Both retinol and carotene are unaffected by most cooking methods but small amounts may be lost during frying or prolonged cooking. Some carotene is lost during slow drying of fruit and vegetables, but in modern, quick drying the losses are very much reduced. During storage, retinol in fatty foods may be lost by oxidation. This may be prevented by the use of antioxidants, by refrigeration and by the exclusion of light, e.g. wrapping fats in foil and storing fish liver oils in dark glass bottles.

None of these losses is sufficiently large to be of practical significance. In all cases the majority of the vitamin A value of the food is retained.

The B vitamins

The B vitamins are a group of vitamins which, although chemically different from each other, are all water soluble and tend to occur in similar foods. They mostly act as co-enzymes in chemical reactions in the body.

Thiamin (vitamin B_1)

Thiamin is a white solid which is soluble in water.

Sources

Thiamin is found in all cereal grains. Most of the thiamin is found in the germ and bran of the grain (see page 204) and therefore white flour contains considerably less thiamin than wholewheat flour. To overcome this deficiency thiamin is added by law to white flour in Britain. Most breakfast cereal manufacturers add thiamin to their products. Brown rice is a good source of thiamin but polished white rice, which is used more extensively, contains very little.

Other sources of thiamin include meat (especially bacon, ham and pork), potatoes, peas, beans, nuts and milk. Brewers' yeast is a particularly rich source since, during the production of beer, the yeast absorbs thiamin from the cereal grain. However, it is not considered to be a food, although it is used by some people as a dietary supplement. Products made from yeast, such as yeast extract, are eaten in such small quantities that they make an almost negligible contribution to the diet. The thiamin content of some foods is shown in Table 8.4.

Table 8.4 *Thiamin content of some foods*

Food	*mg thiamin per 100 g*
Dried brewers' yeast	15.6
Cornflakes	1.0
Peas	0.74
Pork	0.57
Wholemeal bread	0.34
White bread	0.21
Potatoes	0.21
Lamb	0.09
Beef	0.06
Milk	0.04

The most important sources of thiamin in the British diet are bread and other cereal foods, meat, milk and potatoes (see Table 8.5).

Table 8.5 *Contributions made by different foods to the total thiamin content of the average British diet*

Food	*Contribution to total thiamin intake*	
Bread	23%	46% (bread and other cereal foods)
Other cereal foods	23%	
Meat	13%	
Milk	10%	
Potatoes	10%	

Function

Thiamin is involved in the oxidation of nutrients and the release of energy in the body. In the cells of the body, glucose is gradually broken down in a series of reactions which release energy in a controlled manner (see page 144). Each reaction in the series requires a specific enzyme. A complex compound containing thiamin acts as a co-enzyme for two of the reactions in the sequence.

Deficiency

If thiamin is deficient in the diet glucose is only partially oxidized. The breakdown stops at a substance called pyruvic acid. A build-up of pyruvic acid in the blood causes muscular weakness, palpitations of the heart and degeneration of the nerves. These are the main symptoms of a disease called **beriberi** which is common in parts of Asia where the staple food is polished rice. Beriberi develops more readily with carbohydrate-rich diets. There are two main types of beriberi. In wet beriberi the patient suffers from oedema (fluid in the tissues) and in dry beriberi there is severe emaciation and wastage of the tissues. It has been said that a person suffering from the extreme weakness of beriberi will sum up how he feels by the following statements: 'It is better to sit than to stand. It is better to lie down than to sit. It is better to die than to live.'

Beriberi can, to some extent, be prevented by parboiling unpolished rice. If rice grains are parboiled before the bran and germ are removed much of the thiamin is absorbed by the inner part of the grain.

Beriberi rarely occurs with Western diets, though it has been found in anorexics and alcoholics. A high intake of alcohol increases the requirement for thiamin as thiamin is needed to break down alcohol in the body.

Recommended intake

Since thiamin is necessary for the oxidation of glucose the amount required by the body is related to the amount of carbohydrate in the diet; 0.6 mg thiamin is recommended for every 4200 kJ (1000 kcal) derived from carbohydrate. For practical purposes it is more convenient to relate thiamin requirements to total energy intake and the figure 0.4 mg thiamin per 4200 kJ (1000 kcal) is used. For an adult man whose energy requirement is 10,600 kJ per day, the RNI is **1.0 mg** of thiamin, and for a woman who needs 8100 kJ, the RNI is **0.8 mg** per day. Requirements are increased during pregnancy (0.9 mg per day) and lactation (1.0 mg per day).

Losses on cooking and processing

Thiamin, like all other B vitamins, is soluble in water. About 20% of the thiamin is lost when potatoes are boiled. Thiamin decomposes at high temperatures, particularly in alkaline conditions. Meat loses about 40% of its thiamin when roasted and when bread is baked about 25% of the thiamin is destroyed. The loss on baking is greater if an alkaline substance, such as sodium bicarbonate, is used as a raising agent.

Some preservatives have an adverse effect on thiamin. For example, sodium sulphite and sulphur dioxide which are used to prevent the browning of prepeeled potatoes and which are added to many other processed foods including dried fruits and vegetables, speed up the loss of thiamin. Sulphur dioxide is a permitted preservative in meat products, such as sausages and beefburgers, i.e. foods which would otherwise be good sources of thiamin.

Riboflavin (vitamin B_2)

Riboflavin is a yellow, water-soluble compound.

Sources

Good sources of riboflavin include cheese, liver, kidney and eggs. It is also found in milk, meat, potatoes and green vegetables. Liver is a particularly rich source. Riboflavin is found in bread and cereals but to a lesser extent than thiamin, although, like thiamin, it is added to most breakfast cereals. Table 8.6 shows the riboflavin content of some of these foods.

The main sources of riboflavin in the British diet are milk, breakfast cereals and other cereal foods, meat and vegetables (see Table 8.7).

Function

The function of riboflavin is similar to that of thiamin. It forms part of the enzyme system concerned in the oxidation of glucose and the release of energy in body cells.

Table 8.6 *Riboflavin content of some foods*

Food	*mg riboflavin per 100g*
Dried brewers' yeast	3.68
Liver	3.10
Kidney	2.10
Weetabix	1.50
Cornflakes	1.30
Eggs	0.47
Cheese, Cheddar	0.40
Beef	0.23
Milk	0.17
White bread	0.06
Cabbage	0.02
Potatoes	0.02

Table 8.7 *Contributions made by different foods to the total riboflavin content of the average British diet*

Food	*Contribution to total riboflavin intake*	
Milk	35%	
Breakfast cereals	13%	21%
Other cereal foods	8%	
Meat	16%	
Vegetables	6%	

Deficiency

A deficiency of riboflavin affects the eyes, lips and tongue. Cracks appear at the corners of the mouth, the tongue becomes red and swollen and in severe cases blood vessels invade the cornea of the eye. These symptoms, however, are not specific to riboflavin deficiency; they may be caused by a lack of other B vitamins or by other means. A diet deficient in riboflavin will almost certainly be deficient in other nutrients as well.

Recommended intake

Riboflavin requirements are related more closely to body-weight than to energy intake. The RNIs for riboflavin are **1.3 mg** per day for men and **1.1 mg** per day for women with an increase to 1.4 mg per day during pregnancy and 1.6 mg during lactation.

Cooking losses

Riboflavin is only slightly soluble in water and is fairly stable to heat (though it is less stable in alkaline conditions). The overall loss during cooking is small and very much less than the corresponding loss of thiamin.

Effects of sunlight

Riboflavin is sensitive to light. Milk, the most important source of riboflavin in the diet, loses riboflavin at the rate of about 10% per hour if left in direct sunlight. It is best, therefore, not to leave milk in glass bottles on doorsteps for long periods.

Niacin (nicotinic acid)

Niacin is the name used to refer to both nicotinic acid and nicotinamide. Nicotinic acid is a white, crystalline, water-soluble solid, which is converted into its amide, nicotinamide, in the body. Nicotinamide can also be formed in the body from the amino acid, tryptophan. It is convenient to express the niacin content of foods in terms of equivalents.

1 mg niacin equivalent = 1 mg available niacin
= 60 mg tryptophan

Sources

Niacin is widely distributed in plant and animal foods. Foods with a good niacin activity include yeast, meat (particularly offal), fish, cheese, pulse vegetables and cereals. Much of the niacin in wheat is lost during the milling process and therefore, in Britain, niacin is added by law to white flour. It is also added to most breakfast cereals by the manufacturers, although there is no legal requirement to do so. Milk, eggs, potatoes and beer are moderately good sources. Table 8.8 shows the niacin content of a variety of foods.

The most important sources in the British diet are meat, milk, bread and other cereals, and potatoes (see Table 8.9).

Function

Niacin, like thiamin and riboflavin, forms part of an enzyme system concerned in the oxidation of glucose and the release of energy in body cells.

Table 8.8 *Niacin equivalents of some foods*

Food	*mg niacin equivalents per 100 g*
Dried brewers' yeast	62.9
Peanuts, roasted	18.9
Liver	17.9
Beef	8.5
Cheese, Cheddar	6.1
Wholemeal bread	5.9
Cod	4.9
Eggs	3.8
Peas	3.6
White bread	3.4
Potatoes	1.1
Milk	0.8
Beer	0.6

Table 8.9 *Contributions made by different foods to the total niacin content of the average British diet*

Food	*Contribution to total niacin equivalents*	
Meat	32%	
Milk	11%	
Bread	10%	22%
Other cereal foods	12%	
Potatoes and other vegetables	12%	

Deficiency

A prolonged deficiency of niacin gives rise to a disease known as **pellagra.** The symptoms of the disease include diarrhoea, dermatitis (scaling and discoloration of the parts of the skin exposed to the sun) and dementia (mental disorders). Pellagra has, therefore, been called the disease of the three Ds. It exists among communities of people who live mainly on a diet of maize. There are two reasons for this. Firstly, the niacin present in maize is bound in a complex form and is unavailable to the body. Secondly, unlike other cereals, maize is deficient in tryptophan. At one time pellagra was responsible for thousands of deaths every year in the southern states of America. Nowadays, the diet in this part of the world is more varied and pellagra is rare.

In Mexico, maize is still widely eaten in the form of tortillas, but the preparation involves treating the maize with lime and this releases the niacin from its bound form.

Recommended intake

As with thiamin, niacin requirements are related to energy intake with an RNI of 6.6 mg niacin equivalents per 4200 kJ (100 kcal). The RNI for adult men is **17 mg** equivalents and **13 mg** equivalents for women with an increase to 15 mg equivalents during lactation.

Losses on cooking

Niacin is soluble in water but is much more resistant to heat than either thiamin or riboflavin. Small amounts are lost during cooking by leaching into cooking water and by the loss of juices from cooked meats.

Folate (folic acid)

Folic acid is the parent molecule for several related compounds known collectively as folates or folate.

Sources

Foods rich in folate include liver, green leafy vegetables and, to a lesser extent, kidney, nuts, pulse vegetables, flour and cereal foods. Folate is added to many breakfast cereals by the manufacturers. Most meat, dairy products and fruits contain relatively little folate. Table 8.10 shows the folate content of some foods.

Table 8.10 *Folate content of some foods*

Food	*μg folate per 100 g*
Liver	330
Cornflakes	250
Brussels sprouts	135
Kidney	77
Cabbage	75
Hazelnuts	72
Peas	62
Roasted peanuts	52
Eggs	50
Potatoes	35
White bread	29
Baked beans	22
Milk	6

The main sources of folate in the UK diet are breakfast cereals, bread, potatoes, green vegetables, other vegetables and milk as shown in Table 8.11.

Table 8.11 *Contributions made by different foods to the total folate content of the average UK diet*

Food	*Contribution to total folate intake*	
Potatoes	13%	34%
Green vegetables	9%	
Other vegetables	12%	
Breakfast cereals	13%	30%
Bread	12%	
Other cereal foods	5%	
Milk	8%	

Deficiency

Folate is one of the few nutrients likely to be deficient in the British diet. A dietary deficiency causes a characteristic type of anaemia. This may occur as a result of a poor diet as occurs with some elderly people or from increased needs, e.g. during pregnancy. There is evidence that a low intake at the time of conception and in early pregnancy may be associated with neural tube defects (spina bifida) in babies.

Recommended intake

The RNI for folate is **200 μg** per day for adults. During pregnancy this increases to 300 μg and during lactation to 260 μg per day.

It has been recommended by the Chief Medical Officer that all women likely to become pregnant should increase their folate intake by eating more folate-rich foods and foods fortified with folate. It is also recommended that women planning a pregnancy should take a daily supplement of 0.4 mg folic acid from the start of trying to conceive until at least the 12th week of pregnancy.

Cooking losses

Folate is readily lost during most cooking processes. It leaches into cooking water and is also destroyed by heat, particularly in the presence of oxygen and alkalis. Large losses (up to 90%) may occur when green vegetables are boiled. Vegetables should be cooked in only a little water for a short time to minimize losses.

Other B vitamins

Vitamin B_{12} (cyanocobalamin)

Cyanocobalamin is involved in more than one enzyme system in the body and is needed, together with folic acid, for red blood cell formation. It has a complex structure and contains, as the name indicates, the element cobalt. It occurs naturally only in foods of animal origin and in yeasts. Liver is the richest source but it is also found in milk, meat, fish and eggs. It is now added to some manufactured foods such as breakfast cereals. In herbivorous animals the vitamin is synthesized by bacteria present in the gut. A deficiency of cyanocobalamin causes **pernicious anaemia**. This disease is nearly always caused by a failure to absorb the vitamin rather than by a dietary deficiency. A protein, formed in the stomach, and known as the intrinsic factor, must combine with the vitamin before the vitamin can be absorbed. A lack of intrinsic factor is the usual cause of pernicious anaemia. Vegans, very strict vegetarians who eat no animal produce of any kind, are the only people in whom a dietary deficiency of vitamin B_{12} has been observed.

Vitamin B_6 (pyridoxine)

Vitamin B_6 is a mixture of pyridoxine and two other related compounds. It is found in many foods, particularly in meat, liver, fish and some vegetables. It functions in many enzyme systems, especially those concerned in protein synthesis. Deficiency is rare. In America infants fed on a pyridoxine-deficient baby food developed convulsions but responded rapidly to treatment with the vitamin. Recently, vitamin B_6 has been prescribed for various conditions and it is thought to be of benefit to some women who are taking oral contraceptives, or suffering from premenstrual syndrome. However, there is evidence that large doses (more than 50 mg per day) can be harmful.

Biotin

Biotin is needed by the body for the release of energy from fats. It is found in a wide variety of foods, particularly egg yolk, liver and yeast. It can be synthesized by bacteria in the intestine and may not be necessary in the diet. Avidin, a substance present in raw egg white, inhibits the absorption of biotin. One of the few recorded cases of biotin deficiency was an eccentric man whose daily diet consisted of ten raw eggs and six bottles of red wine.

Pantothenic acid

This vitamin is also widely distributed in plant and animal foods and there is no danger of deficiency. It is an essential constituent of enzyme systems involved in the release of energy from carbohydrates and fats.

Vitamin C (ascorbic acid)

Ascorbic acid is a white, crystalline substance which is very soluble in water.

Sources

Vitamin C is not as widely distributed in foods as most other vitamins. It is found almost entirely in vegetable foods, in fresh fruits and vegetables but not in cereals or dried pulse vegetables. Very small amounts may be found in animal foods such as raw liver and kidney. Raw milk contains a little vitamin C and some of this is still retained after pasteurization.

The amount of ascorbic acid in fruits and vegetables is very variable, even within the same variety. Table 8.12 shows the average ascorbic acid content of some foods.

Table 8.12 *Ascorbic acid content of some fruits and vegetables*

Fruits	*mg ascorbic acid per 100 g*	*Vegetables*	*mg ascorbic acid per 100 g*
Blackcurrants	200	Parsley	190
Strawberries	77	Spring greens	180
Kiwi fruit	59	Peppers, green	120
Lemons	58	Brussels sprouts	115
Oranges	54	Broccoli	87
Clementines	54	Cabbage	49
Grapefruit	36	Cauliflower	43
Raspberries	32	Peas	24
Peaches	31	Tomatoes	17
Melons	26	Potatoes, new	16
Blackberries	15	Potatoes, old (average)	11
Gooseberries	14	Carrots	6
Bananas	11		
Apples	6		
Pears	6		
Plums	4		

NB All figures are for raw fruits and vegetables.

The vitamin C content of potatoes drops considerably during storage. Although not very rich in ascorbic acid, potatoes are a very important source because of the quantity in which they are eaten. Blackcurrants, on the other hand, are a very good source but are eaten in insufficient quantity to make a significant contribution to vitamin C intake. Synthetic vitamin C, which is equally valuable, is added to many manufactured foods including some fruit juices and fruit drinks to compensate for losses during processing. Fruit juices now provide one-fifth of our vitamin C and soft drinks (which include squashes and carbonated drinks) provide a further 7%. The most important sources of vitamin C are shown in Table 8.13.

Table 8.13 *Contributions made by different foods to the total vitamin C content of the average British diet*

Food	*Contribution to total vitamin C intake*	
Potatoes	12%	39%
Green vegetables	6%	
Other vegetables	21%	
Oranges	7%	45%
Other fruit	18%	
Fruit juices	20%	
Soft drinks	7%	
Milk	5%	

Functions

1 Ascorbic acid is necessary for the formation of collagen, the main protein of connective tissue. Connective tissue is the 'packaging material' which separates, protects and supports the various organs (see page 147). Vitamin C aids the healing of wounds.

2 Ascorbic acid aids the absorption of iron from the intestine.

3 Vitamin C has antioxidant properties, see page 123.

Man, monkeys and guinea-pigs are among the relatively few species which require a dietary source of vitamin C. Other animals synthesize ascorbic acid from glucose in their body cells.

Deficiency

A person existing on a diet containing insufficient ascorbic acid will eventually develop the condition known as **scurvy.** The main symptoms of scurvy are bruising and spontaneous haemorrhaging under the skin. The gums become black and spongy, and wounds and fractures fail to heal in the normal length of time. These symptoms are caused by a failure to form connective tissue. Another common feature of scurvy is anaemia which is due to a failure to absorb iron and an inability to form red blood cells. Until the eighteenth century, when potatoes became a common food, scurvy was common in the late winter and early spring months due to the scarcity of fresh fruits and vegetables. Nowadays, fresh foods are available all the year round and scurvy is rare. There have been some reports of old people who live on a poor diet with very little fresh fruit or vegetables developing signs of vitamin C deficiency. Also, some long-stay geriatric patients suffering from delayed wound healing and pressure sores may have mild scurvy as a result of eating institutional food in which there is little vitamin C left after cooking (see page 119).

Vitamin C supplements, e.g. vitamin drops, for children under five years have helped to reduce the likelihood of infantile scurvy in the UK.

Recommended intake

Since vitamin C cannot be stored in the body, a regular intake is essential. There are, however, differing opinions as to the amount necessary to maintain health. It has been shown that 10 mg per day is sufficient both to prevent and cure scurvy. The RNI for adults is **40 mg** per day. During pregnancy this is increased to 50 mg and during lactation to 70 mg per day to meet the needs of the baby.

It is claimed by some people that massive doses of ascorbic acid, 1000 mg or more per day, may alleviate some of the symptoms of the common cold but these claims are still being assessed. Mega doses such as these can only be obtained by taking a supplement, e.g. ascorbic acid tablets.

Losses on cooking and storage

Ascorbic acid is readily destroyed during cooking. It is very soluble in water and therefore leaches out into cooking water. It is also readily oxidized. Oxidation is most rapid in alkaline conditions, at high temperatures and on exposure to light, air and traces of metals such as zinc, iron and particularly copper.

Ascorbic acid oxidase is an enzyme, present in plant cells, which increases the rate of oxidation. In intact cells the enzyme is separated from the vitamin but when fruits and vegetables are bruised, cut or chopped the enzyme comes into contact with the ascorbic acid and the ascorbic acid is destroyed. However, the enzyme is inactivated at temperatures above 60°C and is therefore destroyed during cooking. In the absence of the enzyme, oxidation can still take place but the rate is reduced.

The amount of ascorbic acid lost during the preparation and cooking of fruits and vegetables depends very much on the methods used. Unless care is taken losses of ascorbic acid may be very large. Table 8.14 shows a list of recommendations which, if followed, will minimize the losses during the storage, preparation, cooking and service of vegetables and fruits.

Table 8.14 *Recommended methods of minimizing vitamin C losses in vegetables and fruits*

Recommendation	*Reason*
Storage	
1 Store in a cool, dark place	The rate of oxidation is increased by heat and light
2 Avoid bruising or damaging fruits and vegetables	Bruising damages the cells and releases the enzyme
Preparation	
1 Prepare just before cooking	The enzyme is released when the cells are cut
2 Do not soak in cold water	Ascorbic acid is very water soluble.
3 Do not cut or chop more than necessary	The enzyme is released when the cells are cut
4 Tear rather than cut green leaves	Tearing causes the leaves to break around the cells
5 Avoid the use of iron (non-stainless) knives graters, etc.	Iron increases the rate of oxidation
Cooking	
1 Place in boiling water	The enzyme is destroyed by heat
2 Use a minimum quantity of water and a covered pan	Ascorbic acid leaches into cooking water; the greater the volume of water, the greater the ascorbic acid loss
3 Cook for a minimum length of time	Prolonged heating increases the amount of oxidation
4 Do not add sodium bicarbonate to green vegetables	Alkalis increase the rate of oxidation
Service	
1 Serve immediately; do not keep in hot cabinets for long periods of time	Keeping hot for 45 minutes reduces ascorbic acid by 50% or more
2 Avoid mashing and puréeing unless there is some other ascorbic acid source to balance the menu	Mashing and puréeing increase the rate of oxidation

It should be pointed out that in practice, especially in large-scale catering, it is sometimes necessary, as a matter of convenience, to disregard some of the recommendations made in Table 8.14. As long as *reasonable* care is taken, the amount of ascorbic acid lost when green vegetables are cooked will not exceed 70%. This means that 30% will be retained. For example, raw cabbage contains 60 mg of ascorbic acid per 100 g; if 30% is retained, 100 g of cooked cabbage will contain $30/100 \times 60 = 18$ mg of ascorbic acid, i.e. about half of the 40 mg recommended daily intake. In other words, cabbage, even after it is cooked, is still a good source of vitamin C.

Since ascorbic acid is water soluble losses can be reduced by avoiding the use of water during cooking. The average loss of vitamin C when potatoes are boiled is 40%. If potatoes are baked in their skins the loss is only 30% and with fried, chipped potatoes it is only 25%.

The method of peeling potatoes also affects the amount of ascorbic acid lost. Thin hand peeling is preferable to thick hand peeling. Machine peeling damages a large number of cells and causes considerable losses.

Fruits lose less vitamin C when cooked than vegetables because they are more acidic and the rate of oxidation is reduced. The average loss of vitamin C due to cooking fruits is only 10%.

Preserved foods

There is about a 50% loss of vitamin C during the canning of fruits and vegetables but a greater loss during drying. Frozen foods retain most of their ascorbic acid. Frozen vegetables may have more vitamin C than 'fresh' vegetables, since vegetables used for freezing are frozen within a few hours of harvest, whereas so-called fresh vegetables, unless they are home grown, are probably two or three days old when bought. There is a gradual loss of vitamin C in frozen vegetables during storage. For example, peas stored at –18°C for eight months lose about 15% of their vitamin C content.

Vitamin D (cholecalciferol)

Cholecalciferol is a white, crystalline compound which is soluble in oils and fats but is insoluble in water.

There are two distinct forms of vitamin D:

1 Cholecalciferol (vitamin D_3) is the natural form of the vitamin occurring in foods. It is formed by the action of sunlight (ultraviolet radiation) on 7-dehydrocholesterol in the skin of humans and animals.

2 Ergocalciferol (vitamin D_2) is a synthetic form of the vitamin which has the same activity as the natural vitamin. It is produced by the ultraviolet irradiation of ergosterol, a compound which can be extracted from yeast.

Sources

1 *Food*. Vitamin D is found in relatively few foods. It occurs naturally in foods of animal origin. Fish liver oils are very rich sources but are dietary supplements rather than foods. Oily fish, eggs, butter, liver and cheese are good sources of vitamin D. It is important to realize that meats, apart from liver and some other offal, contain only a trace of vitamin D. The vitamin D content of milk varies with the time of year but even summer milk is a relatively poor source. For babies whose diet is largely based on cow's milk, a vitamin D supplement is essential and for children up to the age of five years a supplement is advisable. The vitamin D content of some foods is shown in Table 8.15.

Table 8.15 *Vitamin D content of some foods*

Food	*μg cholecalciferol per 100 g*
Cod liver oil	210.0
Herring	22.5
Margarine	7.9
Sardines, canned	7.5
Tuna, canned	5.8
Cornflakes	2.1
Eggs	1.8
Butter	0.76
Liver	0.50
Cheese, Cheddar	0.26
Milk, whole	0.03
Milk, semi-skimmed	0.01

It can be seen from Table 8.15 that the vitamin D content of margarine is approximately ten times that of butter. In Britain margarine for retail sale is enriched with vitamin D. This law does not apply to margarine sold for catering purposes. Vitamin D is also added, though not as a legal requirement, to most other spreadable fats (e.g. low-fat spreads) and to many breakfast cereals.

The main sources of vitamin D in the British diet are margarine and other fats, oily fish, eggs, fortified breakfast cereals and milk (see Table 8.16).

2 *Sunlight*. Vitamin D is formed in the skin on exposure to sunlight. The amount formed in this way varies with latitude and the amount of time the person spends outside in the sun. The quantity of vitamin D synthesized also depends on the degree of pigmentation of the skin. In darker-skinned people less synthesis occurs.

Table 8.16 *Contributions made by different foods to the total vitamin D content of the average British diet*

Food	*Contribution to total vitamin D intake*	
Margarine	30%	49%
Other fats	19%	
Oily fish	21%	
Eggs	9%	
Breakfast cereals	8%	
Milk and cream	7%	

Functions

Vitamin D is necessary for the growth and maintenance of bones and teeth. It is required for the absorption of calcium from the intestine and for the uptake of calcium and phosphorus by the bones and teeth.

Deficiency

Children receiving an inadequate supply of vitamin D develop **rickets,** a disease which was at one time very common in England. A lack of vitamin D results in a failure to absorb calcium and softening of the bones. The long bones bend under the weight of the body; knock-knees and bow legs are typical symptoms of rickets. Before 1900 about 75% of the children living in the poorer, industrialized regions of Britain had rickets. The main causes were a cheap diet composed mainly of cereal foods devoid of vitamin D and a lack of sunshine in the smoky, urban areas. In this century the improvement in living conditions, the development of smokeless zones, the use of cod liver oil as a supplement for babies and the fortification of margarine with vitamin D have all helped to ensure that rickets is no longer a major problem in this country. There are, however, still cases in large cities, particularly among the Asian population. Some traditional Asian diets are low in vitamin D and this, together with the facts that darker-skinned people synthesize less vitamin D and Asian cultures do not encourage exposure to sunlight, account for the occurrence of rickets in this group of people.

In adults an inadequate supply of vitamin D causes **osteomalacia,** a condition in which the bones become soft, weak and painful. Some cases have occurred in this country, especially among elderly, housebound women.

Excess

Too high an intake of vitamin D is harmful as it leads to excessive amounts of calcium being deposited in the soft tissues such as the kidneys. Hypervitaminosis D can result in kidney damage. Vitamin D intakes should be controlled, particularly in young children, and vitamin supplements used only in recommended amounts.

Recommended intake

Adults living a normal lifestyle obtain sufficient vitamin D by the action of sunlight on the skin. Dietary vitamin D is required only for those unlikely to be outside sufficiently or during periods of growth. The RNI for adults confined indoors and for those over 65 years is 10 μg per day. A daily intake of 10 μg for women during pregnancy and lactation is also recommended. This amount is most easily obtained by taking a supplement. A supplement is also recommended for children up to the age of 3 years. The RNI for 0 to 6 months is 8.5 μg and from 6 months to 3 years is 7 μg cholecalciferol per day.

Effect of cooking

Vitamin D is stable to heat and is insoluble in water. It is therefore unaffected by cooking.

Vitamin E (tocopherols)

A number of related compounds called tocopherols show vitamin E activity, the main one being alpha (α)-tocopherol. Vitamin E is found in many foods, but wheat germ, vegetable oils, nuts, margarine and egg yolk are particularly good sources.

Vitamin E is a natural antioxidant. In vegetable oils it helps to reduce rancidity by preventing the oxidation of unsaturated fatty acids. It may also play a part in protecting ascorbic acid against oxidation in fruits and vegetables.

In the body vitamin E has an important role as an antioxidant. Substances known as free radicals, which are produced as a result of normal chemical reactions in the body, can damage the lipids (fatty compounds) found in cell membranes. The free radicals oxidize the lipids, forming peroxides. This lipid peroxidation can cause damage to the cell membrane and leaking of the cell contents which in turn is thought to increase the risk of inflammatory diseases such as rheumatoid arthritis. Peroxides may also play a part in the formation of 'plaque' in artery walls which can lead to coronary heart disease (see page 85). Vitamin E protects lipids, especially polyunsaturated fatty acids (PUFA), against free radical damage.

Free radicals may also damage molecules inside the cell such as DNA and proteins. Cells with damaged DNA are more prone to cancer. Vitamin E is therefore thought to give some protection against some forms of cancer. Other vitamins, especially beta-carotene and vitamin C, also have antioxidant properties.

The amount of vitamin E required in the diet depends on the amount of PUFA in the body's tissues. The more PUFA eaten the more vitamin E is needed. Fortunately, foods rich in PUFA are usually also good sources of vitamin E.

Deficiency of vitamin E does not normally occur in humans though it has occurred in premature babies fed on an infant formula deficient in vitamin E. It has also occurred in some people unable to absorb and utilize vitamin E adequately. These people developed nervous system problems which improved when they were given suitable vitamin E treatment.

Vitamin K

Vitamin K is found in green vegetables and a variety of other foods. It has been shown to be essential for the normal clotting of blood. A deficiency of vitamin K is rarely seen because the vitamin is synthesized by bacteria present in the intestine as well as being present in a normal diet.

Babies, particularly if they are premature, have low levels of the vitamin in their bodies. Vitamin K is now given routinely to newborn babies in the UK.

9 Mineral elements and water

Mineral elements

The mineral elements are those chemical elements, other than carbon, hydrogen, oxygen and nitrogen, which are required by the body. They are present in food, mostly in the form of inorganic salts, e.g. sodium chloride, but some are present in organic compounds, e.g. sulphur and phosphorus are constituents of many proteins.

Mineral elements account for approximately 4% of body-weight. Some, such as calcium and phosphorus, are present in the body in relatively large amounts and are known as major minerals or macrominerals, whereas others occur in very small quantities and are known as trace elements (see Table 9.1).

Table 9.1 *Mineral elements required by the body*

Major minerals (macrominerals)	*Trace elements*
Calcium	Chromium
Chlorine	Cobalt
Iron	Copper
Magnesium	Fluorine
Phosphorus	Iodine
Potassium	Manganese
Sodium	Molybdenum
Sulphur	Selenium
	Zinc

Minerals have three main functions in the body:

1 Calcium, phosphorus and magnesium are constituents of bones and teeth.

2 Some elements are present as soluble salts which help to control the composition of body fluids. These include potassium and magnesium present inside body cells and sodium and chlorine in the fluid outside the cells.

3 Many of the trace elements are concerned in enzyme systems in the body.

Calcium

Sources

Milk and some milk products, such as cheese and yoghurt, are good sources of calcium. In Britain, calcium, in the form of calcium carbonate (chalk), is added by law to all flour except true wholemeal. Small fish, such as sardines, sprats and whitebait, which are eaten with the bones, contain very useful quantities of calcium. Fruits and vegetables contain variable but usually quite small amounts of calcium. Table 9.2 shows the calcium content of some of these foods. People living in hard water areas obtain a certain amount of calcium from drinking water (200 mg per day on average).

Table 9.2 *Calcium content of some foods*

Food	*mg calcium per 100 g*
Cheese, Cheddar	720
Sardines	550
Soya beans, dried	240
Yoghurt, fruit	150
White flour	140
Milk, semi-skimmed	120
Milk, whole	115
White bread	110
Wholemeal bread	54
Baked beans	53
Cabbage	52
Carrots	25

The most important sources of calcium in the British diet are milk, bread and other cereals, and cheese, as shown in Table 9.3.

Table 9.3 *Contributions made by different foods to the total calcium content of the average British diet*

Food	*Contribution to total calcium intake*	
Milk	45%	
Bread	13%	24%
Other cereal foods	11%	
Cheese	12%	

Functions

1 Calcium is necessary for the formation and development of bones and teeth. Bone is a composite material of cartilage and calcium phosphate. The protein fibres of the cartilage form a network on which the calcium phosphate is deposited. There is more than 1 kg of calcium in the bones of an adult. Teeth are similar in composition to bone.

2 Calcium is one of the essential factors required for the clotting of blood.

3 Calcium is necessary for the normal functioning of muscles and nerves in the body.

Absorption

Only about one-third of the calcium in the diet is absorbed from the intestine; the rest passes through the alimentary canal and is lost from the body in the faeces. There are several factors which determine the actual amount of calcium absorbed. Vitamin D assists absorption and without it little or no calcium would be absorbed. Absorption increases when the diet is low in calcium, though this adaption does not occur as readily with old people. Also, a higher proportion is absorbed by young people during periods of growth and by women during pregnancy. The calcium from milk and milk products is more readily absorbed than from plant sources. It is thought that lactose increases absorption. Dicarboxylic acids such as phytic and oxalic acids interfere with absorption. Phytic acid is found in the bran of cereals. It reacts with calcium in the intestine making it unavailable to the body. Oxalic acid, found in small amounts in many vegetable foods, e.g. rhubarb and spinach, behaves in a similar way.

Deficiency

Since vitamin D is essential for calcium absorption the effects of a dietary deficiency of calcium are the same as a deficiency of vitamin D. Severe calcium deficiency causes **rickets** in children and **osteomalacia** in adults. These diseases have been described in the previous chapter. They are more likely to be caused by a shortage of vitamin D than by a lack of calcium in the diet.

There is considerable concern over another bone condition known as **osteoporosis**. This occurs in older people, particularly in women after the menopause. Calcium is gradually lost from the bones which become porous and fracture more readily. Peak Bone Mass (PBM), when the bones are at their most dense, occurs between the ages of 35 and 40 years. From this age, loss of bone occurs at the rate of 0.3% of PBM per year. In women during the five years following the menopause the loss is greater due to the deficiency of the hormone oestrogen. Oestrogen replacement (hormone replacement therapy or

HRT) has been shown to reduce this loss. Osteoporosis is not thought to be caused by a lack of calcium or vitamin D, but plenty of dietary calcium together with regular exercise are recommended as preventative measures.

Recommended intake

Since it is required for bone development, calcium is a particularly important nutrient for children and for women during pregnancy and lactation. Table 9.4 shows the RNIs for calcium for different age groups.

Table 9.4 *RNIs for calcium*

Age	*mg calcium per day*
0–1 year	525
1–3 years	350
4–6 years	450
7–10 years	550
11–18 years, males	1000
11–18 years, females	800
Adults	700
Women, lactation	1250

No increase in dietary calcium is recommended during pregnancy because absorption increases, and stores of calcium in the mother's body are used.

Effect of cooking

Cooking has little effect on the calcium content of foods, though small amounts may be lost by leaching into cooking water. Vegetables cooked in hard water contain a little more calcium than those cooked in soft water.

Iron

Sources

Liver and kidney are two of the best sources of iron. Other meats, although not containing quite as much iron, are nevertheless good sources. Egg yolks have a high iron content but there is very little iron in the white. Iron is found in cereals but about half of this is lost in milling if the bran and germ are discarded. Iron is added to white flour in the UK; flour must by law contain at least 1.65 mg iron per 100 g. It is also added to most breakfast cereals. Potatoes and other vegetables, particularly pulses, are moderately good sources. Dried fruits have quite a high iron content but the main reason for this is that the removal of water results in a concentration of all other constituents. Milk is a relatively poor source of iron. After weaning, a baby's diet should include foods which contain a reasonable quantity of iron, e.g. eggs, minced meat and sieved green vegetables.

Certain foods such as black pudding, cocoa, black treacle, shell fish and curry powder have a high iron content. They are not, however, important sources in the average diet since they are not eaten very often in any quantity.

Table 9.5 shows the iron content of a variety of foods.

Table 9.5 *Iron content of some foods*

Food	*mg iron per 100 g*
Cocoa powder	10.5
Liver	7.0
Cornflakes	6.7
Kidney	5.7
Peas	2.8
Wholemeal bread	2.7
Spinach	2.1
Beef	2.1
Eggs	1.9
White bread	1.6
Baked beans	1.4
Cabbage	0.7
Potatoes	0.4
Milk	0.05

The most important sources of iron in the British diet are bread, breakfast cereals and other cereal foods, meat and vegetables (see Table 9.6).

Table 9.6 *Contributions made by different foods to the total iron content of the average British diet*

Food	*Contribution to total iron Intake*	
Bread	20%	47% (Bread, Breakfast cereals, Other cereal foods)
Breakfast cereals	14%	
Other cereal foods	13%	
Meat	18%	
Vegetables	16%	

Functions

1 The human body contains about 4 g of iron. The majority of this occurs in haemoglobin, a red pigment present in the red blood corpuscles. Haemoglobin is responsible for transporting oxygen from the lungs to the cells of all body tissues. All cells require oxygen in order to break down nutrients and obtain energy. The life of a red blood corpuscle is about 120 days. When the corpuscles break up the iron is not lost from the body; it is used again to make new red corpuscles in the bone marrow.

2 Iron is also found in myoglobin, a protein which acts as an oxygen carrier in the muscles.

3 Iron is also present, in small amounts, in all body cells where it is involved in various enzyme systems.

Some iron is also stored in the body, in the bone marrow, liver and spleen, as a complex with protein known as ferritin.

Absorption

Only between 5% and 20% of the iron a person eats is absorbed. The absorption of iron is a complex process. The amount of iron absorbed appears to depend very much on the need of the body for iron. A person deficient in iron will be able to absorb more than a person who has adequate stores of ferritin. Absorption increases when requirements are high, e.g. during pregnancy.

Another factor affecting absorption is the form of the iron. Iron is absorbed most readily from meat which contains soluble haem iron and to a lesser extent from foods containing non-haem iron, e.g. eggs, vegetables and cereals. Non-haem iron is present as trivalent (ferric) Fe^{3+} iron but it is absorbed most readily in the divalent (ferrous) Fe^{2+} form and therefore reduction of the ferric form is necessary. Ascorbic acid (vitamin C) aids the reduction and therefore aids iron absorption. Eating iron-rich foods with a source of vitamin C is therefore sensible, e.g. a glass of orange juice with an iron-fortified breakfast cereal.

Phytate, found in wholemeal cereals and pulses, interferes with iron, as well as calcium, absorption. Spinach is often quoted as being an important source of iron. However, it is eaten infrequently and also contains oxalic acid which interferes with iron absorption. Tannins, present in tea, also reduce iron absorption.

Deficiency

A deficiency of iron causes **iron deficiency anaemia.** In an anaemic person the number of red blood corpuscles is reduced and the amount of oxygen carried to the tissues is also reduced. This results in a lack of energy and a feeling of lethargy. Other symptoms of anaemia include headaches and dizziness. Anaemia is the most common deficiency disease in Britain but a dietary deficiency of iron is seldom the sole cause. It has been shown in some surveys that about one-sixth of the women in Britain are anaemic. It also occurs in children. One study in Birmingham showed that one-quarter of the children were anaemic. Anaemia is much more common in women than in men due to blood loss during menstruation. It is usually not possible to treat anaemia merely by increasing the iron content of the diet. Normally, iron tablets are prescribed together with advice on dietary sources of iron.

Anaemia may also be caused by a deficiency of nutrients other than iron, e.g. by folic acid deficiency.

Recommended intake

The DoH figures take into account the fact that women of child-bearing age require more iron due to blood losses during menstruation. Children and adolescents need relatively large amounts of iron because blood volume increases during periods of growth. During pregnancy and lactation the requirement for iron is high to allow for growth of the baby and milk production. However, the RNI is the same as for other women as no iron is lost during pregnancy, since menstruation ceases. Table 9.7 shows the RNIs for iron for some age groups. The full table is shown in Appendix II.

Table 9.7 *RNIs for iron*

Age	*mg iron per day*
4–6 years	6.1
7–10 years	8.7
Males	
11–18 years	11.3
19–50+ years	8.7
Females	
11–50 years	14.8*
50+ years	8.7
Pregnancy	14.8
Lactation	14.8

*Insufficient for women with high menstrual losses (iron supplements recommended).

Effect of cooking

Iron is not destroyed by heat but small amounts may be lost in cooking water or discarded meat juices. The use of iron utensils (knives, graters, mincers, etc.) can increase the iron content of food. Some members of the Bantu tribe in South Africa suffer from a condition known as siderosis, in which iron is deposited in the soft tissues of the body.

They cook maize and other cereals in iron pots and their iron intake is very high.

Sodium (and chlorine)

Sources

Sodium is eaten mainly in the form of common salt (sodium chloride). Most natural foods contain relatively little sodium, but considerable quantities of salt are added during cooking and during the processing and preservation of many foods. For example, salt is added during the production of bacon, smoked fish, bread, butter, cheese, breakfast cereals and canned vegetables. Sodium is also supplied by other chemicals used in processing, for example sodium hydrogen carbonate is used as a raising agent, mono sodium glutamate as a flavour enhancer and sodium nitrate as a meat preservative. About 70% of salt in the diet comes from foods (mostly manufactured foods) and about 30% is added during cooking and at the table. Table 9.8 shows the sodium content of some foods.

Table 9.8 *Sodium content of some foods*

Food	*mg sodium per 100 g*
Yeast extract 'Marmite'	4500
Bacon	1470
Cornflakes	1110
Potato crisps	1070
Kippers	990
Corned beef	950
Butter, salted	750
Cheese, Cheddar	670
White bread	520
Peas, canned	250
Eggs	140
Beef	72
Milk	55
Peas, fresh	1

Function

Sodium and chlorine are present as ions in the fluid surrounding body cells (extracelluar fluid) and are essential in the regulation of the water content of the body. They are also involved in acid-base balance and the functioning of muscles and nerves. In a temperate climate most people require about 3 g of salt per day but the average intake is between 5 g and 20 g per day. Excess salt is excreted in the urine. The kidneys regulate the loss and so control the level of sodium and chlorine ions in the tissue fluids.

Deficiency

Salt is also lost from the body in sweat, but there is no means of regulating the amount of salt lost in this way. In hot climates or during strenuous work or exercise, large amounts of salt may be lost through sweating. This will cause a lowering of the salt concentration of the tissue fluids resulting in weariness and muscular cramps. It may be necessary, therefore, for athletes and people working in hot, heavy industries to take extra salt.

Excess

In certain diseases, e.g. some types of kidney disease, too much salt is retained in the body. The correct concentration of salt is maintained by retaining an equivalent excess of water. This results in oedema (excess fluid in the tissues).

High salt intakes are associated with high blood pressure which is itself associated with coronary heart disease and strokes. It is thought that for people likely to develop high blood pressure, a high salt intake is a contributory factor. Current nutritional guidelines (the 1994 COMA report) recommend a reduction in salt intake from the present level of 9 g per day to 6 g per day. This may be done as follows:

1 Using less salt in cooking. Flavour may be provided by pepper, herbs etc.
2 Not adding salt at the table. A salt substitute (e.g. potassium chloride) may be used if necessary.
3 Eating less high-sodium processed foods, such as cured and canned meats and canned vegetables.
4 Eating less salty snack products, e.g. salted peanuts, crisps.

Babies cannot tolerate high sodium intakes because their kidneys cannot excrete the excess. They, therefore, should not be given salty foods, e.g. meat and yeast extracts. It is also important that bottle feeds are made up with the correct amount of water. If there is too little water, the sodium concentration could be too high.

Potassium

Potassium is found in an ionized form inside body cells (i.e. in the intercellular fluid, whereas sodium is in the extracellular fluid). It is involved in the regulation of the fluid content of cells and the functioning of muscles and nerves. It is found in a wide variety of foods, particularly fruits (especially bananas) and vegetables. Deficiency is rare but may occur if potassium is not absorbed, e.g. as a result of excessive use of laxatives. Symptoms of deficiency include mental confusion and muscular weakness. The effect on the heart muscle can lead to heart failure.

It is thought that taking fairly high intakes of potassium may counteract the effects of a high sodium (salt) intake and reduce the likelihood of developing high blood pressure. Current guidelines, therefore, recommend increasing potassium intake in adults from an average of 3 g per day to 3.5 g.

Phosphorus

Phosphorus, together with calcium, is an essential constituent of bones and teeth. It is also present in all living cells where it is involved in the release of energy. Energy produced by the oxidation of glucose is 'stored' in cells in high-energy phosphate compounds. The breaking down of these compounds releases energy when required (see page 144). Phosphorus is also needed for the formation of the nucleic acids, DNA and RNA.

Since phosphorus occurs in all living cells it is found in most foods and a dietary deficiency has never been recorded.

Magnesium

Magnesium is found together with calcium and phosphorus in bones and teeth. It is also needed in the body for the functioning of some enzymes. It is found in the chloroplasts of green plants and therefore green vegetables are a good source. It is also found in potatoes, milk, fruit and meat. Deficiency of magnesium is rare but has occurred as a result of excessive losses during bouts of diarrhoea. Normally, if intake is low the body conserves magnesium by reducing the amount excreted via the kidneys.

Iodine

Sources

The main sources of iodine in the diet are milk, cereals and vegetables. In the UK, the use of iodine-enriched cattle feeds is now widespread and therefore milk and milk products (cheese, etc.) are now the most important source of iodine in the British diet. The amount of iodine in cereals and vegetables varies considerably and depends on the amount of iodine in the soil. Iodine occurs in very low concentrations in sea-water but organisms living in the sea have the ability to concentrate these small amounts. Sea fish is a good source and seaweed is particularly rich in iodine.

Functions

Iodine is a trace element, needed by the body in very small amounts. It is required by the thyroid gland for the formation of hormones involved in the regulation of the rate of oxidation of nutrients in body cells (see page 167).

Deficiency

An insufficient intake of iodine results in **goitre,** an enlargement of the thyroid gland. This condition is common in certain parts of the world, in areas a long way from the sea where the soil contains little iodine. At one time goitre was common in Derbyshire and was known as 'Derbyshire neck'. Nowadays, goitre caused by a lack of iodine is rare in the UK since a large proportion of foods is imported. If there is any chance of the diet being deficient in iodine, 'iodized salt' may be used to increase the intake of iodine. This is ordinary table salt with a small quantity of potassium iodide added.

Cabbages and some other vegetables, e.g. turnips, contain substances known as goitrogens which reduce the absorption of iodine. An excessive consumption of these vegetables over a period of time can also cause goitre.

Fluorine

Fluorine occurs in the body and foods as fluorides (compounds containing fluorine). Drinking water is the main source of fluoride. Foods, with the exception of sea fish and tea, contain insignificant quantities. By combining with calcium phosphate, fluorine hardens tooth enamel and so helps to guard against tooth decay. Experiments carried out in Britain and the United States have shown that the addition of fluoride to drinking water reduces the incidence of tooth decay, especially in young children. Certain local authorities add fluoride to bring the level up to 1 ppm (part per million). An excess of fluoride in water (levels above 3 ppm) causes mottling of teeth.

Zinc

Zinc is present in a wide variety of foods but the main sources in the diet are meat, milk, bread and other cereals. There is little zinc in fruits and vegetables. Only about one-third of the zinc in the diet is absorbed. Absorption is reduced by phytic acid, present in wholegrain cereals, and by the presence of calcium. Iron tablets also interfere with zinc absorption.

Zinc is involved in a large number of enzyme systems in the body and is essential for normal growth and development. Deficiency causes stunted growth and delayed sexual maturity.

Selenium

Selenium forms part of an enzyme system in the red blood cells. The main sources in the diet are cereals, meat and fish. Deficiency does not normally occur in humans.

Water

Water is essential to life. All living organisms contain water; the human body is about 65% water. The body of an adult man contains about 40 litres of water. About 15 litres are present in the extracellular fluid (3 litres in the blood plasma and 12 litres in the tissue fluid). The remaining 25 litres make up the intracellular fluid, i.e. the fluid found within the cells.

Water is essential since it provides a medium in which nutrients, enzymes and other chemical substances can be dispersed and in which the chemical reactions necessary for maintaining life can take place. It is also necessary as a means of transport within the body. Nutrients are carried to cells and waste products are transported from the cells by blood plasma which is 90% water. Waste products are removed from the blood by the kidneys and excreted in the urine.

Water balance

It is possible to exist for several weeks without food but the body can only survive a few days without water. The normal functioning of the body involves a continual loss of water. Water cannot be stored in the body and therefore a regular intake is essential. Water is taken into the body in foods and drinks. Many foods contain a high percentage of water. Some foods which, because of their cellular structure, appear fairly solid contain large quantities of water, e.g. fruits and vegetables. Some colloids, e.g. jellies, are solid but have a high water content. Table 9.9 shows the water content of a variety of foods.

Water from food and drinks is mostly absorbed into the body from the large intestine. Some absorption takes place in the stomach and small intestine.

Table 9.9 *Water content of some foods*

Food	*% Water*
Melon	92
Cabbage	90
Milk	88
Apples	85
Jelly	84
Cod	82
Potatoes	79
Eggs	75
Beef steak	67
White bread	37
Cheese, Cheddar	36
Butter	16
White flour	14
Cornflakes	3
Sugar	0

Water is formed within the body by chemical reactions. When nutrients are oxidized in the cells in order to release energy, carbon dioxide and water are formed. For example, the oxidation of 100 g of glucose produces 60 ml of water.

The body inevitably loses about 1.5 litres of water daily. The kidneys must form at least 600 ml of urine in order to get rid of toxic waste products. Water is also lost by evaporation from the surface of the body and as water vapour in expired air. A small quantity of water is lost in the faeces. Table 9.10 shows a typical water balance for an adult man in a temperate climate.

Table 9.10 *Typical water balance for an adult man*

Intake		*Output*	
	ml per day		ml per day
Drink	1300	Urine	1500
Food	900	Skin	550
Oxidation of nutrients	300	Expired air	350
		Faeces	100
Total	2500	Total	2500

The amount of water taken into the body is determined mainly by habit and social custom. It is also regulated by thirst. The sensation of thirst arises as a result of the concentration of sodium in the blood, caused by a depletion of water. The kidneys control the output of water from the body (see page 150). The body cannot store water and any excess passes into the urine.

Hard water

In many areas of Britain the water from the tap is hard, i.e. it fails to give a lather with soap but tends to form a scum. Hard water is water which contains dissolved mineral salts. There are two types of hardness:

1 *Temporary hardness*

Temporarily hard water, so called because the hardness can be removed by boiling, contains calcium and magnesium hydrogen carbonates. This type of water is found in chalk and limestone regions. Small amounts of carbon dioxide dissolve in rain water forming carbonic acid, a weak acid.

H_2O	+	CO_2	$\longrightarrow$	H_2CO_3
water		carbon dioxide		carbonic acid

Carbonic acid slowly dissolves calcium carbonate (chalk and limestone) forming soluble calcium hydrogen carbonate.

H_2CO_3	+	$CaCO_3$	$\longrightarrow$	$Ca(HCO_3)_2$
carbonic acid		calcium carbonate		calcium hydrogen carbonate

Small quantities of magnesium hydrogen carbonate are formed in a similar way, from magnesium carbonate in the rocks.

2 *Permanent hardness*

Permanently hard water contains calcium and magnesium sulphates dissolved as rain water percolates through rocks containing these salts. This type of hardness cannot be removed by boiling.

Water in different parts of the country varies in hardness depending on the composition of soil and rocks. Water supplies are classified according to the amount of dissolved calcium ions; hardness is expressed as parts per million (ppm) of calcium carbonate. Soft water has less than 50 ppm. 100 ppm is described as moderately hard, and over 200 ppm as very hard.

Disadvantages of hard water

1 When soap is used in hard water it will not lather easily; instead, it forms a scum. Soap is composed of the sodium salts of fatty acids. When soap is placed in hard water some of it reacts with the calcium

and magnesium salts in the water forming insoluble calcium and magnesium salts of the fatty acids. These insoluble salts cling to the fibres of textiles and form a scum on the surface of the water. Scum formation and the wastage of soap can be overcome by the use of a synthetic detergent. The calcium and magnesium salts of soapless detergents are soluble.

2 When water containing calcium and magnesium hydrogen carbonates is heated or boiled, insoluble calcium and magnesium carbonates are formed. For example:

$Ca(HCO_3)_2$	$\longrightarrow$	$CaCO_3\downarrow$	+	H_2O	+	CO_2
calcium hydrogen carbonate		calcium carbonate		water		carbon dioxide

The insoluble carbonates can be seen as scale or 'fur' inside kettles. Scale can build up inside hot-water pipes and boilers reducing their efficiency and in extreme cases scale can cause a complete blockage which could result in an explosion. Scale or fur can be removed by using an acid. Phosphoric and formic acids are used in descaling agents.

3 Used during food preparation, hard water can have an adverse effect on the colour and texture of vegetables, and on the consistency of bread dough.

Advantages of hard water

1 The dissolved calcium salts in hard water increase the dietary intake of calcium.

2 Hard water is more suitable in certain industries, e.g. the steel and brewing industries. It produces better beer.

3 Hard water is safer in conjunction with lead water pipes. Lead poisoning can result from the consumption of soft water which has passed through lead pipes.

Some methods of removing hardness in water

1 Addition of washing soda

Washing soda (sodium carbonate) reacts with the calcium and magnesium salts in hard water forming soluble sodium salts and insoluble calcium and magnesium salts which remain as a precipitate. For example:

$CaSO_4$	+	Na_2CO_3	$\longrightarrow$	$CaCO_3\downarrow$	+	Na_2SO_4
calcium sulphate (hard water)		sodium carbonate (washing soda)		calcium carbonate (insoluble)		sodium sulphate (soluble)

Sodium carbonate is used in washing powders and bath salts.

2 Ion-exchange process

This method is used in domestic and industrial installations for removing both types of hardness. It involves the use of natural or synthetic resins such as 'permutit' and zeolite. The hard water is passed through a column packed with resin and the calcium and magnesium ions in the water are exchanged for sodium ions in the resin. The resin is regenerated from time to time by flushing the column with a concentrated salt (sodium chloride) solution. This replenishes the sodium ions.

3 Use of sequestering agents, e.g. 'Calgon'

A sequestering agent such as 'Calgon' (sodium hexametaphosphate), when added to hard water, encloses the calcium and magnesium ions in stable complexes which are soluble but which do not react with soap. 'Calgon' is used extensively for domestic purposes but is expensive and is therefore of limited industrial use.

Mineral waters

There has been a sharp increase in the consumption of bottled mineral waters in recent years. Mineral waters come from a spring or well. As rain water percolates through rocks, it picks up mineral salts and then collects when it reaches a layer of impermeable rock. The water may emerge as a spring at a fault in the rock or be brought to the surface through a bore hole or well. The mineral salts dissolved in the water can include chlorides, sulphates and bicarbonates of calcium, magnesium and sodium. The mineral content varies according to the source but is never very high. Mineral waters may be still (labelled 'Natural Mineral Water') or sparkling. If carbon dioxide is added to make it sparkling it is labelled 'Carbonated Natural Mineral Water', but if it is naturally effervescent it must be labelled 'Naturally Carbonated Natural Mineral Water'.

10 Basic physiology

Anatomy is the study of the structure of living organisms; physiology is the study of how organisms work or function. The functioning of an organism involves various changes which maintain the stability of the internal environment and keep the organism alive. Physiology is concerned with the changes that take place, where in the organism these changes occur and how they are regulated. An understanding of basic physiology is a necessary part of the understanding of nutrition.

Cells

All organisms, whether plant or animal, are made up of small units called cells. The human body is composed of thousands of millions of cells which are organized into tissues with specialized functions. For example, muscle is a tissue composed of long, spindle-shaped cells which by contraction and relaxation enable the body to move.

Since food is of either plant or animal origin most natural, unprocessed foods have a cellular structure. Cells themselves, although very small, have a complex structure, as shown in Figure 10.1.

Cell membrane

Surrounding every cell is a non-rigid, selectively permeable membrane which allows small molecules to pass in and out of the cell. The membrane consists of two layers of protein with a lipid (fatty) layer in between.

Cell wall (plant cells)

This is a more rigid structure which surrounds the cell membranes of plant cells. Plant cells tend to have a more definite shape than animal cells. Cellulose is the main component of the cell wall, together with pectins and hemicelluloses.

Nucleus

The nucleus controls the activity of the rest of the cell. It contains nucleic acids which form the chromosomes, the particles which carry the genetically inherited information required for the maintenance of the whole cell.

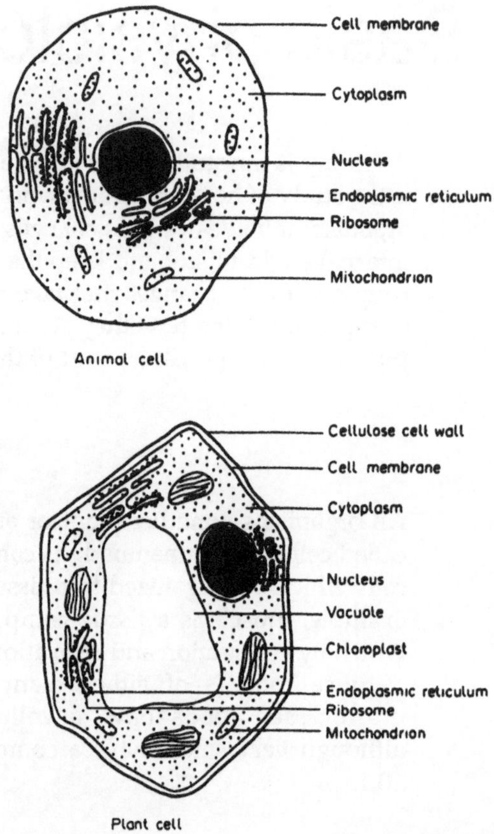

Figure 10.1 *Diagrammatic representations of typical animal and plant cells.*

Cytoplasm

Cytoplasm is a colloidal solution of protein and other substances dispersed in water.

Endoplasmic reticulum and ribosomes

The endoplasmic reticulum is a complex network of tubular cavities which, together with the ribosomes, is responsible for the building up of protein molecules from amino acids (see page 145).

Mitochondria

The mitochondria are sometimes called the 'power houses' of the cell. It is in these structures that nutrients are oxidized and energy is released, i.e. respiration takes place.

Chloroplasts

Chloroplasts occur only in the cells of green plants. They contain the green pigment chlorophyll which can convert light energy into a form that can be used for forming complex organic compounds. Chloroplasts are therefore involved in the process of photosynthesis (see page 59).

Vacuoles

Vacuoles are found only in plant cells. They are spaces filled with a solution of sugars and salts, known as cell sap. They help to maintain the shape of plant cells.

Metabolism

The term metabolism is used to include all the chemical processes involved in maintaining life. It is the total of all chemical reactions by which nutrients are used by the body to produce energy and material for growth and maintenance. Metabolism involves two types of reaction. **Catabolism** is the breakdown of large molecules into smaller molecules and **anabolism** is the synthesis, or building up, of large molecules from smaller molecules. In any one cell of the body catabolic and anabolic processes are carried out simultaneously. Each chemical reaction requires a catalyst. Enzymes are protein substances, produced in cells, which act as biological catalysts. They are studied in more detail in Chapter 11. Two of the most important metabolic processes which take place in cells are energy production and protein synthesis.

Energy production (respiration)

Carbohydrates, fats and proteins contain chemical energy 'locked up' in the molecules. Respiration is the breakdown of these substances and the subsequent release of energy. In order to remain alive, both animals and plants must respire. Respiration normally involves the uptake of oxygen and the release of carbon dioxide and it has become synonymous with breathing. For clarity, therefore, the external signs of respiration (breathing) are termed **external respiration** and the breakdown processes within the cells **internal respiration**.

Energy from carbohydrates

Glucose and glycogen are broken down in the cells of the body into carbon dioxide and water. The breakdown is a complex process which takes place as a series of reactions involving many intermediate products. One of the main intermediate products is pyruvic acid. The following equation represents the breakdown of glucose into pyruvic acid:

$$\underset{\text{glucose}}{C_6H_{12}O_6} \xrightarrow{\nearrow \text{energy}} \underset{\text{pyruvic acid}}{2CH_3COCOOH} + \underset{\text{hydrogen}}{4[H]}$$

This part of the respiratory process is **anaerobic,** i.e. oxygen is not involved. The hydrogen atoms are not released as free hydrogen but are transferred to co-enzymes which act as hydrogen acceptors. (Eventually the hydrogen atoms combine with oxygen to form water.) The breakdown of pyruvic acid is **aerobic**, i.e. oxygen is required.

$$\underset{\text{pyruvic acid}}{2CH_3COCOOH} + \underset{\text{oxygen}}{5O_2} \xrightarrow{\nearrow \text{energy}} \underset{\text{carbon dioxide}}{6CO_2} + \underset{\text{water}}{4H_2O}$$

This stage releases more energy than the first stage.

During periods of strenuous exercise there is insufficient oxygen reaching muscle cells and as a result pyruvic acid is broken down in the anaerobic conditions into lactic acid. A build-up of lactic acid causes muscle fatigue. This reaction also occurs during the hanging of meat (see page 190).

A large number of different enzymes are involved in internal respiration since each reaction in the series requires a specific enzyme. Some of the B vitamins are involved in these enzyme systems.

The energy produced by the oxidation of glucose and other nutrients is not released immediately. Certain organic phosphate compounds are able to store energy until it is required. Two of these compounds of particular importance are:

Adenosine diphosphate (ADP), a compound with two phosphate groups

Adenosine triphosphate (ATP), a compound with three phosphate groups

The addition of one more phosphate group to ADP, to convert it into ATP, requires a relatively large amount of energy. Conversely, the removal of a phosphate group from ATP releases a large amount of energy.

The energy released during the oxidation of nutrients is used to produce ATP from ADP. When energy is needed by the cell ATP is converted into ADP.

Energy from fats

Fat is first of all transferred from the adipose tissue to the liver. In the liver it is hydrolysed to glycerol and fatty acids. The glycerol is converted into pyruvic acid and oxidized by the method already described. The fatty acids are broken down into acetic (ethanoic) acid (CH_3COOH) which joins in with the series of reactions involving the oxidation of pyruvic acid.

Energy from proteins

Proteins in the diet also yield energy, although their main function is growth and maintenance of cells. Amino acids not required for protein synthesis are deaminated in the liver, i.e. the nitrogen-containing part of the molecule is removed. The deaminated molecules are converted into pyruvic acid and other intermediate products which are oxidized and energy is released (see Figure 10.2).

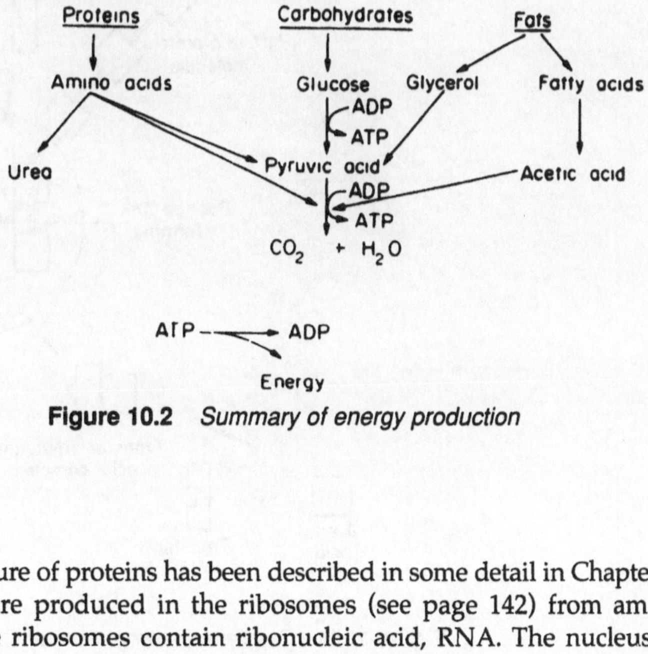

Figure 10.2 *Summary of energy production*

Protein synthesis

The structure of proteins has been described in some detail in Chapter 7. Proteins are produced in the ribosomes (see page 142) from amino acids. The ribosomes contain ribonucleic acid, RNA. The nucleus of the cell which contains deoxyribonucleic acid, DNA, controls protein synthesis. DNA molecules consist of two long chains twined around each other to form a double helix (a spiral-like structure). Cross-links between the chains join sub-units of the molecule called bases. There are four different bases and the order of the bases on the chain determines which proteins are formed in the cell. A sequence of three bases on the chain specifies one individual amino acid. With four different bases available it is possible to produce enough different sequences to cover all the 20 or so amino acids. The DNA molecule does not take part directly in protein synthesis. Instead, the 'coding' on the DNA molecule is transferred to shorter single chains of RNA. These RNA molecules are known as messenger RNA since they transfer the code from the nucleus to the ribosomes. Amino acid molecules present in the cytoplasm of the cell join up with another, even shorter, form of RNA called transfer RNA. There is a different kind of transfer RNA for each type of amino acid. The transfer RNA/amino acid complex is conveyed to the ribosome. Here the amino acids are released from the transfer RNA and arranged in a specific order determined by the sequence of bases on the messenger RNA molecule. The adjacent amino acids combine by forming peptide links and so a polypeptide (protein molecule) is produced. The main stages in protein synthesis are shown diagrammatically in Figure 10.3.

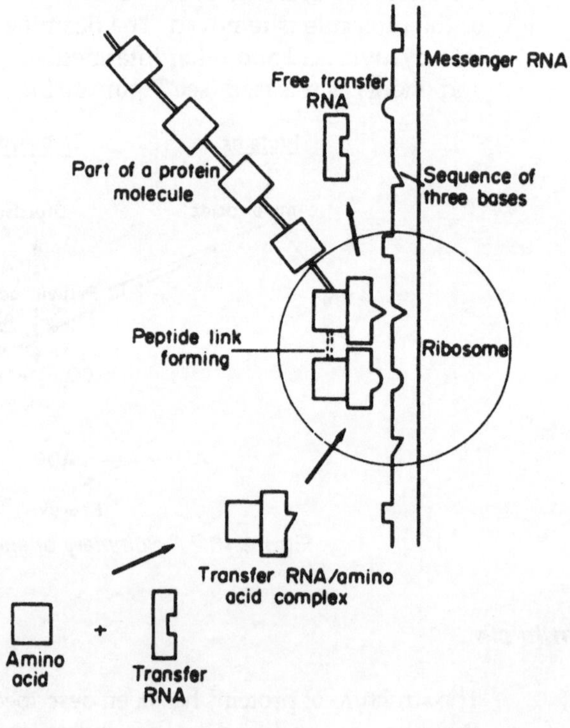

Figure 10.3 *Diagram showing the main stages in protein synthesis.*

Tissues

The millions of cells which make up the human body are not alike. They differ in size, shape and function. Cells are grouped together into tissues, a tissue being composed of a number of cells identical in function and held together by a ground substance or matrix.

There are five basic tissues in the body:

1 Epithelial
2 Connective
3 Muscle
4 Nervous
5 Fluid

Epithelial tissue

This tissue covers the surface of the body and lines internal cavities such as the lungs, mouth and stomach. Epithelial cells touch one another and there is little or no intercellular matrix. The functions of epithelial tissue include protection, e.g. the skin, and secretion and absorption, e.g. the internal lining of the intestines.

Connective tissue

Connective tissue connects and supports other tissues of the body. It consists of relatively few cells within an extracellular matrix. Protein fibres are suspended in the matrix; there are three main types:

(a) white collagen fibres – the most common; made of the protein collagen;
(b) reticular fibres – made of a protein called reticulin;
(c) yellow elastic fibres – composed of the protein elastin. These fibres will stretch but recoil to resume their original length.

The relative proportions of these fibres vary in the different types of connective tissue.

1 *Areolar tissue*. This type of tissue is found under the skin and surrounding internal organs, keeping them in place. It contains many loosely packed collagen fibres.

2 *Adipose tissue*. This is the fatty tissue of the body. It is similar to areolar tissue but the cells are swollen with droplets of fat. This fat represents the main energy reserve of the body. Adipose tissue is also found under the skin and around certain organs. It helps to reduce heat loss from the surface of the body and protects organs such as the kidney.

3 *Fibrous tissue*. This is a form of connective tissue in which collagen fibres are closely packed in bundles or sheets. It is tough and inelastic and forms ligaments and tendons. (Ligaments hold bones together at the joints and tendons attach muscles to bones.) Fibrous tissue also surrounds muscle fibres and bundles of muscle fibres.

4 *Cartilage*. This contains a tough, rubbery organic matrix. Some types contain white collagen fibres and some yellow fibres. Cartilage is found at the ends of the long bones and in the wall of the trachea (windpipe). The discs between the bones of the backbone are cartilage.

5 *Bone*. In bone the matrix is hard due to the deposition of calcium salts, mainly calcium phosphate. These mineral salts constitute about

two-thirds of the weight of bone. When bone is examined under a microscope it can be seen that the bony matrix is present in concentric layers surrounding small central canals which carry blood-vessels. Bone cells are situated in between the layers of bony material.

Muscle tissue

Muscle tissue is composed of elongated cells or fibres. The fibres are surrounded by thin layers of connective tissue. Muscle fibres contract, i.e. become shorter and thicker, in response to stimulation. Contraction of muscle fibres involves the bonding or overlapping of filaments of two proteins, actin and myosin. Energy for this reaction is obtained from the breakdown of ATP into ADP (see page 144).

Nervous tissue

Nervous tissue consists of nerve cells or neurones which have the ability to respond to stimuli (changes in the environment) and to transmit impulses. A neurone has a cell body with many thread-like projections or processes. There is usually a large number of branched processes called dendrites which conduct impulses to the cell body and a single, long process, the axon, which conducts the impulse away. The axon may be a metre or more in length.

Fluid tissue

Blood and lymph may be classified as fluid tissue. They consist of cells which move in a liquid intercellular matrix. See page 149 for further details.

Organs

The various tissues are grouped together to form the organs of the body. There are numerous organs, e.g. heart, lungs, kidneys, brain and spleen. An organ is composed of at least two tissues. For instance, the heart contains epithelial, connective, muscle, nervous and fluid tissue.

Systems of the body

A system is a group of organs which are closely allied to one another and are concerned with carrying out a particular bodily function.

Circulatory system

The circulatory or vascular system consists of the heart, the blood-vessels and the blood. Its function is to transport oxygen, nutrients, hormones and waste products and to maintain a constant composition of tissue fluid, i.e. the fluid surrounding the cells. Blood is contained in an enclosed system of vessels (arteries, veins and capillaries) and is pumped round the body by the heart. The arteries and veins have impervious walls but the capillaries, the very narrow vessels which bridge the arteries and veins, allow water and other small molecules to pass in and out of the blood.

Blood is composed of:

1. red corpuscles – which contain haemoglobin and convey oxygen from the lungs to the rest of the body;
2. white corpuscles – which are concerned with resistance to infection;
3. platelets – which assist in the clotting of blood;
4. plasma – a pale yellow fluid composed of water together with the blood proteins (albumin and globulin), nutrients, salts and other substances.

The lymphatic system is also considered part of the circulatory system. It drains excess fluid from tissue spaces. Lymph is similar in composition to plasma and tissue fluid. The lymphatic system is a one-way system which connects to the blood system. Lymph enters small lymph capillaries which unite to form larger lymph vessels. The vessels then empty their lymph into veins at the base of the neck. Lymph vessels are interrupted by lymph nodes which remove bacteria and other foreign matter from lymph on its return to the blood system. Lymph nodes are grouped in clumps and can be felt as 'glands' in the armpit, groin and neck. They also produce antibodies.

Respiratory system

The function of the respiratory system is to supply the body with oxygen and to get rid of carbon dioxide. During breathing (external respiration) air containing oxygen is brought into close proximity with the blood capillaries in the lungs, and oxygen passes from the lungs into the blood. At the same time carbon dioxide is released from the blood and is eliminated from the body in the air which is breathed out. This exchange of gases takes place at the necessary rate due to the large surface area of the lungs. Air enters through the nose and passes down the trachea or windpipe. The trachea divides into two pipes (bronchi), one leading to each lung. Each bronchus divides repeatedly until, finally, each branch leads into an air sac which has a large number of very small pouches called alveoli. It is through the thin walls of the alveoli that the exchange of gases takes place.

Internal respiration, the release of energy from nutrients in the cells, has been discussed earlier in the chapter.

Digestive system

The digestive system consists of the alimentary canal and its associated glands (salivary glands, pancreas, etc.). Its function is to break down food into a form which can be absorbed into the blood stream. Digestion is covered in some detail in Chapter 11.

Excretory system

The urinary system consists of the kidneys, ureters, bladder and urethra. Its function is to eliminate the waste products that result from metabolic activity and to keep the body fluid composition constant. The kidneys form urine by filtering materials from the blood. They are situated in the abdominal cavity, one on each side of the backbone. Each kidney contains about one million small tubules or filtering units called **nephrons** (see Figure 10.4).

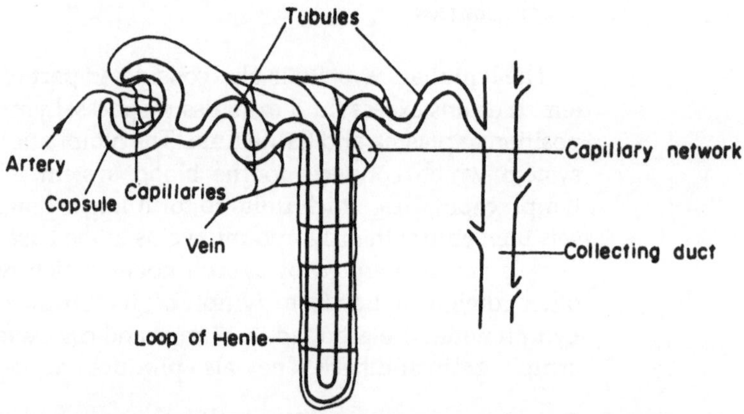

Figure 10.4 *Diagrammatic representation of a nephron.*

The blood-pressure in the capillaries supplying the capsule is high and blood plasma, minus the proteins, is forced through the wall of the capsule into the cavity of the tubule. The main components of the filtrate, i.e. the solution in the tubule, are water, urea, glucose and mineral salts. As the filtrate passes along the tubule many of its constituents are selectively reabsorbed into the blood capillaries surrounding the tubule. All of the glucose and most of the water and mineral salts are reabsorbed. By the time the filtrate reaches the collecting duct it is urine and consists of about 96% water, 2% mineral salts and 2% urea with traces of other nitrogen-containing substances. A constant flow of urine passes from the collecting ducts down the ureters into the bladder. Urine collects in the bladder and is periodically forced along the urethra and eliminated from the body.

The amount of water lost from the body in urine is controlled by a hormone, ADH (antidiuretic hormone), which is produced by the pituitary gland. ADH regulates the quantity of water reabsorbed into the blood stream from the filtrate in the tubules.

The kidneys are not the only organs of excretion. The lungs excrete carbon dioxide and water. Water and salts are lost from the skin in sweat and some other excretory products are passed into the alimentary canal and expelled from the body in the faeces.

Nervous system

The function of the nervous system is to control and coordinate the activities of the body by enabling the body to perceive changes in the environment (stimuli) and to respond accordingly. The nervous system consists of the sense organs, the nerves, the brain and the spinal cord. The spinal cord is a column of nervous tissue which is continuous with the brain and is enclosed in a channel inside the backbone. The sense organs (eyes, ears, skin, etc.) perceive stimuli and electrical impulses pass along sensory nerve fibres to the brain and spinal cord. In the brain and spinal cord action is determined and impulses are sent along motor nerve fibres to the organs which make the required response. Most nerves are made up of both sensory and motor fibres.

The brain and spinal cord constitute the central nervous system. There is a second system, outside conscious control, called the autonomic nervous system. This system regulates the organs of blood circulation, breathing, digestion, excretion and reproduction entirely by reflex action, i.e. by involuntary responses to stimuli.

The senses of sight, taste and smell play an important role in the appreciation of food and in stimulating the secretion of digestive juices.

The eye

The eye consists of a more or less spherical capsule, the main structures of which are illustrated in Figure 10.5. The outer layer consists of a tough, opaque membrane called the sclera which is replaced in the front of the eye by the transparent cornea. The cornea is covered by a thin moist membrane known as the conjunctiva. Behind the cornea is the lens which is held in position by ligaments. Lining the sclera is the choroid layer and inside this is the retina. The retina is pigmented and consists of many nerve endings which combine to form the optic nerve, the link between the eye and the brain. In front of the lens the choroid layer is modified to form a thin muscular sheet, the iris, which has a hole in the centre, the pupil. The iris is the coloured part of the eye. The space between the cornea and the lens contains a watery, colourless fluid, whereas the part of the eyeball behind the lens is filled with a thick, colourless fluid.

Light rays enter the eye through the cornea and pupil and are focused by the lens so that they converge on the retina, where an image is formed. When the eye is at rest distant objects are in focus. In order to focus closer objects the shape of the lens is altered by means of the ciliary muscles. This process is known as accommodation. The amount of light entering the eye is controlled by the iris diaphragm. In dim light the pupil is large; in bright light the pupil constricts.

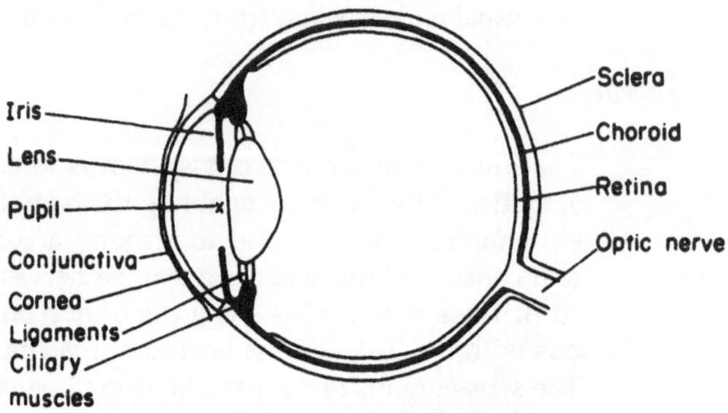

Figure 10.5 *Diagram of the eye.*

The retina has two types of nerve ending: rods and cones. These are both sensitive to light and impulses are conveyed from them, along the optic nerve, to the brain. The rods contain the pigment rhodopsin (visual purple) and are concerned with black and white vision in dim light. A deficiency of vitamin A depletes the supply of rhodopsin and night blindness results. The cones contain other pigments and are concerned with colour vision in daylight.

The sense of taste

The receptors of taste are the taste buds which are situated on the tongue and soft palate, the back part of the roof of the mouth. Each taste bud is a round cluster of spindle-shaped cells from which nerve fibres lead to the brain, as shown in Figure 10.6.

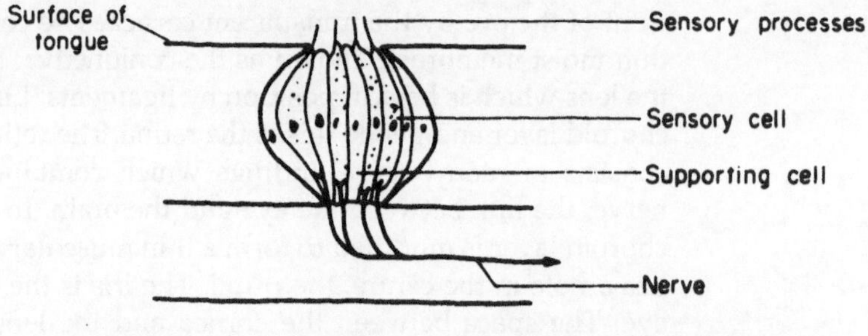

Figure 10.6 *Diagrammatic representation of a taste bud.*

The sensation of taste depends on water, either from food or from saliva, to carry the stimulating substances to the taste buds. The taste buds are capable of recognizing four basic or fundamental tastes, namely, sweet, sour, salt and bitter. These different tastes are transmitted along the nerves by different patterns of impulse. Some parts of the tongue are more sensitive than others to particular tastes, see Table 10.1.

Table 10.1 *The four basic tastes*

Basic taste	*Substances responsible*	*Area of tongue where detected*
Sweet	Sugars, saccharin, aspartame	Tip
Sour	Acids, e.g. citric, malic, tartaric	Tip and sides
Salt	Chlorides, especially sodium chloride (common salt)	Sides
Bitter	Alkaloids, e.g. quinine (tonic water) caffeine (coffee)	Back

The **threshold** of taste is the minimum concentration of a substance which can be detected. People are more responsive to bitter tastes than to sweet tastes, i.e. the threshold for bitterness is lower than for sweetness. The sense of taste tires or shows adaption. For example, if a sucrose solution is held in the mouth for two minutes the threshold for sucrose may be increased by as much as ten times. This explains why sweet drinks seem less sweet the more you drink. Interactions between different tastes can change threshold values. Sour substances will increase the threshold for sweetness, e.g. lemon juice can mask the presence of sugar.

Taste is a very crude sensation. The subtlety of the flavour of food depends on a combination of the four basic tastes, with a variety of odour or smell sensations. The texture and temperature of food also affect its flavour.

The sense of smell (olfaction)

The olfactory organs, the organs responsible for the sense of smell, are found in the upper part of the nose and are somewhat similar in structure to the taste buds. The actual mechanism of olfaction is not clearly understood, but it appears that the hair-like sensory processes of the olfactory cells are stimulated by molecules of volatile (easily evaporated) substances dissolved in the fluid bathing the cells and that the size and shape of the molecule determines the type of impulse which passes along the nerve to the brain. Sniffing directs air to the olfactory area. There are about 4000 different odours recognized by man.

The sense of smell is very acute. The threshold for smell being much lower than for taste. For example, alcohol can be detected by smell at a concentration of over 20,000 times less than can be detected by taste. Vanillin, the volatile compound responsible for the smell of vanilla, can be detected at a concentration of only 2×10^{-10} grams per cubic metre of air.

Smell receptors adapt to prolonged contact with volatile substances. This may sometimes be of benefit, for example, for people working in an unpleasant-smelling environment.

The pleasant smells produced by food during cooking (baking bread, roasting meat, etc.) occur as a result of volatile substances being formed by chemical reactions. These smells tempt the appetite and stimulate the release of digestive juices.

Endocrine system

There are two systems concerned with the control and coordination of the activities of the body. They are the nervous system and the endocrine system. The endocrine system is made up of various glands which release secretions, known as **hormones**, into the blood stream. Endocrine glands are ductless and are distinct from exocrine glands which release their secretions (e.g. sweat, digestive juices) into a duct to be used locally.

Hormones are sometimes called 'chemical messengers' since they are substances produced in one organ or region of the body, but they control or regulate the function of another organ or region of the body.

Some of the more important endocrine glands together with some of their hormones and functions are shown in Table 10.2.

Table 10.2 *Endocrine glands and their functions*

Gland	*Position*	*Hormone*	*Function*
Pituitary	Base of skull	ADH (vasopressin)	Controls water reabsorption in kidney tubules
		Growth hormone	Stimulates growth
Thyroid	Neck	Thyroid hormones	Control basal metabolic rate. Regulate growth
Parathyroids (4 glands)	Embedded in thyroid	Parathyrin	Regulates blood calcium level
Adrenals (2 glands)	Above each kidney	Adrenalin	Increases heart rate and output of glucose from liver in response to fear and stress
		Corticosteroids	Regulate water balance and influence metabolism
Pancreas	Behind the stomach	Insulin	Converts glucose from blood into glycogen (stored in liver and muscles)
Ovaries (female)	Each side of uterus	Oestrogens	Regulate sexual development and functions
Testes (male)	Groin	Androgens	Regulate sexual development and functions

There are many interactions between hormones and a disturbance in one gland can interfere with other hormones and upset the whole balance of the endocrine system.

Reproductive system

The function of the reproductive system is to procreate or reproduce the species. Human life begins as a single-celled embryo formed by the fusion of a sperm from the testes of a male and an ovum (egg) from the ovaries of a female.

11 Enzymes and digestion

Enzymes are substances which control all the chemical reactions in living organisms. They are proteins, produced by living cells, and are often called **organic catalysts** because they speed up (catalyse) reactions which otherwise would occur only very slowly, if at all, but are themselves unchanged at the end of the reaction.

Some enzymes have the effect of changing a single-stage reaction requiring a large amount of energy into a multi-stage process involving only small amounts of energy. All cells produce a large number of enzymes (a typical cell contains about 3000 different enzymes); the function of a cell is determined by the nature of the enzymes present in it. Some cells release enzymes which act outside the cell, e.g. the cells lining parts of the alimentary canal produce enzymes which digest food.

Names of enzymes

Most enzymes are named by adding the suffix **-ase** either to a word indicating the nature of the substrate (i.e. the substance affected by the enzyme) or to the name of the type of chemical reaction which the enzyme catalyses.

Hydrol**ases** catalyse hydrolytic reactions. For example:

carbohydr**ases** break down carbohydrates
lip**ases** break down lipids (fats and oils)
prote**ases** break down proteins

Oxid**ases** bring about oxidation reactions. For example, ascorbic acid oxid**ase** is responsible for the oxidation of ascorbic acid (vitamin C).

Some enzymes, e.g. pepsin and rennin, still retain their original or trivial names.

Mode of action

It appears that enzymes function as catalysts by providing within their molecules 'active sites' which receive molecules of the reacting compounds and at which reactions readily take place.

The action of enzymes is highly specific. In general, a given enzyme will catalyse only one reaction. For example, maltase hydrolyses the sugar maltose (to produce two glucose molecules), but it has no effect on other disaccharides. Maltose is the only molecule which will 'slot into' the active site on the maltase molecule. The reaction between an enzyme and its substrate has been likened to a lock and key action. Figure 11.1 shows diagrammatically the action of the enzyme maltase.

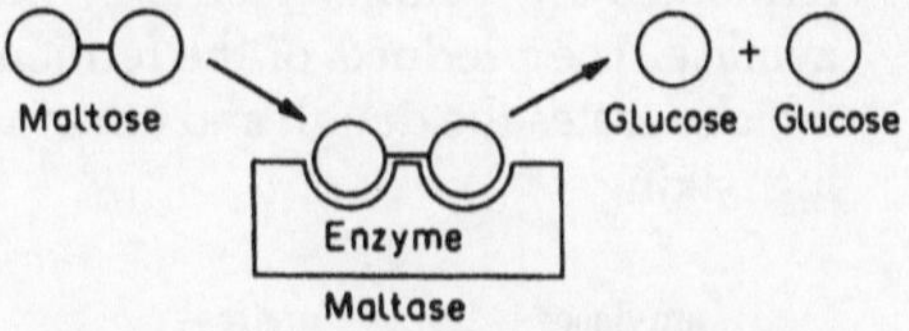

Figure 11.1 *The action of maltase.*

Factors affecting enzyme action

The activity of enzymes is affected by temperature and pH. Some enzymes are affected by the presence of other substances known as co-factors.

1 Effect of temperature

The activity of enzymes is greatly affected by temperature. For animal enzymes the optimum temperature is between 35°C and 40°C, i.e. body temperature. At temperatures above and below the optimum, enzyme activity is reduced. Above 50°C enzymes are gradually inactivated since being proteins they are denatured. At 100°C all enzymes are destroyed. At very low temperatures they are not actually destroyed but their activity is very greatly reduced.

2 Effect of pH

For each enzyme there is an optimum pH. Most enzymes function in a range of pH 5–9, being most active at pH 7 (neutral). If the medium becomes strongly acid or alkaline the enzyme is inactivated Some enzymes, however, only operate in acid or alkaline conditions. For example, pepsin, an enzyme released into the stomach, can only function in acid conditions; its optimum pH is 2.

3 Presence of co-factors

Enzymes often require the help of another substance in order to function effectively. **Co-enzymes** are non-protein compounds which aid enzyme activity. Many co-enzymes are vitamins or vitamin derivatives. Certain mineral ions, e.g. zinc, iron and magnesium, are **enzyme activators**. They must be mixed with the reacting substances before some enzymes will work.

Other substances act as **enzyme inhibitors**. For example, cyanide is a poison because it inhibits respiratory enzymes, resulting in death.

Some enzymes of importance in food production

1 Enzymes in breadmaking

Enzymes play a very important role in breadmaking. Flour contains **amylases** (diastase) which, in the presence of water, convert starch into maltose. The enzyme **maltase** which is secreted by yeast continues the breakdown by splitting maltose into glucose. Glucose is subsequently fermented by a number of enzymes in yeast, known collectively as **zymase**. The products of the fermentation process are carbon dioxide which aerates the dough and ethanol (alcohol) which is driven off during baking.

$$\text{Starch} \xrightarrow[\text{in flour}]{\text{amylases}} \text{maltose} \xrightarrow[\text{in yeast}]{\text{maltase}} \text{glucose} \xrightarrow[\text{in yeast}]{\text{zymase}} \text{carbon dioxide and ethanol}$$

Proteases, present in flour and yeast, are also important in breadmaking. They act on the protein in flour, gluten, making it more extensible and capable of retaining the carbon dioxide produced by the fermentation.

2 Production of alcoholic drinks

The fermentation of glucose by yeast enzymes is also the essential process in the production of beers and wines. In this case the alcohol is retained and the carbon dioxide is allowed to escape or is only partly retained.

Enzymes are used to remove cloudiness in wines and fruit juices. For example, hazes brought about by the presence of pectin in the product can be removed by the addition of small quantities of **pectinase**, an enzyme which breaks down pectin.

3 Cheese production

Rennet, the essential constituent of which is the enzyme **rennin**, is used in cheese manufacture to coagulate the protein in milk and so form the curd.

4 Meat tenderizing enzymes

During the hanging of meat, proteases, naturally present in meat, break down the connective tissue thus making the meat more tender. Meat is sometimes treated before cooking with artificial tenderizers. These tenderizers contain protein-splitting enzymes such as **papain**, which is obtained from the papaya plant, and **bromelin**, extracted from pineapple juice.

5 Tea production

During the drying of tea leaves important chemical changes take place. Colourless phenolic compounds are oxidized and brown-coloured compounds (including tannins) are formed. The oxidation is brought about by naturally occurring **oxidases**, e.g. polyphenoloxidase.

Some undesirable effects of enzymes in foods

1 Autolysis

Enzymes naturally present in the tissues of plants and animals continue to act after the harvesting of plants and the slaughter of animals and may bring about undesirable chemical changes in food during storage. This destruction of plant and animal cells by their own enzymes is known as **autolysis** and is one cause of food spoilage.

2 Microbial spoilage

Spoilage of food also results from the activities of micro-organisms such as bacteria and moulds. Enzymes contained within the micro-organisms break down the constituents of food and produce unpleasant end products. For example, the smell of stale fish is due to a nitrogen-containing compound called trimethylamine which is produced by the enzymic breakdown of protein.

3 Enzymic browning

When the cells of apples, potatoes and some other fruits and vegetables are cut and exposed to the air, enzymes present in the cells bring about an oxidation reaction; colourless compounds are converted into brown-coloured compounds. This is similar to the changes which occur during the drying of tea leaves, but in this case the changes are undesirable. Browning does not occur in cooked fruits and vegetables since the enzymes are destroyed by heat.

4 Oxidation of ascorbic acid (vitamin C)

The enzyme **ascorbic acid oxidase** is responsible for oxidation of vitamin C (see page 118).

Digestion

Food taken into the mouth is of no use to the body until it has been absorbed through the lining of the digestive tract (alimentary canal) and carried by the blood to the cells. Digestion is the breakdown of complex nutrient molecules into molecules small enough to be absorbed through the lining of the intestine. Certain components of food, monosaccharides, salts, vitamins, water and alcohol, do not need to be digested since they are composed of small soluble molecules. Digestion is mainly a chemical process of hydrolysis. Hydrolytic enzymes are produced in various organs and are released into the alimentary canal in digestive juices. The nutrients hydrolysed by digestive enzymes are shown below:

Disaccharides ⟶ Monosaccharides
Polysaccharides

Fats and oils ⟶ Fatty acids and glycerol

Proteins ⟶ Amino acids

Digestion is also, in part, a physical process. Food particles are reduced in size by the grinding and chewing action of the teeth and by the muscular action of the alimentary canal, e.g. stomach contractions.

The digestive system consists of the digestive tract, together with various associated organs such as the pancreas. The digestive tract can be thought of as a continuous tube, about 8 metres long, open at both ends, the upper opening being the mouth and the lower opening the anus. The various parts of the digestive system are shown in Figure 11.2.

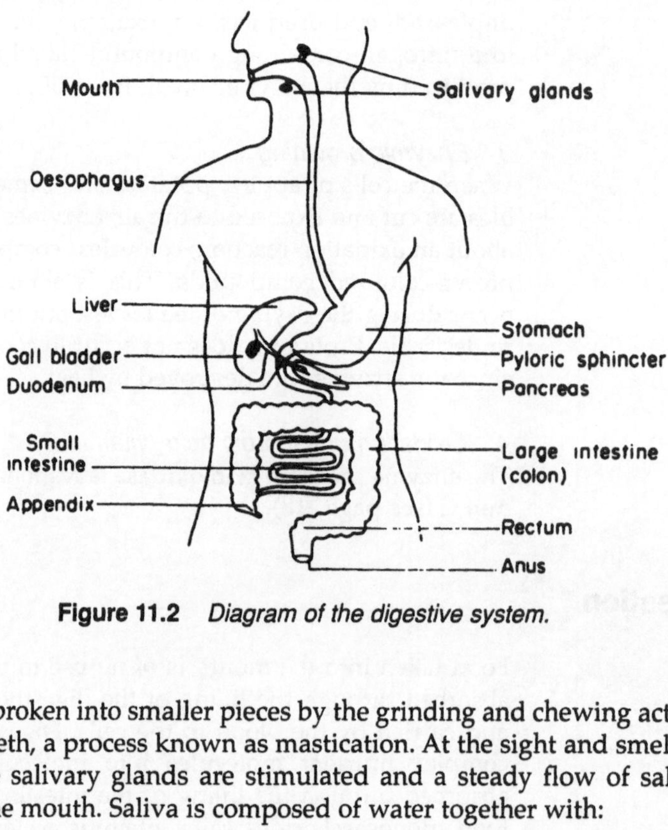

Figure 11.2 *Diagram of the digestive system.*

Mouth
Food is broken into smaller pieces by the grinding and chewing action of the teeth, a process known as mastication. At the sight and smell of food the salivary glands are stimulated and a steady flow of saliva enters the mouth. Saliva is composed of water together with:

1 **mucin** – a slimy, protein substance which lubricates food and makes it easier to swallow;
2 **salivary amylase** – an enzyme which initiates the breakdown of starch into maltose.

Food is mixed with saliva and reduced to a soft mass or bolus by the action of the tongue and jaws before it is swallowed. After being swallowed it is carried down the oesophagus by **peristalsis**, rhythmic contractions of the muscles in the wall of the oesophagus.

Stomach

The stomach acts as a reservoir, so that, rather than eating continually, food need only be consumed at intervals. It is also the site of some digestion. The cells lining the stomach produce gastric juice. Secretion of gastric juice is stimulated by the sight, smell and taste of food and also by the presence of food in the stomach. Gastric juice contains:

1 **pepsin** – an enzyme which breaks down some proteins into smaller molecules called polypeptides;
2 **hydrochloric acid** – which activates pepsin and kills bacteria;
3 **rennin** – an enzyme which coagulates milk protein, important only in babies;
4 **intrinsic factor** – a substance needed for the absorption of vitamin B_{12}.

Waves of muscular contractions in the stomach walls mix the food with the gastric juice producing a mixture known as **chyme**. At intervals small portions of chyme pass through a valve called the pyloric sphincter into the small intestine.

Small intestine

The majority of digestive processes take place in the small intestine. As chyme enters the duodenum, the first part of the small intestine, it is acted on by three digestive juices:

1 *Pancreatic juice* which, as its name suggests, is produced in the pancreas and which contains:

(a) **trypsin and chymotrypsin** – enzymes which continue the digestion of proteins;
(b) **pancreatic amylase** – an enzyme which breaks down starch into maltose. It is more effective than salivary amylase;
(c) **lipase** – an enzyme which hydrolyses lipids (fats and oils) into fatty acids and glycerol. Some fats are only partially hydrolysed to diglycerides and mono glycerides.

2 *Bile* which is a yellow-brown fluid produced in the liver and stored in the gall bladder. The presence of fat and other foods in the duodenum brings about contraction of the gall bladder and the flow of bile into the duodenum. Bile does not contain an enzyme but contains **bile salts** which aid pancreatic lipase by emulsifying fats and oils.

Both pancreatic juice and bile are alkaline and they neutralize the acidic chyme entering the duodenum from the stomach.

3 *Intestinal juice* which is secreted by the cells lining the small intestine and which contains:

(a) **peptidases** – a group of enzymes which complete the breakdown of proteins by splitting polypeptides into their constituent amino acids;
(b) **disaccharide-splitting enzymes** – maltase, sucrase (invertase) and lactase which hydrolyse maltose, sucrose and lactose into their respective monosaccharides.

Digestion takes place not only in the duodenum but also in the jejunum and ileum, the remaining sections of the small intestine. Some of the final stages of digestion occur in the cells of the intestinal wall. Absorption of nutrients takes place along the whole length of the small intestine. Any food which is not digested and absorbed passes from the ileum into the large intestine.

Large intestine (colon)

The main function of the large intestine is to remove water from the fluid mixture which enters from the small intestine. Water is absorbed through the lining of the colon so that undigested food leaves the body in a semi-solid state. The large intestine contains a very large number of bacteria which break down some of the cellulose and other components of undigested food by their own enzymes and which synthesize certain vitamins, e.g. some B vitamins and vitamin K. The vitamins can be absorbed into the bloodstream.

Undigested food materials, residues from digestive juices, dead cells from the lining of the digestive tract, bacteria and water form the faeces which are passed out of the body through the anus.

Table 11.1 gives a summary of the digestive processes.

Absorption

Some nutrients are absorbed from the stomach, but most absorption takes place in the small intestine. The small intestine is very long, about 6 metres, and its inner lining is folded into finger-like projections called villi. These two factors mean that the surface area over which absorption can take place is very large, about 20 m^2 (square metres).

Each villus is supplied with a network of blood capillaries and a lymph vessel, and nutrients are absorbed into the blood- or lymph-system. Non-fatty nutrients, which include monosaccharides, amino acids, water-soluble vitamins and mineral salts, are absorbed directly into the blood-system. Fatty nutrients, such as fatty acids and fat-soluble vitamins, pass into the lymph-vessels and enter the bloodstream at veins in the base of the neck.

Table 11.1 *A summary of the digestive processes*

Part of digestive tract into which juice is released	*Digestive juice*	*Main components*	*Action*
Mouth	saliva	mucin	aids mastication and swallowing
		amylase	starch → maltose
Stomach	gastric juice	pepsin	protein → polypeptides
		HCl	activates pepsin, kills bacteria
Small intestine	pancreatic juice	trypsin and chymotrypsin	split polypeptides and proteins
		amylase	starch → maltose
		lipase	lipids → fatty acids and glycerol
	bile	bile salts	emulsify fats and oils
	intestinal juice	peptidases	polypeptides → amino acids
		maltase	maltose → glucose
		sucrase	sucrose → glucose and fructose
		lactase	lactose → glucose and galactose

Digestibility

The terms 'digestible' and 'indigestible' are normally used subjectively to describe the effect foods have on the digestive system. Indigestible foods are those which cause digestive discomfort. The ease of digestion of a food is of practical importance only in the cases of people with weak or defective digestive systems.

In the stricter scientific sense, the digestibility of a food or nutrient is a measure of the amount which is digested and absorbed. It is normally expressed as a percentage.

$$\text{Digestibility of a food or nutrient} = \frac{\text{weight of food/nutrient digested and absorbed}}{\text{weight of food/nutrient eaten}} \times 100$$

Normally, the digestibility of carbohydrates is about 95% and of proteins and fats about 90%.

12 Food and energy

All living organisms require a source of energy. The earth's primary source of energy is the sun, without which there could be no life. Plants, by the process of photosynthesis (see page 59), are able to convert the sun's energy into chemical energy. Animals are unable to utilize the sun's energy directly and so they eat plants or other animals in order to obtain energy. The chemical energy in food is released in the cells of animals by oxidation; this process is known as internal respiration and is explained in some detail in Chapter 10. Some of the energy released is used to maintain metabolic processes in the cells; some is converted into heat to maintain body temperature and some is converted into mechanical energy which is used for physical activity.

Units of energy

As described in Chapter 1, the unit of energy is the **joule**. Since the joule is too small for practical nutrition the kilojoule (kJ) is used. The kilojoule has replaced the kilocalorie (kcal), sometimes written 'Calorie'.

1 kcal = 4.18 kJ

An even larger unit, the megajoule (MJ) is also used.

$$\begin{aligned} 1\text{ MJ} &= 1{,}000{,}000\text{ joules } (10^6\text{ J}) \\ &= 1000\text{ kJ} \end{aligned}$$

Energy value of nutrients

The three groups of nutrients which provide the body with energy are carbohydrates, fats and proteins.

1 g of carbohydrate provides 17 kJ (4 kcal)
1 g of fat provides 37 kJ (9 kcal)
1 g of protein provides 17 kJ (4 kcal)

Alcohol makes a significant contribution to the energy value of beers, wines and spirits.

1 g of alcohol provides 29 kJ (7 kcal)

Energy value of foods

The energy value of a food depends on the quantities of carbohydrate, fat and protein in the food. Since 1 g of fat provides 37 kJ, approximately twice the number of kJ from 1 g of carbohydrate or protein, it follows that fatty foods supply the most energy. Foods containing a high percentage of water, and therefore a smaller proportion of energy giving nutrients, provide the least energy.

Table 12.1 shows the energy value of a selection of foods.

Table 12.1 *Energy value of some foods*

Food	*kJ per 100 g*	*kcal per 100 g*
Sunflower oil	3696	899
Cooking fat	3674	894
Butter	3031	737
Cheese, Cheddar	1708	412
Sugar	1680	394
Cornflakes	1535	360
Bacon	1473	352
White flour	1450	341
White bread	1002	235
Beef	736	176
Eggs	612	147
Chicken	508	121
Bananas	403	95
Peas	344	83
Cod	322	76
Potatoes	318	75
Milk, whole	275	66
Apples	199	47
Beer	132	32
Melon	119	28
Cabbage	109	26
Lettuce	59	14

It should be pointed out that the figures in this table are for 100 g of food, not for portions of the foods. To compare the energy values of, say, an egg and a glass of milk the weights of the foods must be taken into account. A small egg weighs approximately 50 g and therefore one egg provides 306 kJ (50/100 × 612); a glass of milk weighs about 200 g and provides 550 kJ (200/100 × 275).

There are two methods by which the energy value of foods can be determined. Firstly, if the composition of the food is known its energy value can be calculated as shown in the following example.

100 g of milk contains:		
4.8 g carbohydrate which provides 4.8 × 17 kJ	=	81.6 kJ
3.9 g fat which provides 3.9 × 37 kJ	=	144.3 kJ
3.2 g protein which provides 3.2 × 17 kJ	=	54.4 kJ
		280.3 kJ

Secondly, if a weighed portion of food is placed in oxygen and ignited the heat produced by the combustion of the food is a measure of its energy value. This process is carried out in a calorimeter.

Main sources of energy in the British diet

The most important sources of energy in the average British diet are bread and other cereal foods, meat, fats, dairy produce and sugar (see Table 12.2).

Table 12.2 *Contribution made by different foods to the total energy content of the average British diet*

Food	*Contribution to total energy intake*	
Bread	13%	31%
Other cereal foods	18%	
Meat	14%	
Butter, margarine and other fats	13%	
Milk, cream and cheese	13%	
Vegetables	10%	
Sugar, preserves and confectionery	7%	

Use of energy by the body

Energy is required by the body for basal metabolism, i.e. for maintaining basic body processes, for physical activity and for additional needs during growth, pregnancy and lactation.

1 Basal metabolism

Basal metabolism is the term used to describe the basic metabolic processes which keep the body alive. Energy is needed to keep the heart beating and the lungs functioning, to maintain body temperature and muscle tone and for the numerous chemical reactions taking place in body cells. The rate at which energy is used up in maintaining basal metabolism is called **basal metabolic rate** (BMR).

BMR varies from person to person and is measured when a person is lying down, relaxed, still and warm and at least 12 hours after a meal. It can be measured by determining the amount of heat given out by the body. This is done by enclosing the person in an insulated chamber and measuring heat output. Another simpler method used for measuring BMR is for the person to breathe into specially designed apparatus which monitors either oxygen uptake or carbon dioxide output. Since oxygen is used up and carbon dioxide is released during the oxidation of nutrients in the body, a measure of either oxygen uptake or carbon dioxide output can be used to determine the rate of energy production in the body.

There are various factors which affect the BMR of an individual.

(a) *Body size.* It is obvious that a large person uses up more energy in maintaining basic body processes than a smaller person. The most critical factor is not total body-weight but lean body mass, i.e. the weight of the body excluding fat. Women have lower metabolic rates than men, partly because they are lighter but also because they have proportionally less lean body tissue and proportionally more body fat.

BMR of an average 70 kg man is 290 kJ per hour (70 kcal per hour)
BMR of an average 55 kg woman is 250 kJ per hour (60 kcal per hour)

In conditions of undernutrition or starvation lean body mass is reduced and this therefore reduces BMR. This partly explains why people are able to exist on diets considerably lower in energy than is normally recognized as adequate.

(b) *Age.* Children have a lower BMR than adults because their body size is smaller but proportionally their BMR is higher, i.e. their BMR per kilogram of body weight is greater. In adults the BMR of both men and women falls with increasing age. The average fall in BMR for a 70 kg man is from 290 kJ per hour at the age of 20 years to 260 kJ (62 kcal) per hour at 70 years of age.

(c) *Activity of the thyroid gland.* The thyroid gland secretes into the bloodstream iodine-containing hormones which control metabolic rate. Thyroxin is the major one of these hormones. In normal healthy people there can be a considerable difference in thyroid gland activity between one person and another. However, in certain cases the thyroid gland may be abnormally active or inactive. An overactive thyroid gland increases BMR by 20% or sometimes more. The person tends to be underweight, very active and excitable, and usually has protruding eyeballs. This condition can be treated by removal, by surgery, of part of the thyroid gland. A person with an abnormally underactive thyroid has a very low BMR and tends to be overweight and slow moving. Administration of thyroxin will help to alleviate this condition.

(d) *Thermogenic effect of food.* The intake of food stimulates metabolism and after a meal metabolic rate increases. The extra energy appears in the form of heat. This stimulation of BMR is known as the thermogenic effect of food.

2 Physical activity

In addition to basal metabolism, energy is used by the body for muscular activity. The energy requirements for various activities have been determined by measuring oxygen uptake during different activities. Average values of some of these figures are shown in Table 12.3.

Table 12.3 *Energy expenditure for various activities*

Activities	*kJ/ min (average)*
Sitting, watching TV, reading, eating	5.5
Playing piano, driving, washing up, ironing, office work	7.5
Housework, cooking, snooker, bowling	9.5
Walking (3—4 km/hr), cricket, painting and decorating, making beds	13
Walking (4–6 km/hr), gardening, table tennis, bricklaying	17
Walking (6–7 km/hr), chopping wood, volleyball	22
Walking uphill, climbing stairs, jogging, cycling, football, tennis	31

Activities which involve moving the body about, particularly those involved in moving the body upwards, e.g. walking upstairs, require a large amount of energy.

A woman working in an office might in one day use up energy in the following manner:

			kJ
8 hours sleeping (BMR)	8 ×250	=	2000
1 hour walking	60 × 17	=	1020
1 hour housework	60 × 9.5	=	570
6 hours sitting (eating, etc.)	6 × 60 × 5.5	=	1980
7 hours office work	7 × 60 × 7.5	=	3150
1 hour gardening	60 × 17	=	1020
			9740

The body is unable to completely convert chemical energy from food into mechanical energy; the efficiency of conversion is only 15–20%. The energy which cannot be used for physical activity is converted into heat and is used to maintain body temperature. Any excess heat is lost from the body in sweating and this explains why hard work or exercise makes a person hot.

3 Growth, pregnancy and lactation

Extra energy is needed during periods of growth to provide for extra body tissue. About one-third of the total energy needs of a new born baby is used in forming new body tissue. This decreases as the child gets older. Extra energy is also needed during pregnancy for the growth of the baby and during lactation (breast-feeding) for the production of milk.

Energy requirements

The amount of energy a person requires depends on age, body size and activity. In adults the degree of activity is largely determined by occupation. For example, a farm worker will need more energy than a computer operator. However, energy requirements are also affected by leisure activities; playing football or tennis uses more energy than reading or watching television.

The DoH figures for Estimated Average Requirements (EARs) for energy for men and women are shown in Table 12.4

Table 12.4 *Estimated Average Requirements (EARs) for energy*

	Male		*Female*	
Age	*kJ/day*	*kcal/day*	*kJ/day*	*kcal/day*
19–50 years	10 600	2550	8100	1940
51–59 years	10 600	2550	8000	1900
60–64 years	9930	2380	7990	1900
65–74 years	9710	2330	7960	1900
75+ years	8770	2100	7610	1810
Pregnancy (last 3 months)			+800	+200
Lactation			+1900–2400	+450–570

In women during pregnancy and lactation, recommended energy intakes are higher in order to meet the energy requirements of the growing baby.

Energy requirements for children, when related to body-weight, are higher than in adults since BMR when related to body size is higher in children than in adults. Also, children tend to be more active than adults. Babies and young children have proportionally higher energy needs than older children due to rapid growth in the first years of life and to proportionally greater heat losses from the surface of the body (the younger the child the greater the ratio of surface area to body-weight).

The complete table of EARs published by the DoH is shown in Appendix II.

If energy input (food intake) is equal to energy output (energy used for basal metabolism and physical activity), body-weight remains constant. If energy input is greater than output, the excess food is converted into fat and obesity results.

In adults a useful way of measuring body fatness is to use the Body Mass Index (BMI) which is a measure of a person's body-weight in kilograms divided by the square of their height in metres.

$$\text{BMI} = \frac{\text{body weight (kg)}}{\text{height (m}^2\text{)}}$$

People can then be divided into categories according to their weight status:

BMI
under 20 = underweight
20–25 = normal (desirable) weight
25–30 = overweight
above 30 = obese

Table 12.5 shows the increase in incidence of overweight and obesity in men and women in England between 1980 and 1991.

Table 12.5 *Percentage of overweight and obese adults in England, 1980 and 1991*

		1980		*1991*	
Weight status	*BMI*	*Men*	*Women*	*Men*	*Women*
Overweight	25–30	35	24	40	26
Obese	30+	6	8	13	15

Obesity is one of the major nutritional problems of the Western world and is one of the commonest causes of ill-health in the UK. It reduces life-expectancy and is a factor in coronary heart disease and various other conditions including high blood pressure, gall-bladder disease and varicose veins. It also increases the chances of developing diabetes in middle life.

Causes

The development of obesity results from both environmental and genetic factors but inevitably follows an energy intake in excess of energy expenditure. The main sensations regulating food intake are hunger, appetite, satiety and satiation. Hunger is the physiological need to eat and is controlled by the hypothalamus, a region at the base of the brain. Appetite is the psychological desire to eat and is triggered by the sight and smell of palatable food. Satiety is a reluctance to start eating and satiation is a feeling of fullness at the end of a meal which limits the size of the meal.

These regulating mechanisms may be influenced by a number of factors with the effect that energy input is greater than energy output. Some of the factors involved include:

1 *Heredity*. Body type and structure tend to be inherited. Overweight parents often have overweight children, but it can be argued that this is as much due to family eating habits as to inherited characteristics.

2 *Reduced physical activity*. Obesity is seldom found in people who lead active lives and have jobs involving hard physical work. It is thought that the control of food intake by hunger and appetite works well in active people, but that it fails when activity falls below a certain level so that the normal balance between energy input and output is no longer maintained. This results in a food intake greater than is needed.

Also, people tend to adopt patterns of eating when young and as they get older they continue to eat the same amount, but their physical activity and energy output are reduced. As a result they put on weight.

3 *Eating habits*. People often eat more than they need. This applies particularly to highly palatable fat-rich, sugary foods such as chocolate, biscuits, and cakes which have a high energy density. It has been shown that people spontaneously have a higher energy intake when offered a high fat diet.

4 *Psychological factors*. People with psychological or emotional problems tend to find solace in food and often overeat.

5 *Endocrine factors*. Many overweight people tend to blame their glands. However, endocrine disorders rarely cause obesity. Very occasionally obesity may be the result of defective hormone production by the thyroid, pituitary or sex glands. Obesity is more likely to be due to a disorder of the hypothalamus, which in turn may affect the functioning of the endocrine glands.

Treatment

In order to lose weight it is essential to reduce energy intake below the level of energy output so that body fat is used as an energy source. This can be done either by reducing intake, i.e. going on a slimming diet, or by increasing output, i.e. increasing physical activity.

1 *Diet*. The contributions made by the three major nutrients to the total energy intake of the average British diet are as follows:

	Contribution to total energy intake
Carbohydrate	46%
Fat	40%
Protein	14%

In order to reduce energy intake it is not advisable to cut down on protein since it is an essential nutrient and intake must be maintained even on a reducing diet. It is sensible to restrict fat intake by cutting down on the intake of fried foods, butter, cream, full-cream milk, fatty meat, etc. Carbohydrate intake should also be reduced but by restricting non-milk extrinsic sugars (NMES) rather than starch or intrinsic sugars in fruit. Sugar, being 100% carbohydrate, contains no vitamins or minerals, i.e. provides 'empty calories' (see page 71). Foods such as sugar itself, sweets, soft drinks and jams should therefore be reduced as much as possible. Many highly palatable manufactured foods are rich in both fat and sugar, e.g. cakes, biscuits, chocolates, ice cream and other desserts, and should be severely restricted. Alcoholic drinks in excess can lead to obesity and it is sensible to restrict drinking to lose weight.

2 *Activity*. An increase in activity by a sedentary overweight person should have quite a marked effect since increased activity will not only use up more energy but will also help the appetite control function more efficiently. For a moderately active overweight person exercise alone is not sufficient to bring about a significant loss of weight. For example, taking a walk which lasts three-quarters of an hour is only equivalent to using up the energy produced by a packet of potato crisps. Also increased activity stimulates the appetite and therefore with increased exercise there is a tendency to increase food intake to balance the extra energy output. The best method of weight reduction is to combine a reduced food intake with regular daily exercise.

A further argument in favour of exercise is that if a person loses weight by restricting intake alone they tend to lose both lean body tissue and body fat, but if they exercise as well they lose fatty tissue only.

Eating Disorders

There are several psychological disorders in which normal eating patterns break down. These include:

1 **Anorexia nervosa**. This is characterized by severe weight loss as a result of avoidance of food and fear of being overweight. It most often affects adolescent girls and young women.

2 **Bulimia nervosa**. This is characterized by bouts of gross

overeating, usually followed by self-induced vomiting and/or large doses of laxative drugs. It often follows a period of anorexia nervosa and most sufferers are women between the ages of 15 and 30 years.

Treatment for both conditions includes supervision of eating habits, psychotherapy and antidepressant drugs.

13 Nutrition in practice

Nutritional considerations of groups of people

Nutrient and energy requirements vary according to the age, sex, activity and type of work of the person concerned. There are certain groups of people within the community, for example old people and some ethnic groups, who may have particular nutritional problems and whose diets need particular attention.

Infants and young children

Some of the energy and nutrient requirements of infants and young children are shown in Table 13.1. For the first few months of life these requirements are met by a single food, milk. Babies may be either breast-fed or bottle-fed. There are various dried products on the market available for infant feeding; these infant formulas are based on modified cow's milk. However, there are several advantages of breast-feeding. Human milk is the natural food for babies and it contains nutrients in the correct proportions. Cow's milk contains more protein but less fat, lactose and vitamins A and C. There is the possibility that dried milk products may be unhygienically prepared or made up to incorrect concentrations with water. The Health of the Nation report in 1992 set a target of 75% of babies to be breast-fed by the year 2000.

Milk is a satisfactory food for the first few months of life but from about four months, solid foods, such as infant cereal products, should be introduced into the diet. Babies are born with a store of iron which lasts for four to six months. Milk is a poor source of iron, and iron-containing foods, such as pureed fruit and vegetables, egg yolk and minced meat, should be included in the diet from this age. The recommended daily intake of vitamin D for children up to five years is very high and a vitamin D supplement is advised, especially since milk is also a poor source of vitamin D. Supplements of vitamins A and C are also recommended.

Cow's milk may be introduced into the diet from the age of one year, but this should be whole milk and not skimmed or semi-skimmed, which are both too low in energy and vitamin A for infants and very young children. Semi-skimmed milk may be introduced after the age of 2 years. Young children have high energy needs in relation to their small size since they are active and growing fast. Food should, therefore, be of fairly high energy density, i.e. in the region of 10 kJ per gram of food.

Table 13.1 *EARs for energy and RNIs for nutrients for children aged up to six years*

	Age range		
	0–3 months	*1–3 years*	*4–6 years*
Energy (kJ)*	2280	5150	7160
(kcal)*	545	1230	1715
Protein (g)	12.5	14.5	19.7
Vitamin A (μg retinol equivalents)	350	400	300
Thiamin (mg)	0.2	0.5	0.7
Riboflavin (mg)	0.4	0.6	0.8
Niacin (mg equivalents)	3	8	11
Vitamin C (mg)	25	30	30
Vitamin D (μg)	8.5	7	—
Calcium (mg)	525	350	450
Iron (mg)	1.7	6.9	6.1

*These figures are for boys only; figures for girls are slightly lower.

Important foods in the diet of children include lean meat, fish, eggs, fruits, vegetables, bread and cereal products. Cereals need not be all wholegrain. A mix of 'white' and wholegrain is best since excessive intakes of fibre can cause toddler diarrhoea.

School children

Recommended energy and nutrient intakes for boys and girls aged seven to ten years and 15 to 18 years are shown in Table 13.2. The full table, for all age groups, is given in Appendix II.

Energy requirements are high in relation to body-weight since children are normally very active and are growing fast. The rate of growth accelerates before and during adolescence, but growth usually stops at 14 to 16 years in girls and 16 to 19 years in boys. Although energy requirements are high, meals should not be too bulky since children have smaller stomachs than adults. Also, obesity among school children and adolescents is becoming more of a problem in developed countries and therefore overeating should be discouraged.

Children should be taught to eat sensibly from an early age. Foods such as meat, liver, fish, cheese, bread, potatoes and other vegetables, fruits and milk are good sources of many nutrients. Encouragement should be given to eat proper meals and not to exist on snack foods. Many of the foods eaten as snacks are not nutritious and displace other more nutrient-rich foods from the diet. These include sweets, crisps, sweet biscuits and soft drinks.

Table 13.2 *EARs for energy and RNIs for nutrients for boys and girls aged seven to eight years and 15 to 18 years*

	Age range (years)			
	Boys 7–10	*Girls 7–10*	*Boys 15–18*	*Girls 15–18*
Energy (kJ)	8240	7280	11 510	8830
(kcal)	1970	1740	2755	2110
Protein (g)	28.3	28.3	55.2	45.0
Vitamin A (µg retinol equivalents)	500	500	750	600
Thiamin (mg)	0.7	0.7	1.1	0.8
Riboflavin (mg)	1.0	1.0	1.3	1.1
Niacin (mg equivalents)	12	12	18	14
Vitamin C (mg)	30	30	40	40
Calcium (mg)	550	550	1000	800
Iron (mg)	8.7	8.7	11.3	14.8

Girls during adolescence should be encouraged to eat plenty of iron-rich foods since iron losses occur due to menstruation and therefore requirements are high.

Adults

The energy requirements of adults vary depending on their age, sex, the type of work they do and their leisure activities. Average figures for energy needs for adults are shown in Table 12.4. People's leisure time and recreational activities may make very varied demands on their energy needs. For example, a man spending his evening watching television is obviously using less energy than one playing football or squash. It is important that energy intake does not exceed energy needs since this will lead to obesity. People with sedentary occupations are probably most likely to overeat. Meals and portion sizes should be varied according to energy needs. For example, the diet of an office worker could include plenty of salads and fruit with moderate amounts of potatoes, cereal products, meat and fish, whereas someone doing heavy manual work will need to fill up with plenty of potatoes, bread and other cereal products and have larger portions of meat, fish, etc.

Pregnancy and lactation

Energy and nutrient requirements are increased during pregnancy and lactation (breast feeding), as shown in Table 13.3.

Table 13.3 *EARs for energy and RNIs for nutrients for non-pregnant, pregnant and lactating women (19–50 years)*

	Non-pregnant women	*Pregnant women*	*Lactating women*
Energy (kJ)	8100	8900	10 300
(kcal)	1940	2140	2460
Protein (g)	55.5	61.5	66.5
Vitamin A (μg retinol equivalents)	600	700	950
Thiamin (mg)	0.8	0.9	1.0
Riboflavin (mg)	1.1	1.4	1.6
Niacin (mg equivalents)	13	13	15
Folate	200	300	260
Vitamin C (mg)	40	50	70
Vitamin D (μg)	–	10	10
Calcium (mg)	700	700	1250
Iron (mg)	14.8	14.8	14.8

The mother's diet must provide for the laying down of extra tissue in her body and the growth and development of the foetus during pregnancy, and the provision of milk during lactation. Nutrients of particular importance during this period are vitamins C, D and folic acid, together with iron and calcium. The intake of foods rich in these nutrients such as milk, cheese, eggs, fruits and vegetables should be increased to meet these higher requirements. Folate is particularly important during the early weeks of pregnancy and prior to conception (see page 114). Energy intakes should not be excessive, but should be such as to ensure optimum weight gain during pregnancy (about 12.5 kg). During the last three months of pregnancy, when a large transfer of iron from the mother to the foetus occurs, an iron supplement (e.g. iron tablets) is advisable. Constipation is common during pregnancy and increased amounts of NSP (fibre) together with adequate fluid intake are recommended.

Pregnant women are advised not to eat liver. Liver is extremely rich in vitamin A and too much vitamin A, especially in the first 3 months of pregnancy, is associated with certain birth defects. Other foods which should be avoided during pregnancy include soft cheeses and pâtés because of the risk associated with *Listeria monocytogenes* (see Chapter 16).

The recommended energy and nutrient intakes for older men and women are shown in Table 13.4. Older people do not need as much energy as younger people since they are less active and since basal metabolic rate declines with age. However, nutrient requirements are similar to, or only slightly less than, those for younger people. This means that they need less food but that the food they do eat must be rich in nutrients.

Some old people, particularly those living on their own, do not obtain an adequate diet. There are a variety of reasons for this, one of the major ones being financial. Other reasons include apathy, poor appetite, ignorance of nutritional values, difficulty in chewing foods and physical disabilities which make shopping and cooking a problem.

Older people who do not get outside much in summer months need plenty of dietary vitamin D (from foods such as margarine, eggs and oily fish) or a vitamin D supplement.

Table 13.4 *EARs for energy and RNIs for nutrients for older men and women*

	Age range (years)			
	Men		*Women*	
	65–74	*75+*	*65–74*	*75+*
Energy(kJ)	9710	8770	7960	7610
(kcal)	2330	2100	1900	1810
Protein (g)	53.3	53.3	53.3	53.3
Vitamin A (μg retinol equivalents)	750	750	750	750
Thiamin (mg)	0.9	0.9	0.8	0.8
Riboflavin (mg)	1.3	1.3	1.1	1.1
Niacin (mg equivalents)	16	16	12	12
Vitamin C (mg)	40	40	40	40
Vitamin D (μg)	10	10	10	10
Calcium (mg)	700	700	700	700
Iron (mg)	8.7	8.7	8.7	8.7

Nutritious foods are not necessarily the most expensive or those which need elaborate cooking. Relatively cheap foods which need little preparation include milk (fresh or dried), eggs, cheese, canned fish (e.g. tuna and sardines), fruit juices, potatoes (fresh or dried), breakfast cereals, bread and margarine or low fat spread.

Maintaining an interest in food is important for old people. Luncheon clubs and eating with friends are ways of increasing morale and stimulating the appetite of those who live alone. Many old people receive 'Meals on Wheels' on one or more days a week. The 'Meals on Wheels' scheme aims to supply old people with a nutritionally balanced, hot midday meal. This is organized locally by the Women's Royal Voluntary Service.

Vegetarians and vegans

Vegetarians, for a variety of reasons, do not eat meat but many do consume other animal products such as milk, cheese and eggs. The term 'lactovegetarian' is used to describe a person whose diet includes milk and cheese but not meat, poultry, fish or eggs. An 'ovo-lactovegetarian' consumes milk, cheese and eggs but not meat, poultry or fish. Generally speaking, there are few nutritional problems with these types of diets. The nutrient most likely to be deficient is iron. This can be supplied by eggs (if eaten), cereals, pulses and green vegetables.

The term 'vegan' is used to describe a person who chooses, usually for humanitarian or health reasons, a very much stricter diet that contains no foods of animal origin. Nutrient requirements, with the exception of vitamin B_{12}, can be met by a diet composed only of plant foods, but this requires careful planning and the inclusion of a wide variety of foods. In the average British diet the nutrients provided largely by foods of animal origin include protein, riboflavin, vitamin D and iron. For vegans protein needs can be met by cereals, pulses, nuts, mycoprotein (quorn) and TVP (textured vegetable protein); riboflavin requirements can be met by nuts, cereals, potatoes and soya; vitamin D requirements by margarine and exposure to sunlight; and iron requirements by pulses, green vegetables, cereals and cocoa. There are fortified breakfast cereals and yeast extract products available which contain vitamin B_{12}.

The calcium content of vegan diets is sometimes low but there is no evidence of calcium deficiency among vegans. It is thought that their ability to absorb calcium is increased. Sometimes vegan diets have a low energy density, particularly if they contain a lot of watery fruit and vegetables. Energy density can be kept at a satisfactory level by eating plenty of cereals, nuts and pulses. If well planned, a vegan diet is healthy and adheres to many of the current nutritional guidelines. Obesity and coronary heart disease are less common among vegans than the rest of the population.

Ethnic and religious groups

In general, the traditional diets of the various ethnic communities and different religious groups in the UK are nutritionally adequate. There is, however, some concern about low vitamin D intakes in Asian vegetarian groups. Because exposure to sunlight, particularly by women and children, may also be low (because of customs and the wearing of enveloping clothes) rickets and osteomalacia sometimes occur. In addition, the iron content of some traditional diets is low and iron deficiency anaemia sometimes occurs among women and children, particularly in the Asian community.

There are various dietary restrictions practised by different religious and ethnic groups. Some of these are as follows:

Jews. Jews eat no pork; other meat must be kosher, i.e. slaughtered by a licensed person and then soaked and salted. Only fish with scales and fins may be eaten. Meat and dairy foods must not be prepared or eaten together.

Hindus. Hindus do not eat beef and most are vegetarian. Fish is rarely eaten and no alcohol is allowed.

Muslims (Islam). Muslims do not eat pork or shellfish. Meat must be 'Halal' i.e. slaughtered according to Muslim law. Regular fasting is required including the month of Ramadan.

Rastafarians. Rastafarians eat no animal products except milk and avoid processed foods, salt, coffee and alcohol.

Meal planning

Meals

It is traditional in Britain to have three meals a day, together with one or more snacks between the main meals.

Breakfast

This is an important meal of the day but one that is sometimes missed. The body needs food first thing in the morning since it is generally about 12 hours since the last meal. Research has shown that people who eat breakfast are more efficient, alert and less accident-prone during the morning than those who do not. It is not essential though to have a full, cooked 'English' breakfast. Cereals and milk, toast and marmalade with tea or coffee to drink is sufficient for the majority of people.

Midday meal

For many people this is a cooked 'meat and two veg.' type of meal eaten in an industrial canteen or at school. However, it is not essential to have a hot midday meal. Cold meals or packed lunches, if carefully planned, can be equally or more nutritious. Sandwiches with fillings of meat, eggs, fish or cheese together with fruit or salad provide the basis of a well-balanced meal.

Evening meal

Depending in part on what is eaten in the middle of the day, this may be a full cooked meal (i.e. dinner) or a simpler meal. In certain parts of the country 'high tea', which usually consists of a cooked dish or salad with bread and butter and cakes, is still very popular. Many older people prefer their main meal at midday and a lighter meal in the evening.

Snacks

Between-meal snacks may consist simply of a cup of tea or coffee perhaps with biscuits, mid-morning, mid-afternoon and bedtime, or they may be something more substantial. Many of the foods commonly eaten as between-meal snacks, e.g. sweets, chocolates, cakes, biscuits, crisps and soft drinks, are low in essential nutrients but high in energy. They tend to reduce the appetite for the more nutritious main meals. Foods high in sugar are also harmful to teeth, particularly if eaten frequently. If snacks are eaten between meals more nutritious foods, such as fresh and dried fruit, unsalted nuts, raw vegetables, yoghurt and fruit juices, should be encouraged.

Selection of foods

It is obviously impractical to calculate in detail the nutrient and energy contents of normal menus. It is important, however, that meals are nutritionally balanced, or at least that the food consumed over the period of a day and certainly over a week should be balanced nutritionally.

A balanced meal is one which contains adequate amounts of protein, vitamins, minerals, fibre and energy but with limited amounts of fat, sugar and salt. Most foods contain a wide variety of nutrients and most nutrients are found in many different foods. The simplest way, therefore, to have a balanced meal is to include a wide variety of foods. Foods may be divided into five groups and included in the diet as follows:

1 **Meat, fish and alternatives** (cheese, eggs, pulses) which provide protein, energy, B vitamins and iron (meat and eggs). Include lower fat alternatives whenever possible.

2 **Milk and milk products** (cheese, yoghurt) which provide calcium, protein, B vitamins, vitamin A and energy. Use lower fat alternatives when possible.

3 **Bread and other cereals** (pasta, rice, breakfast cereals) which provide energy, protein, B vitamins, iron, calcium and fibre. Include plenty of these and use high fibre varieties where possible.

4 **Fruits and vegetables** which provide vitamin C, vitamin A, minerals and fibre. Include plenty and choose a wide variety.

5 **Butter, margarine and fat spreads** which provide vitamin D, vitamin A and energy. Include small amounts only and use low-fat spreads when possible.

It will be noticed that sugary and fatty foods (such as cakes, biscuits, crisps, sweets, jams and soft drinks) are not included. These types of foods should be kept to a minimum and included only to make the diet more palatable. Their inclusion in the diet should not be at the expense of other more nutritious foods.

In addition to nutritional value there are a number of other factors which should be considered when planning meals and menus. The factors include:

1 *Cost and availability*. Both overall food costs and costs in relation to nutritional value should be considered. In institutional catering (hospitals, schools, etc.), for example, food costs must be kept to a minimum while nutritional standards are maintained. Cheaper cuts of meat have practically the same nutritional value as more expensive cuts, though they may take longer to cook. Fat spreads are more nutritious than butter and also cheaper. Bread and potatoes are relatively cheap in relation to the nutrients they contain. Seasonal foods such as fruits and vegetables are obviously cheaper when bought in season. Table 13.5 shows some of the cheaper sources of energy and nutrients.

Table 13.5 *Cheaper sources of energy and nutrients (in order of cheapness)*

	Foods
Energy	Vegetable oil, sugar, margarine, butter, white bread, pulses
Protein	Pulses, white bread, wholemeal bread, liver, pasta, baked beans, eggs
Vitamin A	Liver, carrots, margarine, butter, eggs, milk
Thiamin	Potatoes, fortified breakfast cereals, pulses, bread, frozen peas, liver
Riboflavin	Liver, fortified breakfast cereals, eggs, yoghurt, wholemeal bread, cheese
Niacin	Liver, pulses, canned tuna, fortified breakfast cereals, nuts, white bread, chicken
Vitamin C	Fortified dried potato, oranges, fruit juices, fresh soft fruits, potatoes, frozen peas
Vitamin D	Margarine, low-fat spreads, oily fish, eggs, fortified breakfast cereals, butter, liver
Calcium	Milk, white bread, cheese, wholemeal bread, ice cream, eggs
Iron	Pulses, liver, fortified breakfast cereals, bread, frozen peas, potatoes, eggs
Fibre (NSP)	Pulses, wholemeal bread, high-fibre breakfast cereals, baked beans, frozen peas, potatoes

Food choice is limited by availability, though in Britain wholesalers and retailers stock a wide variety of foods.

2 *Time and labour for food preparation.* A caterer must consider preparation times and the amount of labour required when planning menus. Labour costs must be included in the overall costs of food preparation. On the domestic side, people such as working mothers will aim to keep food preparation time to a minimum. This may necessitate the use of more expensive 'convenience' foods.

3 *Variety and appearance.* Meals should be varied and appetizing. There should be variation in the colour, texture, flavour and types of foods. For example, a meal consisting entirely of white foods (such as baked cod, boiled cauliflower, mashed potatoes and rice pudding) is not attractive.

4 *Consumer preferences.* The likes and dislikes of the consumer must be taken into account. There is little point in preparing meals which, although they may be cheap, nutritious and attractive, contain foods disliked by the consumer.

5 *Religious and cultural food habits.* Food choice may be limited by cultural or religious food habits. (see page 180).

Portion sizes

Portion sizes vary according to the energy needs of the consumer. Table 13.6 shows average portion sizes of a variety of foods.

Diet and health

Nutritional knowledge has increased and ideas about what constitutes a healthy diet have changed considerably in recent years. Scientific investigations and research have shown relationships between certain diseases and various factors in the diet. The typical 'Western' diet is high in fat and refined carbohydrate (white flour and sugar) and low in fibre. There are strong links between this type of diet and coronary heart disease, strokes, obesity, bowel disorders and tooth decay. It is now realized that by modifying the diet we can reduce the risk of developing these conditions. Various government reports have been published which recommend changes to our dietary pattern in order to reduce the risk of developing these diseases. The main reports are:

1 **The NACNE report, 1983**. 'Proposals for Nutritional Guidelines for Health Education in Britain' by the National Advisory Committee on Nutrition Education.

This was the first of the reports to give guidelines for improving the diet and figures for target intakes of certain nutrients. The main recommendations were:

(a) To reduce total fat intake from about 40% to 30% of total dietary energy with saturated fat 10% of total energy.

(b) To reduce sucrose (sugar) intake to 20 kg per person per year.
(c) To increase fibre intake by about 50%.
(d) To reduce salt intake from about 12 g per person per day to 9 g per person per day.
(e) To reduce alcohol intake by two-thirds to 4% of total energy.
(f) To eat more vegetable protein at the expense of animal protein.
(g) To eat sufficient food and increase exercise to maintain optimum body weight.

Table 13.6 *Average portion sizes of a variety of foods*

Food	*Quantity*	*Weight*
		g
Roast beef	average serving	100
Fish, cooked	average serving	100
Sausage, cooked	1 large	40
Bacon, cooked	1 rasher	25
Cheese	2.5 cm^3 (1 inch cube)	25
Eggs	1	60
Milk	for 1 cup of tea	25
Milk	1 glass	200
Peas	average serving	80
Tomato	1	70
Potatoes, boiled	average serving	150
Potato chips	average serving	150
Boiled rice	average serving	150
Pasta, boiled	average serving	200
Apple, orange	1	125
Bread	1 slice (large loaf)	35
Biscuits	1	10–15
Fruit cake	average portion	70
Butter, margarine	for 1 slice of bread	7
Jam	for 1 slice of bread	15
Breakfast cereals	average serving	30
Soup	average serving	200
Shepherd's pie	average serving	250
Yoghurt	1 carton	125
Ice cream	average serving	80
Apple pie	average serving	125
Sugar	1 teaspoon	5
Coffee, instant	for 1 cup	2

2 **The COMA report, 1984.** A report on 'Diet and Vascular Disease' by the Committee on Medical Aspects of Food Policy.

This report states that coronary heart disease and cerebrovascular disease (stroke) account for more than one-third of deaths in the UK and that dietary changes could reduce this figure. The main recommendations are:

(a) To decrease total fat intake to 35% of energy intake with saturated fats 15% of energy. The ratio of polyunsaturated fatty acids to saturated fatty acids should be increased to 0.45.
(b) Not to increase sugar intake.
(c) To find ways of reducing salt intake.
(d) To avoid excessive intake of alcohol.
(e) To compensate for a reduced fat intake by increasing the intake of fibre-rich carbohydrates (bread, cereals, fruit and vegetables).
(f) To avoid obesity by a combination of appropriate food intake and regular exercise.
(g) Not to smoke cigarettes.

3 **The Health of the Nation White Paper, 1992**. This identified five key areas for immediate action. These included coronary heart disease and stroke and cancers. The nutrition targets to be achieved by the year 2005 included:

(a) To reduce the food energy derived from saturated fat by 35% (from 17% in 1990 to 11%).
(b) To reduce average food energy from total fat by at least 12% (from about 40% to no more than 35%).
(c) To reduce the proportion of adults who are obese (20% or more overweight) by 25% for men and 33% for women (from 8% for men and 12% for women).

As a result of this report the Nutrition Task Force was set up which published the Eat Well programme to help implement these targets. This covers proposals for areas such as education, advertising, nutrition labelling, nutrition training for caterers and health professionals, and product development in the food industry.

4 **The COMA report, 1994**. 'Nutritional Aspects of Cardiovascular Disease' by the Committee on Medical Aspects of Food Policy.

This report confirms nutritional targets of earlier reports but discusses options for dietary change and considers specific foods. The general recommendations include:

(a) People should maintain a desirable body-weight through regular physical activity and eating appropriate amounts of food.
(b) People should be more physically active.
(c) People should not smoke.

The nutrient recommendations include:

(a) Total fat intake should be reduced to 35% of dietary energy.
(b) Saturated fat intake should be reduced to 10% of dietary energy.
(c) No further increase in average intake of n-6 PUFA (from vegetable oils, spreads, etc.).

(d) Average intake of n-3 PUFA (from oily fish, etc.) should be increased from 0.1 g per day to 0.2 g per day.
(e) Trans fatty acids (from hardened oils, etc.) should provide no more than 2% of dietary energy.
(f) Complex carbohydrates (e.g. starch) and sugars in fruits and vegetables should restore the energy deficit following a reduction in fat intake. Carbohydrates should provide approximately 50% of dietary energy.
(g) A reduction in average salt intake from 9 g per day to 6 g per day.
(h) An increase in average potassium intake to about 3.5 g per day.

Table 13.7 *Healthy eating in practice*

EAT MORE:	
Poultry and fish	
Bread, Breakfast cereals, Pasta and rice } especially wholegrain	
Fresh and dried fruit	
Pulse vegetables, e.g. baked beans	
Potatoes and other vegetables	
EAT LESS:	HEALTHIER ALTERNATIVE:
Meat, especially fatty meats, pies, sausages, etc.	Poultry, fish, pulses
Whole milk	Skimmed or semi-skimmed milk
Butter, Hard margarine	Polyunsaturated margarine, Low fat spread
Fried foods	Grilled foods
Cream	Yoghurt, fromage frais
High fat cheeses, e.g. Cheddar	Low fat cheeses
Chips, roast potatoes	Jacket, boiled potatoes
Salt	Herbs, spices
Soft drinks, Alcoholic drinks	Fruit juices, 'diet' drinks, Low alcohol drinks
Crisps, salted nuts	Unsalted nuts
Sugar	Artificial sweeteners
Cakes, biscuits, Sweets, chocolates, Ice cream and other desserts	Fresh and dried fruit

The main food recommendations are that people should:

(a) Eat at least two portions of fish, of which one should be oily fish (mackerel, herring, etc.), per week.
(b) Use reduced fat spreads and dairy products, e.g. semi-skimmed milk, low fat yoghurt, half fat cheese.

(c) Replace fats rich in saturated fatty acids with oils and fats rich in monounsaturated fatty acids (e.g. olive oil).
(d) Increase consumption of vegetables, fruit, potatoes and bread by at least 50%.

More details on the effects of fat, sugar, fibre and salt on health are given in earlier chapters.

So that individuals may choose a healthier diet, or caterers provide healthier meals, or food manufacturers produce healthier products, the recommendations need to be converted into practical measures. It is important, however, that meals and foods are attractive and appetizing as well as healthy. The major changes needed involve reducing the amounts of fatty, animal foods eaten, such as meat, butter, whole milk and cream, and eating more cereal foods and starchy vegetables, e.g. bread, breakfast cereals, pasta, rice and potatoes (particularly wholegrain cereals). Table 13.7 lists items we should be aiming to eat more of or less of, and some of the more healthy alternatives.

14 Commodities

Meat

Structure

Meat is the flesh or muscle of animals. It is composed of microscopic fibres, each fibre being an elongated cell. The fibres are held together by connective tissue to form bundles, which are clearly visible in most meats. The whole muscle is also surrounded by connective tissue (see Figure 14.1). Fatty deposits, known as 'marbling', and blood vessels are found between bundles of fibres. The fibrous nature of muscle gives rise to what is known as the 'grain' of meat. It is easier to cut or chew meat with the grain, i.e. in the direction of the fibres, rather than across the fibres.

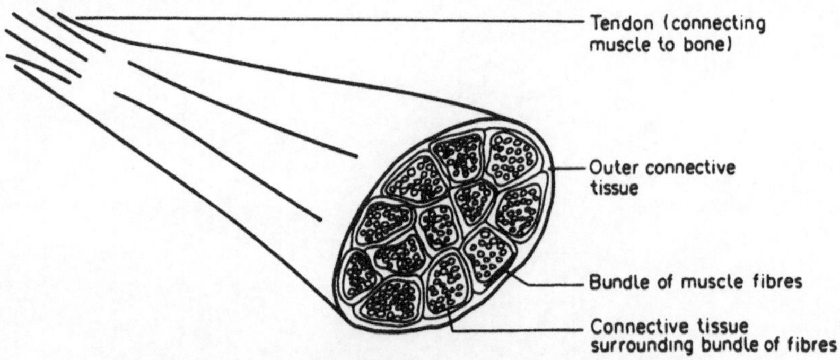

Figure 14.1 *Diagram showing the structure of meat.*

Composition

The composition of meat is very variable. The fat content varies from 10% to 50%, depending on the animal and the part of the animal from which the meat has come. Water content is inversely proportional to fat content, i.e. a meat with a high fat content has a low water content and vice versa. Table 14.1 shows the average percentage composition of raw beef, pork and lamb.

Table 14.1 *Composition of raw beef, pork and lamb*

	Beef %	Pork %	Lamb %
Protein	17	16	15
Fat	23	30	30
Carbohydrate	0	0	0
Water	59	53	54
Vitamins and minerals	1	1	1

Meat proteins

The cells of the muscle fibres contain two soluble proteins, **actin** and **myosin**, which are responsible for the contraction of muscles. Connective tissue contains the proteins **collagen, elastin** and **reticulin** (see page 147). Collagen is found in skin and tendons as well as around muscle fibres. During cooking it is gradually converted into gelatin. Elastin is a tough, insoluble protein and is found in blood vessel walls and ligaments. Reticulin is fibrous and is found between muscle fibres. Neither elastin nor reticulin is affected by cooking. Elastin is very tough and is commonly known as 'gristle'.

Fat

Deposits of fat, marbling, are found in the connective tissue between bundles of fibres. Fat is also stored in the bodies of animals under the skin and around certain organs, e.g. suet around the kidneys. A certain amount of fat in meat is desirable since it keeps meat moist during cooking. Yellow fat normally indicates that the meat has come from an old animal. The yellowness is due to the deposition of carotene.

Food value

Meat is a valuable protein food and an important source of B vitamins (especially niacin) and iron. It is a poor source of calcium. Although liver and kidney contain vitamins A and D, meat does not. Table 14.2 shows the contribution made by meat to the total intake of certain nutrients in the average British diet.

There is no significant difference in nutritional value between expensive and cheaper cuts of meat, or between fresh and frozen meat. Canned meats contain less thiamin than cooked, fresh meat.

Tenderness

The tenderness of meat depends on:

1 *Size of muscle fibres.* Meat composed of small, narrow fibres is more tender than meat made up of larger fibres.

Table 14.2 *Contribution made by meat to the total content of certain nutrients in the average British diet*

Nutrient	*Contribution made by meat to total intake*
Niacin equivalents	32%
Protein	29%
Iron	18%
Riboflavin	16%
Thiamin	13%

2 *Amount of connective tissue.* Tough meat contains more connective tissue than tender meat. The older the animal and the greater its activity during life, the greater the amount of connective tissue.

3 *Activity of the animal before death.* Animals must be rested before slaughter. If they are not, the supplies of glycogen in the muscle tissues are reduced and less lactic acid is produced during hanging (see point 4).

4 *Length of hanging.* After slaughter meat is hung for several days in order to make it more tender. During hanging glycogen, present in muscle tissue, is converted into lactic acid and the pH of the meat falls from about 7.4 to 5.5. The reduction in pH brings about partial denaturation of the fibre proteins. Also during hanging, enzyme action causes a partial breakdown of the proteins which increases tenderness and contributes to the flavour of meat.

Meat may be further tenderized before cooking in the following ways:

1 Physically, e.g. pounding with a steak hammer, cutting or mincing. This helps to break up fibres and connective tissue.

2 Chemically, by using:

(a) acid marinades, e.g. lemon juice, vinegar, wine. These help to coagulate proteins;

(b) enzymes, which break down proteins, e.g. meat tenderizing powders contain papain, a protein-splitting enzyme extracted from the papaya plant.

Colour

The red colour of fresh meat is mainly due to **myoglobin**, a purplish-red pigment somewhat similar in chemical structure to haemoglobin. This pigment reacts under various conditions to form other compounds. When meat is cut and the surface layer exposed to air, bright red oxymyoglobin is formed. During the storage or ageing of meat myoglobin is converted into brownish-red metmyoglobin. When meat is cooked myoglobin is converted, at temperatures above 60°C, into a brown compound called hemichrome. Nitrites which are used in the curing and processing of many meat products, convert myoglobin into pink-coloured nitrosomyoglobin. This accounts for the pink colour of products such as ham, bacon and luncheon meat. These reactions are summarized in Figure 14.2.

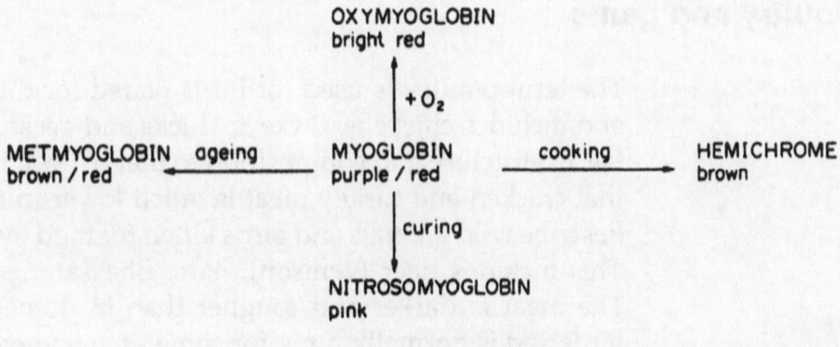

Figure 14.2 *Meat pigments*

Effect of cooking

Meat is cooked in order to increase palatability and tenderness. Also, normal, thorough cooking kills most, if not all, food poisoning organisms that might be present. Various changes occur in meat during cooking.

1 Muscle fibre proteins coagulate and the meat shrinks.

2 Shrinkage results in a loss of juices from the meat. The juices contain water, water soluble salts and vitamins, and peptides (short chains of amino acids). Meat juices, together with fat, are largely responsible for the flavour of meat.

3 Collagen in the connective tissue is converted into gelatin. This makes meat more tender. Moist cooking methods, e.g. stewing and braising, result in a greater breakdown of connective tissue than dry methods, such as roasting, and are therefore more suitable for cheaper cuts which contain greater quantities of connective tissue.

4 Certain nutrients are lost or destroyed during the cooking of meat. B vitamins, being water soluble, are lost in the juices. Thiamin is destroyed by heat and losses during cooking vary from 30% to 50%. Riboflavin and niacin are more heat stable and losses are smaller.

Offal

Certain organs of animals, such as the liver, kidney and heart, can be eaten and are known collectively as offal. Other types of offal include tripe (the tissues of the stomach) and sweetbreads (the pancreas). Most offal has a high nutritional value. Liver, for example, is a very good source of iron, riboflavin, niacin, folate and vitamin A. Although it is eaten relatively infrequently it provides one-third of the vitamin A in the average British diet. Liver is also a good source of protein, thiamin and vitamin D.

Poultry and game

The term poultry is used for birds reared for their meat and/or eggs and includes chickens, turkeys, ducks and geese. Poultry meat is similar in structure and composition to that of beef, lamb and pork except that chicken and turkey meat is much lower in fat. 'Game' is used to describe wild animals and birds killed for food by hunting or shooting. This includes deer (venison), hare, pheasant, partridge and grouse. The meat is darker and tougher than in domesticated animals and birds and is normally hung for some time to develop flavour and tenderness.

Fish

There are many species of both freshwater and sea-water fish used for human consumption. One of the main differences between meat and fish is that fish deteriorates rapidly and should be eaten as soon as possible after being caught.

Structure

The typically flaky texture of fish is due to the fact that fish muscle consists of blocks of short fibres, called myotomes, rather than the long fibres of animals. The myotomes are separated by thin sheets of connective tissue. Fish has less connective tissue than meat and no elastin, and is, therefore, much more tender.

Composition

There are two main types of fish. Oily fish, such as herring, mackerel, salmon and sardines, contain between 10% and 20% unsaturated oil. White fish, which includes cod, haddock and plaice, contains less than 2% oil. The compositions of raw cod and herring are shown in Table 14.3.

Food value

Fish is a good source of protein but it does not make a significant contribution to total protein intake in Britain since fish consumption is low. Oily fish contains n-3 PUFA (see page 85) and vitamins A and D, and all fish provides B vitamins. Small fish, such as sardines, which are eaten with the bones are a good source of calcium. Fish is therefore a nutritious food and its consumption should be encouraged.

Table 14.3 *Composition of raw cod and herring*

	Cod %	*Herring* %
Protein	17	17
Fat	1	19
Carbohydrate	0	0
Water	82	64
Vitamins and minerals	1	1

Eggs

Structure

A hen's egg weighs about 60 g and is made up of three major parts: shell, white and yolk. The porous shell is composed mainly of calcium carbonate. The colour of the shell does not indicate the quality of the egg but depends on the breed of hen. Inside the shell two thin membranes separate the shell from the white. The white is divided into regions of thick and thin white and accounts for about 60% of the total weight of the egg. The yolk is suspended in the white and is held in position by strands of protein called chalazae (see Figure 14.3).

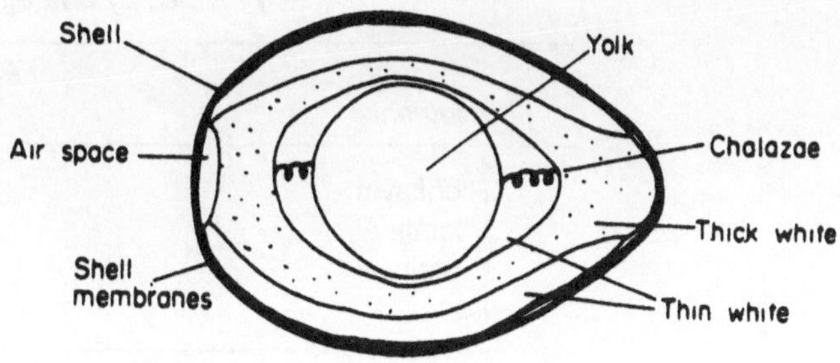

Figure 14.3 *The structure of a hen's egg.*

Composition

The white of an egg is basically a colloidal solution of protein (mainly **albumin**) in water, together with small quantities of vitamins and mineral salts. The yolk is a fat-in-water emulsion and is approximately one-third fat, one-half water and one-sixth protein. The main protein is **vitellin**. The yolk also contains vitamins and mineral salts. Table 14.4 shows the approximate percentage composition of the whole egg, the white and the yolk.

Table 14.4 *Composition of egg*

	Whole egg (excluding shell) %	*White %*	*Yolk %*
Protein	13	9	16
Fat	11	trace	31
Carbohydrate	0	0	0
Water	75	88	51
Vitamins and minerals	1	1	1

Food value

Since an egg supplies a developing chick with all its essential nutrients its food value is high, but it is not a complete food for humans. Eggs are normally considered as protein foods but they also provide substantial quantities of iron, vitamins A and D, and riboflavin. They provide smaller amounts of other B vitamins. Table 14.5 shows the percentage of the Reference Nutrient Intake of certain nutrients (for an adult) provided by one 60 g egg.

Eggs contain saturated fat and cholesterol and are, therefore, not recommended in large numbers for people at risk from coronary heart disease.

Table 14.5 *Percentage of the RNI of certain nutrients provided by one egg*

Nutrient	*Percentage of RNI*
Riboflavin	22
Vitamin A	16
Protein	14
Iron	10

Changes during storage

Various physical and chemical changes take place in an egg during storage:

1 The air space increases in size. This is due to the loss of water through the porous shell and its replacement by air.

2 Water passes from the white to the yolk due to the osmotic pressure exerted by the yolk. The yolk becomes enlarged and the membrane surrounding it weakens.

3 Thick white is gradually converted into thin white.

4 The pH of both the white and yolk increases. This is due to a loss of carbon dioxide through the shell. A solution of carbon dioxide in water is weakly acid and, therefore, a loss of carbon dioxide increases alkalinity.

5 If eggs are stored for a long time bacterial spoilage occurs. Bacteria enter the egg through the porous shell. One of the most noticeable effects is the presence of hydrogen sulphide produced by bacterial breakdown of protein; this gives rise to the typical 'bad egg' smell.

When comparing a fresh egg and a stale egg it will be noticed that the stale egg, when cracked open and placed on a plate, is much flatter and spreads much further than the fresh egg. The stale egg is flatter due to the weakened yolk membrane and it spreads further because it contains more thin white.

Effect of cooking

When eggs are heated the proteins in the white and yolk coagulate. Egg white proteins coagulate first at about 60°C and the white becomes opaque and forms a gel. The yolk proteins coagulate at 66°C and the yolk thickens. The rate of coagulation is increased by the presence of salts and acid. Salt and vinegar can be added to the water used for poaching eggs to bring about rapid coagulation of the white. When eggs are boiled, salt or vinegar in the water coagulates any white which escapes if the shells are cracked.

Iron sulphide is formed in eggs during cooking and sometimes causes a black discoloration around the yolk of hard-boiled eggs. The sulphur is derived from sulphur amino acids in egg white proteins and the iron from the yolk. The reaction occurs more readily in stale eggs than fresh ones. Discoloration can be reduced by placing eggs in cold water immediately after cooking.

There is a small loss of between 5% and 15% of the thiamin and riboflavin in eggs as a result of cooking.

Uses of eggs in cooking

In addition to increasing the nutritional value of dishes, eggs are important in cookery because they have several useful physical properties.

1 *Thickening and binding*. Since egg proteins coagulate when heated, eggs are very useful thickening and binding agents. Egg is used as

a thickening agent in dishes such as egg custard and as a binding agent in such products as rissoles.

2 *Emulsifying.* Egg yolk contains lecithin, an emulsifying agent (see page 54), and is used in the preparation of mayonnaise and other emulsions.

3 *Foaming.* When egg white is beaten, air is incorporated and the protein partially coagulates, forming a foam. This is the basis of meringue (see page 57).

Milk

Since, in this country, 'milk' normally implies cow's milk, the following section covers the composition and food value of cow's milk only. In other countries, milk from other animals, such as ewes, goats and even camels and buffalo, is often an important constituent of the diet.

Composition

Milk is composed of a variety of nutrients either dissolved in water or dispersed in the form of a colloid. The colloidal system is complex but is basically a fat-in-water emulsion (see page 53). Table 14.6 shows the average percentage composition of whole milk with skimmed and semi-skimmed (half fat) for comparison.

Table 14.6 *Composition of milk*

	Whole %	*Semi-skimmed* %	*Skimmed* %
Protein	3.2	3.3	3.3
Fat	3.9	1.6	0.1
Carbohydrate	4.8	5.0	5.0
Water	87.8	89.8	91.1
Vitamins and minerals	0.6	0.6	0.6

The composition of milk varies depending on the age and breed of the cow, the type of food fed to the cow and the time of year. Milk leaving the farm must reach legal standards of quality; it must contain a minimum of 3.0% butterfat and 8.5% solids-not-fat (SNF).

Proteins

The proteins in milk are colloidally dispersed in the water phase. The most important proteins are **caseinogen** and the whey proteins, **lactalbumin** and **lactoglobulin**. During digestion caseinogen is converted by the action of rennin into a coagulated form called casein.

Fat

The fat in milk is in an easily digestible, emulsified form. In milk fresh from the cow the fat droplets are uniformly dispersed, but when milk is allowed to stand the droplets rise to the top of the milk and form a layer of cream. Milk can be treated to prevent the formation of a cream layer. This type of milk is known as **homogenized** milk and is prepared by forcing milk under pressure through very small holes. The fat is broken down into smaller droplets which remain evenly dispersed and the milk has the same composition throughout.

Carbohydrate

The carbohydrate in milk is the disaccharide, **lactose**, which is less sweet than other sugars.

Food value

Milk, being a complete food for young calves, is of high nutritional value. It is a valuable source of protein, riboflavin and calcium and provides important quantities of other B vitamins and vitamin A. It is not, however, a complete food for humans as it is relatively deficient in iron, vitamin C and vitamin D. Table 14.7 shows the contribution made by milk to the total intake of certain nutrients in the average British diet.

Table 14.7 *Contribution made by milk to the total content of certain nutrients in the average British diet*

Nutrient	*Contribution made by milk to total intake*
Calcium	46%
Riboflavin	35%
Protein	17%
Vitamin A (retinol equivalents)	12%
Niacin equivalents	11%
Thiamin	10%

568 ml (1 pint) of milk provides 680 mg of calcium, i.e. almost the recommended daily intake of calcium for an adult. It also provides one-half of the riboflavin and one-quarter of the protein and vitamin A requirements.

Average milk consumption in Britain is 300 g (more than half a pint) per person per day. An increasing proportion of this is low fat milk, i.e. skimmed or semi-skimmed. Low fat milks are a useful way of reducing saturated fat intake while maintaining intake of protein, calcium and B vitamins. However, skimmed milk is not suitable for babies and children under five years due to its lower energy and vitamin A content.

Effect of cooking

When milk is heated, the whey proteins coagulate and a skin forms on the surface. The skin holds steam and is responsible for the ease with which milk 'boils over'. During prolonged cooking caramelization of the lactose may occur; this contributes to the characteristic flavour of sterilized milk and oven-cooked milk puddings. Some of the thiamin and vitamin C in milk is destroyed by cooking.

Effect of processing

Milk is an ideal medium for bacterial growth and, therefore, in order to make it safe and to improve its keeping quality, it is normally processed before being sold. In Great Britain about 50% of the milk produced is sold as liquid milk; 95% of this is heat treated. (Heat treatment is described in Chapter 18.) The remaining 50% is used to manufacture milk products such as evaporated milk, dried milk, cheese and butter. During processing there is a loss of heat-sensitive vitamins (thiamin and vitamin C). Table 14.8 shows the percentage loss of these two vitamins resulting from the production of various types of milk.

Table 14.8 *Percentages of thiamin and vitamin C lost during the processing of milk*

Type of milk	*% loss of thiamin*	*% loss of vitamin C*
Pasteurized	10	20
Sterilized	30	50
Spray dried	10	20
Evaporated	20	60
Sweetened, condensed	10	15

The greater the severity of heat treatment the greater the loss of vitamins. Pasteurization is a mild heat treatment compared with sterilization. Condensed milk does not require the same degree of heat treatment as evaporated milk because of its high sugar content.

Dried skimmed milk contains only a trace of fat and, therefore, lacks vitamins A and D. It should not, therefore, be used for feeding babies. However, it is a useful protein supplement since it is approximately 37% protein. It also has a high calcium and riboflavin content.

Cream

Cream is a fat-in-water emulsion. It is separated from milk by centrifugation, a process which involves spinning milk in a centrifuge so that the heavier particles are forced to the outside and the lighter particles, which make up the cream, remain nearer the centre.

Composition

Cream contains all of the fat and a proportion of the protein and lactose in milk. Table 14.9 shows the approximate compositions of single and double cream.

By law single cream must have a minimum fat content of 18% and double cream of 48%. Single cream will not whip since only cream with a fat content greater than 30%, will whip. Cream which is sold as 'whipping cream' generally contains 35% to 40% fat.

Clotted cream has a very high fat content (at least 55%, and often as much as 70%) and is produced by heating milk in special pans and skimming off the cream.

Table 14.9 *Composition of single and double cream*

	Single cream %	Double cream %
Protein	2.5	1.5
Fat	19.0	48.0
Carbohydrate	4.0	2.5
Water	74.0	47.5
Vitamins and minerals	0.5	0.5

Food value

All types of cream contain useful quantities of vitamins A and D. Double cream has a higher energy value than single cream since it has a higher fat content.

Butter

Butter is made by churning cream. The conversion of cream into butter is described in Chapter 6. Butter is a water-in-fat emulsion.

Composition

The precise composition of butter is variable, though it must, by law, contain at least 80% milk fat. Table 14.10 shows the composition of an average butter. The composition of margarine and other fat spreads are included for comparison. There are now many spreadable fats on the market (e.g. dairy spreads, low fat spreads). These vary considerably in their composition.

Table 14.10 *Compositions of butter, margarine and fat spreads*

	Butter %	Margarine %	Dairy spread %	Low fat spread %
Protein	0.5	0.1	0.5	6.0
Fat	81.5	81.5	73.5	40.5
Carbohydrate	0.0	1.0	0.0	0.5
Water	15.5	16.0	22.0	50.0
Vitamins and minerals	2.0	2.0	2.5	2.5

Food value

Both butter and margarine are valuable sources of vitamins A and D, though the actual vitamin content of butter varies considerably, being lower in the winter months when there is a shortage of fresh foods for the cows. Butter provides 5% of the vitamin A and 2% of the vitamin D in the average British diet. Margarine is fortified with these two vitamins by law and contains approximately ten times as much vitamin D as butter. It provides 9% of the vitamin A and 30% of the vitamin D in the average diet.

Butter and margarine both have a high fat content and therefore a very high energy value; 100 g (3.5 oz) butter provides 3031 kJ (737 kcal).

Yoghurt

Yoghurt is made by souring milk, using a pure culture of bacteria. The two species of bacteria normally used are *Lactobacillus bulgaricus* and *Streptococcus thermophilus*. They convert the lactose in milk into lactic acid which together with a variety of minor products is responsible for the characteristic flavour of yoghurt. The acid also brings about coagulation of the milk proteins and helps to preserve the product.

Since it is made from milk the composition and food value of yoghurt are similar to milk. Low fat yoghurt is produced from skimmed milk. Fruit yoghurts are normally higher in carbohydrate since, as well as fruit, they usually contain added sugar.

Cheese

Cheesemaking is a traditional method of preserving surplus summer milk. There are more than 400 different varieties of cheese but the basic principles of manufacture are the same for all of them.

Principles of cheesemaking

1 Milk is pasteurized and cooled to about 20°C.

2 A 'starter' culture of souring bacteria is added which converts lactose into lactic acid.

3 Rennet is added and in the acid conditions it rapidly coagulates the protein, forming a curd or 'coagulum' which, as well as casein, contains fat, fat-soluble vitamins, calcium and most of the water-soluble vitamins.

4 The curd is left to harden and is then cut into small pieces to promote the drainage of whey (the fluid which remains when the curd forms). Whey contains only 2% solids which includes the whey proteins (lactalbumin and lactoglobulin) together with lactose and some of the water-soluble vitamins from the milk.

5 The curd is pressed to give a firmer texture and salt is added.

6 The salted cheese is packed into moulds, pressed and left to ripen or mature. During this stage micro-organisms grow in the cheese and the flavour develops.

English cheeses such as Cheddar and Cheshire are ripened by the activity of bacteria already present in the cheese. Other cheeses, such as Camembert and Brie, are allowed to develop mould on their outer surfaces. Cheeses such as Stilton and Danish Blue are mould ripened but are pierced with copper wires to encourage mould growth throughout the cheese.

The holes or 'eyes' in cheeses such as Gruyère are a result of the production of carbon dioxide by certain species of bacteria. Cream cheese is prepared from cream rather than whole milk, while cottage cheese is made from skimmed milk and is, therefore, very low in fat. Low fat soft cheese is also made from skimmed milk but with a small amount of cream added.

Vegetarian cheeses are made without rennet (an animal product) but with other enzymes, e.g. a fungal enzyme.

Composition

In some respects cheese can be thought of as a concentrated form of milk (1 litre of milk produces approximately 100 grams of cheese). However, unlike milk, cheese does not contain carbohydrate; the lactose is partly converted into lactic acid and the remainder is lost in the whey.

Table 14.11 shows the composition of Cheddar cheese (a high fat hard cheese), Brie (a medium fat soft cheese) and cottage cheese (a low fat soft cheese).

Table 14.11 *Composition of Cheddar, Brie and cottage cheese*

	Cheddar %	*Brie* %	*Cottage cheese* %
Protein	26.0	19.0	14.0
Fat	34.0	27.0	4.0
Carbohydrate	0.0	0.0	0.0
Water	36.0	49.0	79.0
Vitamins and minerals	3.5	3.5	3.0

Food value

Since cheese has a lower water content than milk it is a more concentrated source of nutrients. Cheese is particularly rich in calcium and is a good source of protein, vitamin A and riboflavin. It also provides useful quantities of other B vitamins and vitamin D but contains no vitamin C and is a relatively poor source of iron.

Effect of cooking

When cheese is subjected to mild heat the fat melts but there is no significant effect on the nutritive value. Prolonged cooking causes 'stringiness' which is due to over-coagulation of the protein and its separation from the fat and water.

Cereals

Cereal grains are the seeds of cultivated grasses. Cereals are the most important source of food for man and they form the staple food in most countries. In some countries they provide 70% or more of the total energy intake. Cereals may be used as the whole grain, e.g. rice, or they can be ground into a flour, e.g. wheat flour. The most important cereals are wheat, rice, maize (corn), barley, oats and rye.

Wheat

Wheat is grown in Europe, North America and parts of Asia and Australasia where the climate is temperate.

Structure of a wheat grain

A grain of wheat is covered by tough, fibrous layers of pericarp and seed coat which are called the **bran** or husk. Inside is the **germ** which is the actual seed or embryo and which is situated at the base of the grain (see Figure 14.4). By far the largest component of the grain is the

endosperm, a starchy food reserve for the germ. The outer layer of the endosperm is called the aleurone layer. The germ is separated from the endosperm by the scutellum.

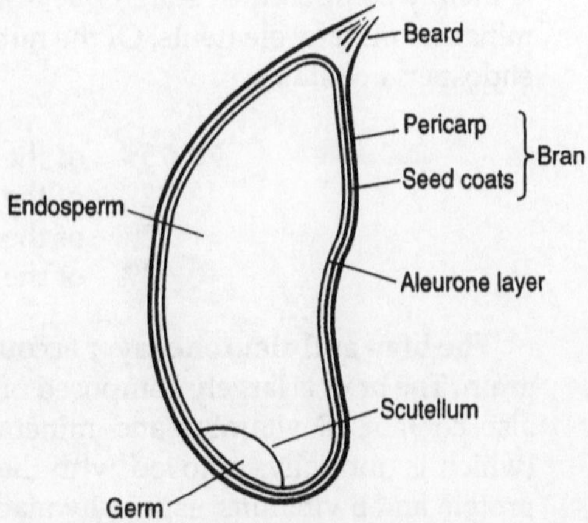

Figure 14.4 *Vertical section through a grain of wheat.*

Composition

The composition of wheat varies depending on the variety. For example, hard Canadian wheats have a high **gluten** (protein) content, whereas the gluten content of soft English wheats is considerably less. The terms 'hard' and 'soft' refer to milling properties of the wheats and should not be confused with 'strong' and 'weak' which refer to the baking properties of a flour. The strength of a flour depends on the quality rather than the quantity of gluten. A strong flour is one which produces a dough that is difficult to stretch and has good gas-retaining properties. Strong flours are suitable for breadmaking, whereas weak flours make better cakes and biscuits. In general, hard wheats produce strong flours and soft wheats produce weak flours.

Table 14.12 shows the average composition of a Canadian wheat (Manitoba) and English wheat.

Table 14.12 *Compositions of Manitoba and English wheats*

	Manitoba %	*English* %
Protein	13.5	9.0
Fat	2.5	2.0
Carbohydrate	69.0	74.0
Water	13.5	13.5
Vitamins and minerals	1.5	1.5

Distribution of nutrients within the grain

Nutrients are not uniformly distributed within a grain of wheat.

The **endosperm** forms about 83% of the total weight of the grain. It is mainly composed of starch but also contains protein, some B vitamins and mineral elements. Of the nutrients in the grain as a whole the endosperm contains:

70–75%	of the protein
32%	of the riboflavin
12%	of the niacin
3%	of the thiamin

The bran and aleurone layer account for 14.5% of the weight of the grain. The bran is largely composed of indigestible cellulose (fibre) but also contains B vitamins and mineral elements. The aleurone layer (which is normally removed with the bran during milling) is rich in protein and B vitamins, especially niacin. Of the nutrients in the whole grain the bran and aleurone layer contain:

86%	of the niacin
42%	of the riboflavin
33%	of the thiamin
19%	of the protein

The germ (including the scutellum) accounts for only 2.5% of the weight of the grain. The germ is rich in fat, protein, iron and B vitamins (the scutellum is particularly rich in thiamin). Of the nutrients in the whole grain the germ contains:

64%	of the thiamin
26%	of the riboflavin
8%	of the protein
2%	of the niacin

Milling of wheat

In order to turn wheat into a more digestible form it is milled into flour. The bran and germ are removed as flakes and the endosperm is ground into a fine powder. In the 1870s steel roller mills were introduced; they replaced revolving flat stones.

There are three main stages in flour milling.

1 Cleaning and conditioning

The wheat is first passed through a series of machines which remove dirt, chaff and other impurities. It is then 'conditioned', i.e. brought to the optimum moisture level for milling, by a process involving moistening and drying of the grain. Conditioning toughens the bran so that it is more easily removed during milling and makes the endosperm more friable (easily crumbled) so that it is more easily ground into flour.

2 *Breaking*

The cleaned and conditioned wheat is passed through five pairs of corrugated steel rollers known as break rolls. One roller of each pair rotates at two and a half times the speed of the other so that the grain is sheared open and the endosperm is separated from the bran. After passing through each set of rolls the product is sieved and separated into three fractions:

1 Coarse particles of bran with attached endosperm. This is passed on to the next set of break rolls.

2 Coarse endosperm particles known as semolina. Bran particles mixed with the semolina are separated by a current of air, bran being less dense than semolina.

3 A small quantity of fine endosperm particles or flour.

The gap between the break rolls is made progressively narrower so that at each stage a little more endosperm is removed from the bran.

3 *Reduction*

The semolina obtained from the break rolls is passed through ten or more reduction rolls. These are smooth rollers and one roller of each pair rotates one and a half times as fast as the other. The endosperm particles are gradually reduced in size by the crushing action of the rolls and damage to the starch granules is minimized. After passing through each set of rolls the product is sieved and separated into fine particles of flour, larger particles which are passed to the next set of reduction rolls and coarse particles which are returned to a previous set of rolls. As with the break rolls, the reduction rolls are set progressively closer together and at the end of the process fine white flour is obtained. The germ is flattened rather than ground by the reduction system and is removed by sieving.

Extraction rate

The extraction rate is the percentage of the whole grain which is converted into flour:

Wholemeal flour	100%
Brown flour (wheatmeal)	85–90%
White flour	73%

Wholemeal flour consists of the whole grain including the bran and germ, wheatmeal contains the endosperm and germ but only the inner layers of bran, and white flour contains only the endosperm.

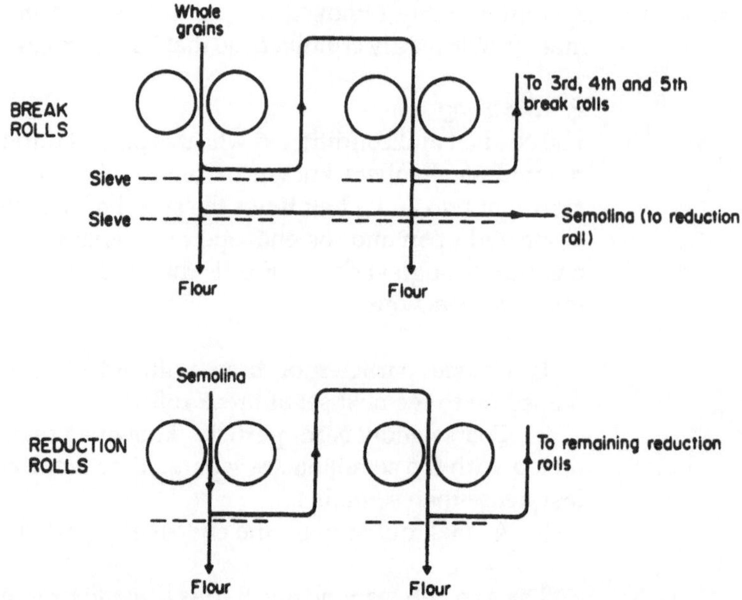

Figure 14.5 *Simplified diagram of the milling process.*

Fortification of low extraction rate flours

Because low extraction rate flours contain little or no bran or germ, they have less protein, fat, B vitamins, minerals and fibre. The composition of flour in the UK is controlled by the **Bread and Flour Regulations 1984** which require all flours to contain minimum quantities of thiamin, niacin and iron. By law all flour must contain at least:

0.24 mg thiamin per 100 g
1.60 mg niacin per 100 g
1.65 mg iron per 100 g

These quantities occur naturally in flours with an extraction rate of 80% or more.

A further legal requirement involves the addition of calcium carbonate (chalk) to all flours except true wholemeal (100% extraction) at the rate of 235–390 mg calcium carbonate per 100 g flour. (This is equivalent to 94–156 mg calcium per 100 g flour.)

Bread

Bread is made from a dough of wheat flour, water, salt and yeast. When water is added to flour the wheat proteins, glutenin and gliadin, form gluten which is elastic. Kneading develops a network of gluten in the dough. Before being baked the dough is left to rise. During this stage the dough increases in size due to production of carbon dioxide, a result of the fermentation of sugars by the yeast present in the dough (see page 218). The gluten network traps the gas and during baking the gluten coagulates, thus fixing the size and shape of the loaf.

Much of the bread now made in Britain is produced using the Chorleywood Bread Process in which the initial fermentation stage is replaced by a short period of intense mechanical agitation using special high-speed mixers. Another modern method of breadmaking is the Activated Dough Development (ADD) process. In this method the dough is chemically developed with ascorbic acid and the amino acid cysteine and the fermentation period is reduced.

Composition

The composition of bread is similar to that of flour except that it contains considerably more water. Table 14.13 shows the percentage composition of white, brown (wheatmeal) and wholemeal bread.

Table 14.13 *Composition of white, brown and wholemeal bread*

	White %	*Brown* %	*Wholemeal* %
Protein	8.0	8.5	9.0
Fat	1.5	2.0	2.5
Available carbohydrate (starch and sugars)	49.0	44.0	42.0
Fibre (NSP)	1.5	3.5	6.0
Water	38.0	40.0	38.0
Vitamins and minerals	1.5	1.5	1.5

Food value

Bread is one of the most important foods in the British diet. It provides important quantities of protein, B vitamins, iron and calcium. Table 14.14 shows the contribution made by bread to the total intake of certain nutrients in the average diet.

Table 14.14 *Contribution made by bread to the total content of certain nutrients in the average British diet*

Nutrient	*Contribution made by bread to total intake*
Thiamin	23%
Carbohydrate	21%
Iron	20%
Protein	14%
Calcium	13%
Niacin equivalents	9%

Although consumption of brown and wholemeal bread is increasing, white bread is still more popular. The main reason for this is that white flour has better baking properties and produces a loaf with a more open texture which many people prefer. Also, white flour is more acceptable with millers and bakers since, due to its lower fat content, it is less prone to rancidity during storage, i.e. it has better keeping qualities.

In recent years, though, particularly since the recommendations by the NACNE and COMA Reports to eat more fibre, the consumption of wholemeal bread has increased. The fibre content of wholemeal bread is more than three times that of white bread. Wholemeal bread also contains more B vitamins and minerals, though white flour does have some of these nutrients 'added back' after milling. Some minerals, although present in larger amounts in wholemeal bread, may not be as readily absorbed due to the presence of phytic acid in the fibre.

There are now various 'soft grain' and 'bran-enriched' breads on the market. These are basically white bread with added cereal grains (wheat, rye and maize) or added bran (sometimes pea bran). The advantage of this type of bread is that it has the texture of white bread but with a fibre content equivalent to wholemeal bread.

Pasta

Pasta is made from hard, durum wheat which is milled into semolina, mixed with water and dried. It may be enriched with egg yolk. It is produced in a variety of shapes and sizes, e.g. spaghetti (thin rods), macaroni (tubes), lasagne (sheets) and farfallette (butterfly-shaped). Pasta provides a good basis for a meal by supplying starch, protein, B vitamins and minerals. When served with meat or vegetable sauces it forms a nutritionally well-balanced meal. Wholemeal pasta is also available; this is a good source of dietary fibre.

Rice

Rice grows best in damp tropical climates and is the staple food in many parts of Asia. A grain of rice has approximately the same structure as a grain of wheat. Mechanical milling or 'polishing' removes the bran and germ leaving only the white endosperm. The endosperm represents over 90% of the grain but contains only 9% of the thiamin. In many parts of the East where the staple food is polished rice, thiamin deficiency is common. A deficiency of thiamin causes the disease beriberi which is described in Chapter 8. In some mills the rice is parboiled prior to polishing. If this process is carried out the majority of the thiamin, instead of being lost in the bran, remains in the polished grains. If all rice was parboiled in this way beriberi could be almost completely eradicated.

Brown rice is not polished but contains the whole grain. It takes longer to cook than white rice but is higher in fibre as well as thiamin.

Vegetables

Vegetables have no common biological structure. They are obtained from different parts of many plants. Some vegetables, like cabbage and lettuce, are leaves; others, such as carrots and radishes, are roots; cucumbers and tomatoes are fruits; celery is a stalk; cauliflower is a flower and peas and broad beans are seeds. However, all vegetables possess some similar nutritional properties. They usually have a high water content and, therefore, their contribution to the total energy intake of the diet is low. They are important in the diet because of their content of indigestible carbohydrate (mostly cellulose) which provides fibre. Also many vegetables are good sources of vitamin C, beta-carotene and mineral elements, particularly iron.

Table 14.15 shows the composition of potatoes, cabbage, peas, tomatoes and carrots, the vegetables consumed in the largest quantities in Britain.

Table 14.15 *Compositions of some vegetables*

	Potatoes %	*Cabbage* %	*Peas* %	*Tomatoes* %	*Carrots* %
Protein	2.0	1.5	7.0	0.5	0.5
Fat	0.0	0.5	1.5	0.5	0.5
Available carbohydrate (starch and sugars)	17.0	4.0	11.5	3.0	8.0
Dietary fibre	1.5	2.5	4.5	1.0	2.5
Water	79.0	90.0	75.0	93.0	90.0
Vitamins and minerals	0.5	0.5	0.5	0.5	0.5

Potatoes

The potato is a cheap and popular food in Britain. The average intake is 150 g (5.5 oz) per day. A potato is a swollen underground stem or tuber which acts as a food reserve for the plant. Potatoes have a higher starch content than most other vegetables and provide 318 kJ (75 kcal) per 100 g. They yield more kilojoules per hectare than cereal crops.

Potatoes are an important source of vitamin C in the British diet. Their ascorbic acid content is variable since vitamin C is lost during storage; old potatoes may have only one-quarter the vitamin C content of new potatoes. They are also good sources of folate and potassium. Table 14.16 shows the contribution made by potatoes to the total intake of certain nutrients in the average diet.

Table 14.16 *Contribution made by potatoes to total content of certain nutrients in the average British diet*

Nutrient	*Contribution made by potatoes to total intake*
Folate	13%
Potassium	13%
Vitamin C	12%
Thiamin	10%
Niacin equivalents	4%
Iron	4%

Green vegetables

These are of particular value in the diet because of their content of vitamin C, folate, iron, beta-carotene (the precursor of vitamin A) and fibre. Green vegetables are best as a source of vitamin C when eaten raw in salads, etc., since their ascorbic acid is readily lost during cooking (see page 118). The beta-carotene content varies in different vegetables but increases in proportion to the greenness of the vegetable. Spinach is often quoted as being a good source of iron but, although it has a high iron content, the availability of the iron to the body is reduced by the presence of oxalic acid (see page 130).

Pulse vegetables

Pulse vegetables are the seeds of leguminous plants and include peas, beans and lentils. The crops can be harvested, as they are in Britain, before the seeds are fully mature and dry or, as in the tropics, the seeds can be allowed to mature and can be stored dry, like a cereal crop. In the East, pulses make a larger contribution to the diet than in the West. Soya beans, lentils and dhals (split peas) are important foods in countries such as China and India.

In Britain, green peas and baked beans in tomato sauce are eaten in considerable quantities, though various dried beans, e.g. kidney, borlotti and haricot beans, are becoming more popular, particularly in vegetarian cooking. All pulses contain significant quantities of protein and some, e.g. peas, contain useful amounts of thiamin. Vitamin C and beta-carotene are found in fresh pulse vegetables.

Soya beans are particularly rich in protein; dried soya beans are about 36% protein. The importance of soya beans as a meat substitute has been considered in Chapter 7.

Root vegetables

Root vegetables, like all vegetables, provide dietary fibre and a variety of minerals. Carrots are an important source of beta-carotene and account for 13% of the total vitamin A content of the average British diet. All root vegetables contain some vitamin C but generally not in such large quantities as are found in green vegetables.

Effect of cooking on vegetables

When vegetables are cooked they become more tender and more digestible. This is due to the softening or partial breakdown of the cellulose cell walls and the gelatinization of the starch. During cooking the green colour of leafy vegetables is intensified, although overcooking results in yellowness.

The major effect of cooking on the nutritive value of vegetables is the loss or destruction of vitamin C; this is considered in Chapter 8.

Fruits

Fruits, like vegetables, contain a high percentage of water and are therefore low in energy value. Also, like vegetables, they are an important source of dietary fibre. One of the main differences between fruits and vegetables is in the nature of the carbohydrates present. In general, fruits have a higher sugar content than vegetables and ripe fruits contain little or no starch. Grapes, for example, contain 15% sugar and oranges about 8%; neither fruit contains any starch. The sugar in fruit is usually a mixture of glucose and fructose. Fruits also contain a variety of organic acids, in particular citric, malic and tartaric acids. These acids are responsible for the sourness of unripe fruit. During ripening the concentration of these acids falls and that of sugar rises.

The main importance of fruit in the diet is as a source of vitamin C. Fruits and fruit products provide 44% of the vitamin C in the average British diet. However, only certain fruits, e.g. blackcurrants, citrus fruits and strawberries, contain valuable quantities. The vitamin C content of many fruits does not compare very favourably with that of vegetables. Apples, pears and plums are among the fruits with a relatively low vitamin C content.

Commercial fruit juices are now one of the major sources of vitamin C, providing one-fifth of the vitamin C in an average diet. They are usually made from concentrated juices which are diluted and preserved by the UHT (ultra heat treatment) process (see page 289).

Dried fruits have a high energy value due to the removal of water but they do not contain any vitamin C.

15 An introduction to microbiology

Microbiology is the study of micro-organisms (microbes). Micro-organisms are very small, usually single-celled, organisms which are not individually visible to the naked eye. They can only be seen with the aid of a microscope. They are widely distributed in the environment and are found in foods. Certain of them, if present in food in large enough numbers, can cause food poisoning. Micro-organisms are the main cause of food 'going off', i.e. food spoilage. However, not all micro-organisms are undesirable. In fact, they are essential to all forms of life since they break down complex organic matter and return nutrients to the soil. Micro-organisms are used by man in the production of certain foods, e.g. bread and yoghurt.

Although some of the effects of micro-organisms have been known and utilized for thousands of years, these microscopic organisms were first seen and studied only 300 years ago. In 1675 a Dutch lens grinder, van Leewenhoek, made a microscope with lenses of sufficiently good quality that he was able to observe micro-organisms in a variety of materials such as teeth scrapings and pond water. The significance of his findings was not appreciated at the time. It was nearly 200 years later that a Frenchman, Louis Pasteur, studied fermentation processes and demonstrated that it was micro-organisms which caused an undesirable sour taste in some wines. He developed a process of heating wine to kill the micro-organisms which caused the souring. This process is still used today to kill undesirable organisms in many food products and is known as pasteurization. While Pasteur was working in France, Robert Koch, in Germany, demonstrated that anthrax, a fatal disease of sheep and cattle, was caused by a bacterium. From this time onwards great advances were made in the field of microbiology. The organisms responsible for a large number of diseases were identified. In Scotland, Joseph Lister introduced the idea of antiseptic surgery and greatly reduced the incidence of infection in patients during and after surgery.

Classification of micro-organisms

Micro-organisms can be classified into five biological types:

1 Protozoa	4 Microscopic fungi – moulds and yeasts
2 Algae	
3 Viruses	5 Bacteria

(Each group is described under the appropriate heading later in the chapter.)

This list classifies micro-organisms according to their structure. It is sometimes more convenient to classify them according to their role in relation to human beings. In this functional classification there are four groups:

1 Pathogens

These are micro-organisms which cause disease. All viruses are pathogenic but only some are pathogenic to man. Certain bacteria also cause disease in man. Some of these diseases can be transmitted by food, e.g. food poisoning, cholera and typhoid (see Chapter 16).

2 Spoilage organisms

These micro-organisms do not cause disease but they spoil food by growing in the food and producing substances which alter the colour, texture and odour of the food, making it unfit for human consumption. Examples of food spoilage include the souring of milk, the growth of mould on bread and the rotting of fruits and vegetables. Food spoilage and the methods of preventing it (i.e. food preservation) are covered in Chapter 18.

3 Beneficial organisms

Many micro-organisms have a beneficial effect and play an important part in everyday life.

(a) Micro-organisms are essential to life since they are responsible for the rotting or decay of organic matter. The complex organic components of dead plants and animals are broken down by microbial activity into simpler, inorganic compounds which are made available for new plant growth, and the whole cycle of life is able to continue.

In the treatment of sewage, micro-organisms are used to break down complex organic compounds.

(b) Micro-organisms are used at various stages during the manufacture of certain foods. Their activities are essential in the production of foods such as bread, beer, wine, cheese and yoghurt.

(c) Antibiotics, such as penicillin, are substances used to destroy bacteria in the body. Many are produced as a result of microbial activity. For example, penicillin is obtained from a mould called *Penicillium*.

4 Inert organisms

This group includes those organisms which are neither harmful nor beneficial to man. *Commensals* are organisms which live in humans but which do not cause disease in the part of the body where they are normally present. For example, *Streptococcus faecalis* is a bacterium which is harmless in its normal habitat, the large intestine. However, some commensals can be pathogenic if they spread to areas of the body where they are not normally found. *Streptococcus faecalis*, for example, causes disease if it infects the kidneys.

Although it is convenient to use a functional classification, it must be emphasized that this is not a hard and fast division. An individual organism may, in differing circumstances, fall into each of the four groups. For example, the bacterium *Escherichia coli* is generally considered to be inert. However, in some cases it may be pathogenic since it can cause food poisoning. Certain strains can cause food spoilage without causing illness. It has been used for removing glucose from egg white prior to drying, so may therefore be considered useful.

Protozoa

Protozoa are small single-celled animals. They are motile, i.e. capable of independent movement. They mostly live in water, for example in ponds, rivers and the sea and in the water in soil. A common example is *Amoeba*, see Figure 15.1.

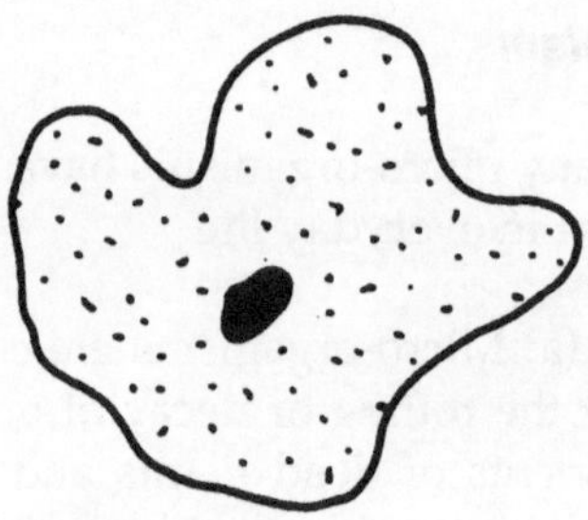

Figure 15.1 *Amoeba.*

They feed by engulfing tiny food particles and reproduce by binary fission, i.e. dividing into two halves.

The majority of protozoa are non-pathogenic but there are a few pathogenic species of some importance. For example, *Entamoeba histolytica* causes amoebic dysentry, a type of dysentry common in the tropics. Malaria is caused by the protozoan *Plasmodium* which is transmitted by mosquitoes. *Toxoplasma gondii* is an organism sometimes found in animals which may be transmitted to man during the handling of raw meat (particularly pork and mutton). It is estimated that there are one million people in the world infected with the organism and the disease (known as toxoplasmosis) has recently become of more concern in this country.

Algae

Algae are simple plants. Some are macroscopic (large), e.g. seaweeds, but many are microscopic. They contain chlorophyll or a similar pigment which enables them to photosynthesize (see page 59). This means that they do not require complex organic substances as food but can utilize carbon dioxide and water. Microscopic algae usually live in water. Although each cell is capable of an independent existence they tend to grow in a mass and are often visible as green slime, e.g. on the surface of ponds.

Viruses

These are the smallest of all micro-organisms, varying in size from 10 to 300 nm (1 nm = 10^{-9} metre). Most viruses are not visible under the light microscope but can be observed and photographed with the aid of an electron microscope. Viruses are acellular, i.e. they do not have a cellular structure. They are made up of a central core of nucleic acid (see page 145) surrounded by a protein coat. They cannot feed, grow or multiply in isolation; they must always live as parasites in larger living cells. A virus particle attaches itself to a cell and the core of the virus penetrates and directs the life of the cell so that many more virus particles are formed. These new particles are then set free to attack other cells. The host cell is injured or even destroyed by the invading virus. Therefore, viruses are always pathogenic; they cause disease in man, animals, plants and other micro-organisms. Table 15.1 gives some examples of virus diseases.

Most virus diseases in man are transmitted by contact, but some are known to be transmitted by contaminated food or water, e.g. hepatitis A. Some diseases may be transmitted to man from animals, for example rabies from dogs and psittacosis from parrots.

Most virus diseases of man confer immunity, i.e. an attack of the disease confers resistance to a subsequent attack. This is due to the production of antibodies, substances formed in the body in response to infection. Artificial immunity may be conferred by means of vaccination. A vaccine consists of a weakened or dead form of a pathogen and when it is injected into the body it is practically harmless yet it induces antibody production.

Table 15.1 *Some examples of virus diseases*

Host	*Virus disease*
Man	Common cold, Influenza, Measles, Mumps, Chickenpox, Smallpox, Poliomyelitis, AIDS
Animals	Foot-and-mouth disease, Rabies, Distemper, Myxomatosis, Psittacosis
Plants	Mosaic diseases

Many virus diseases of animals and plants are of economic importance. Thousands of pounds are lost annually due to destruction of crops and livestock by virus diseases.

Bovine spongiform encephalopathy (BSE) or 'mad cow disease' is a disease which affects the brain of cattle. The BSE epidemic in the UK which started in 1986 was thought to be due to cattle being fed on cattle feeds containing meat-and-bone meal from sheep infected with a similar disease, scrapie. Since 1988 all cattle suspected of having BSE have been compulsorily slaughtered and since 1989 there has been a ban on the use of specified bovine offals (including the brain) in human food and animal feeds. The agent responsible for BSE is **prion** which consists of a single protein molecule and is even simpler in structure than a virus.

Microscopic fungi

Fungi are plants but, unlike green plants, they do not possess any chlorophyll. They are therefore unable to photosynthesize and require complex organic compounds as food. Those that grow and feed on dead organic material are termed **saprophytes,** while those feeding on living plants and animals are **parasites.**

1 Moulds

Moulds are usually multicellular, i.e. each mould growth consists of more than one cell. However, each cell is capable of independent growth and therefore moulds may be classified as micro-organisms. Moulds consist of thin thread-like strands called **hyphae** (sing. hypha). The hyphae grow in a mass on or through the medium on which the mould is growing. This mass of hyphae is known as the mycelium. There are basically two types of mould:

(a) **non-septate moulds** – these do not possess cross walls (septae). The hyphae are continuous tubes containing many nuclei dispersed throughout the cytoplasm and are therefore considered to be multicellular;

(b) **septate moulds** – these possess septae or cross walls (see Figure 15.2) which divide the hyphae into separate cells, each cell containing a nucleus.

Reproduction

Reproduction in moulds is chiefly by means of asexual spores. In non-septate moulds the spores are normally formed within a spore case, or sporangium, at the tip of a fertile hypha. Most septate moulds reproduce by forming unprotected spores known as conidia. Conidia are cut off, either singly or in chains, from the tip of a fertile hypha. Both types of sporing bodies are shown in Figure 15.2.

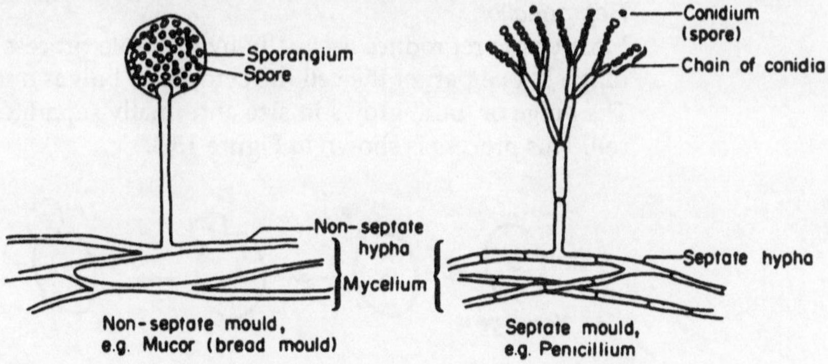

Figure 15.2 *Asexual reproduction in moulds.*

When ripe the spores are released into the air. If they find their way to a suitable substrate (food) they germinate and produce a new growth of mould. Some moulds also produce sexual spores, by the fusion of two hyphae.

Many moulds cause food spoilage. Spoilage may occur even in refrigerated foods. However, certain moulds are used in food production, particularly in cheesemaking; Danish blue, Roquefort and Camembert are mould-ripened. Moulds are also used in the manufacture of soy sauce and some products used in the food industry, e.g. citric acid.

Although most moulds are harmless, a few are pathogenic and cause diseases in plants, such as potato blight, and skin infections in man, such as 'athlete's foot' and ringworm. Certain moulds are capable of causing illness by producing toxins in foods known as **mycotoxins.** (Mycology is the study of fungi.) The mould *Aspergillus flavus* produces aflatoxin. This has been found in groundnuts (peanuts), figs, cereals and some other foods. There is considerable concern over levels of aflatoxin in some of these foods and in animal feeds. High levels of aflatoxin are associated with cancer of the liver. Ergot is a fungus which attacks rye and it can cause a serious illness (known as ergotism) in people who eat bread made from infected grain.

One of the most spectacular developments in medicine in this century was the discovery of penicillin and other antibiotics produced by moulds.

2 Yeasts

Yeasts are simple single-celled fungi. They are mainly saprophytic and usually grow on plant foods. Yeast cells may be oval, rod-shaped or spherical. They are larger than bacteria and under a high-power microscope a distinct nucleus is visible.

Reproduction

Most yeasts reproduce asexually by a simple process known as 'budding'. In one part of the cell the cytoplasm bulges out of the cell wall. The bulge or 'bud' grows in size and finally separates as a new yeast cell. This process is shown in Figure 15.3.

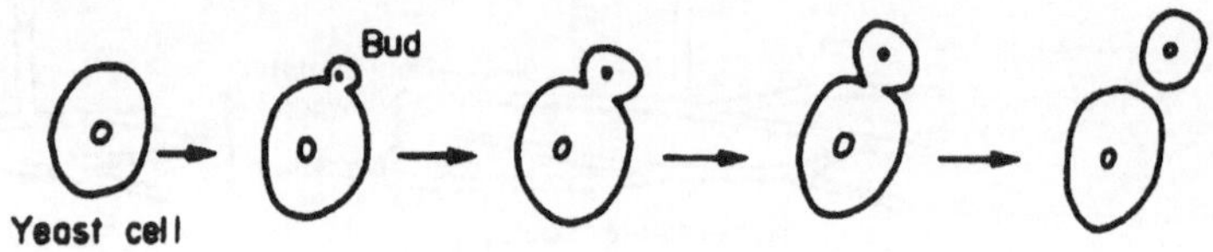

Figure 15.3 *Budding in yeast.*

Yeasts may cause spoilage in certain foods, e.g. fruit juices, jams and meat. These yeasts are normally referred to as 'wild yeasts' in order to distinguish them from those used commercially in the production of alcoholic drinks and bread.

The economic importance of yeast lies in its ability to break down carbohydrate foods into alcohol and carbon dioxide. This process, known as **alcoholic fermentation**, is anaerobic, i.e. takes place in the absence of oxygen. Yeast contains a collection of enzymes known as zymase which is responsible for the fermentation of sugars, such as glucose, into ethanol (ethyl alcohol) and carbon dioxide. Alcoholic fermentation may be represented by the following equation:

$$\underset{\text{glucose}}{C_6H_{12}O_6} \xrightarrow{\text{zymase}} \underset{\substack{\text{ethanol} \\ \text{(ethyl alcohol)}}}{2C_2H_5OH} + \underset{\substack{\text{carbon} \\ \text{dioxide}}}{2CO_2}$$

If a plentiful supply of oxygen is available, yeast cells will respire aerobically. In this case, yeast enzymes are able to break down sugars more completely, and carbon dioxide and water are produced.

$$\underset{\text{glucose}}{C_6H_{12}O_6} + \underset{\text{oxygen}}{6O_2} \longrightarrow \underset{\text{carbon dioxide}}{6CO_2} + \underset{\text{water}}{6H_2O}$$

More energy is obtained from aerobic than from anaerobic respiration. It is important when yeast is being grown commercially that it is supplied with plenty of air so that sufficient energy is available for growth.

The two most important industrial uses of yeast are in breadmaking and for the production of alcohol. The species generally used in these processes is *Saccharomyces cerevisiae*.

Production of alcoholic beverages

All alcoholic beverages, such as beers, wines and spirits, are produced by the anaerobic fermentation of a carbohydrate material by yeast. A large range of starting materials can be used; the carbohydrate may be in the form of starch, e.g. in wheat, barley, rice or potatoes, or in the form of sugars, e.g. in fruits, molasses or added sugar (sucrose). In addition, the following substances may be added:

1 *Amylase*. Yeast cells are not able to produce enzymes capable of breaking down starch. Therefore, if starch is used, a substance containing amylase (diastase) must be added. Amylase is an enzyme which catalyses the breakdown of starch into maltose. Malt (germinating barley) has a high amylase content and is used in the brewing of beer.

2 *Available nitrogen*. This is necessary for the synthesis of protein during the growth and multiplication of the yeast cell. This nitrogen may be provided by protein present in the carbohydrate-containing food used, e.g. by the wheat, or it may be added in the form of ammonium salts or nitrates.

3 *Water*. Water is necessary for the growth of the yeast and also to increase the volume of the mixture.

The mixture is enclosed in a container and oxygen is excluded; this ensures that respiration is anaerobic rather than aerobic. It is then held at a warm temperature in order to encourage the yeast cells to grow and multiply. Fermentation is allowed to continue until the desired concentration of alcohol is obtained. The maximum concentration which can be achieved by fermentation is 16%, since if it increases further the yeast cannot grow. The alcohol content of fortified wines, spirits and liqueurs is increased by distillation.

Breadmaking

The main ingredients used in breadmaking are flour, water, yeast and salt. These are made into a dough and fat, milk and sugar may also be added. The flour provides starch, amylase and protein and is an excellent food for the yeast. The bread dough is allowed to ferment prior to baking and the carbon dioxide produced causes the dough to rise. During baking the carbon dioxide expands causing the loaf to rise further.

A more detailed description of breadmaking is given on page 206. An account of the various enzymes of importance in breadmaking is given on page 158.

Bacteria

Bacteria (sing. bacterium) are a very important group of micro-organisms because of both their harmful and their beneficial effects. They are widely distributed in the environment. They are found in air, water and soil, in the intestines of animals, on the moist linings of the mouth, nose and throat, on the surface of the body and on plants.

Bacteria are the smallest single-celled organisms, some being only 0.4 μm (micrometre) in diameter. The cell contains a mass of cytoplasm and some nuclear material. It does not have a distinct nucleus, but just a single strand of DNA. The cell is enclosed by a cell wall and in some bacteria this is surrounded by a capsule or slime layer. The capsule consists of a mixture of polysaccharides and polypeptides. Figure 15.4 shows a generalized picture of a single bacterium.

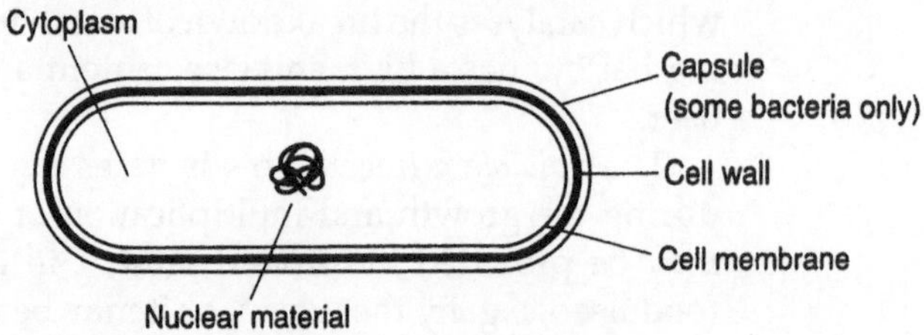

Figure 15.4 *A bacterial cell.*

Bacteria are classified into four basic groups depending on the shape of the cells:

1 Coccus (pl. cocci) – spherical
2 Bacillus (pl. bacilli) – rod-shaped
3 Vibrio – short, curved rods
4 Spirillum (pl. spirilli) – long, coiled threads

When bacteria are grown on a culture medium in the laboratory the cells may be grouped together. Cocci, for example, may be joined in chains (Streptococci) or arranged in clusters (Staphylococci). The four basic shapes of bacteria are shown in Figure 15.5.

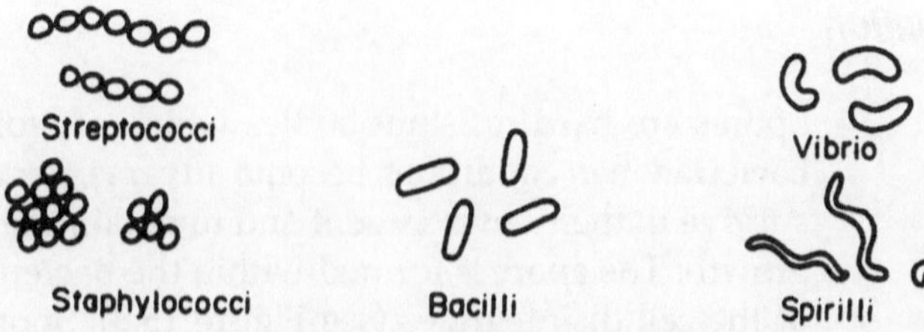

Figure 15.5 *Shapes of bacteria.*

Motility

Some bacteria are motile, i.e. capable of movement. These bacteria possess long thread-like structures called flagella (sing. flagellum) which originate from inside the cell membrane. The flagella move in a whip-like manner and help to propel the bacteria through liquid, such as water. Bacteria can be classified further according to the number of flagella they possess and the position of the flagella on the bacterial cell (see Figure 15.6).

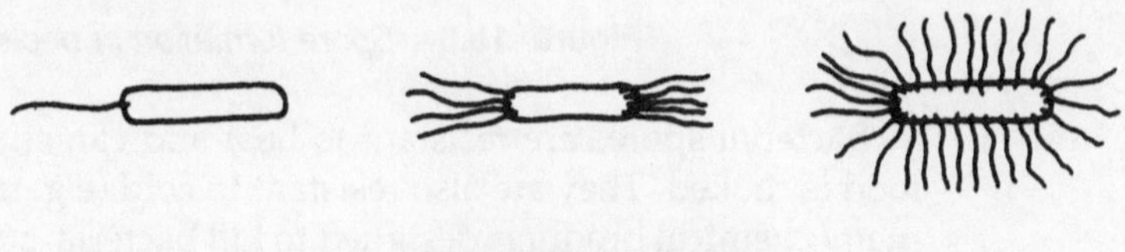

Figure 15.6 *Flagella.*

Reproduction

Bacteria reproduce by a process known as **binary fission**. The nuclear material reproduces itself and divides into two separate parts and then the rest of the cell divides, producing two daughter cells which are equal in size. This process is shown in Figure 15.7.

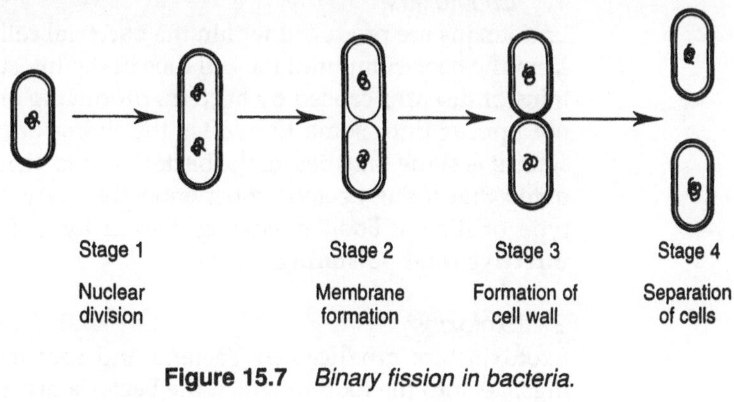

Figure 15.7 *Binary fission in bacteria.*

Spore formation

Spores are hard resistant bodies which are formed by some types of bacteria when conditions become adverse, i.e. when they are unable to survive in their environment and to obtain the materials necessary for growth. The spore is formed within the bacterial cell and then the rest of the cell disintegrates (see Figure 15.8). Spores can survive adverse conditions for very long periods of time. When conditions become favourable the spore germinates producing a new bacterial cell. Spore formation occurs in only certain types of bacteria. The two groups of bacteria which form spores (*Bacillus* and *Clostridium*) are both rod-shaped.

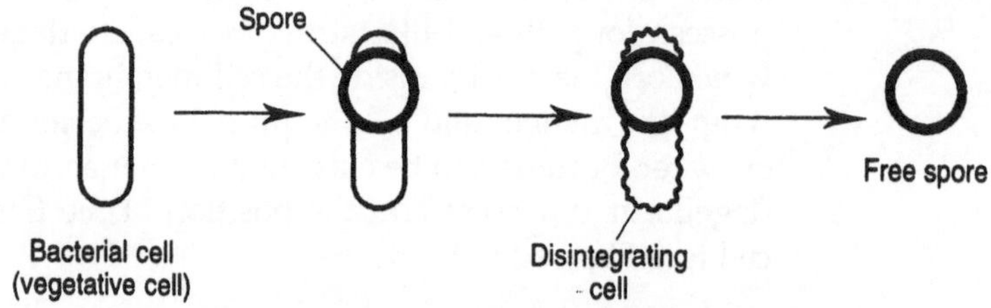

Figure 15.8 *Spore formation in bacteria.*

Bacterial spores are resistant to heat and can survive in food when food is cooked. They are also resistant to cold (e.g. refrigeration) and to many chemical products designed to kill bacteria, such as disinfectants.

The normal cells of bacteria are described as **vegetative cells** to distinguish them from spores.

Toxins

Bacteria produce a variety of substances as a result of their metabolism. Some of these substances are harmful to humans and are known as toxins (i.e. poisons). There are two types of toxins:

1 Endotoxins

Endotoxins are produced within the bacterial cell and are not released from the bacterium until the cell dies in the intestinal tract. The symptoms of diseases caused by bacteria producing endotoxins usually do not appear until some time after the living bacteria enter the body, since it is some time before the bacterial cells disintegrate. It should be noted that living bacteria must enter the body in order to cause this type of illness. Food poisoning caused by endotoxins is known as **infective food poisoning**.

2 Exotoxins

Exotoxins are produced by bacteria and secreted into the surroundings, i.e. into the food in which the bacteria are growing. It is not necessary to ingest living bacteria; the illness is caused by the toxin alone. Some types of food poisoning illnesses are caused by eating a food containing an exotoxin which has survived, even though the bacteria which produced it have died. The symptoms of the illness usually appear soon after the exotoxin enters the body. Food poisoning caused by exotoxins is known as **toxic food poisoning**.

Both types of toxins may be described as enterotoxins, i.e. substances which have a harmful effect on the digestive system.

Bacterial taxonomy

Taxonomy is the science of classification applied to living things and it involves their identification, naming and arrangement. The system of classification devised by Linnaeus (1707–1798), a Swedish botanist, has now been accepted universally as a means of reference. In this system each individual type of organism is called a **species**. Species or organisms having close similarities are arranged in a group known as a **genus** (pl. genera). Genera with similar characteristics are put in the same family, similar families into orders and orders into classes. This system uses two Latin names to describe each organism. The generic name refers to its genus and is written with a capital letter and the specific name indicates its species and is written with a small letter. For example, the name *Clostridium perfringens* refers to species of bacteria known as *perfringens* belonging to the genus *Clostridium*. The generic name is often abbreviated to one or two letters, e.g. *B.* for *Bacillus, Cl.* for *Clostridium*. Most animals and plants can be classified according to their morphology, i.e. according to their shape, in conjunction with evidence obtained from fossils. However, the classification of bacteria is more difficult, because fossils of bacteria do not exist and it is difficult to distinguish more than four basic shapes with the aid of a microscope. It is possible to classify bacteria using other criteria and some of the more simple means of classification are given in the following list:

1 Motility and possession of flagella
2 Pigment production
3 Spore formation
4 Heat resistance of vegetative cells and spores
5 Selective staining techniques
6 Selective culture techniques
7 Biochemical tests

Selective culture techniques involve the use of a variety of media. Some media contain substances which suppress the growth of most bacteria but allow particular types to grow. Biochemical tests make use of the fact that different species of bacteria use widely differing materials as food and produce different substances as a result of their metabolism.

It is possible to stain either the whole of the bacterial cell or a part of the cell with various stains or dyes. The ability to retain the stain depends on the species of bacteria. The most common stain used is the Gram stain. Bacteria which retain the stain, becoming violet when viewed under the microscope, are Gram positive. Other bacteria which do not retain the stain are Gram negative and appear pink.

Some of the more important genera of Gram positive and Gram negative bacteria known to cause food spoilage and food poisoning are listed below.

GRAM POSITIVE BACTERIA

BACILLUS – Aerobic, spore-forming rods. Often cause problems in the canning industry because the spores are very resistant to heat. *B. anthracis* causes anthrax in man and animals. *B. subtilis* (*B. mesentericus*) causes a type of spoilage known as ropiness in bread. *B. cereus* may cause food poisoning.

CLOSTRIDIUM – Anaerobic, spore-forming rods. Cause problems in the canning industry due to heat resistance of spores. *Cl. perfringens* causes food poisoning. *Cl. botulinum* causes a rare but lethal form of food poisoning.

CORYNEBACTERIUM – Aerobic rods, do not form spores. Cause food spoilage. *C. diphtheriae* causes diphtheria.

LACTOBACILLUS – Long rods, do not form spores, usually anaerobic. Often cause spoilage of dairy products and processed meat products. Are used in the manufacture of yoghurt and cheese. *L. bulgaricus* is used in yoghurt production. *L. thermophilus* may cause spoilage of milk.

LEUCONOSTOC – Cocci. Often cause spoilage in dairy products and foods with a high sugar content. Produce characteristic slimy growth.

LISTERIA – Rods, do not form spores. *L. monocytogenes* is responsible for the illness 'listeriosis'.

MICROCOCCUS – Can tolerate high levels of salt and grow fairly well at low temperatures. Often cause spoilage of preserved or refrigerated meats. Some species produce characteristic pink or orange-red pigment.

MYCOBACTERIUM – Rods. *M. tuberculosis* causes bovine TB. Unpasteurized milk from infected cattle can transmit the disease to humans.

SARCINA – Cocci, may be aerobic or anaerobic. Cause spoilage of wide range of unrefrigerated foods. Often produce yellow pigments.

STAPHYLOCOCCUS – Large cocci. Found in the nasal cavities of man and certain other animals as well as on the skin. *Staph. aureus* infects wounds and may cause boils and carbuncles. It is also one of the common causes of food poisoning.

STREPTOCOCCUS – Some species occur in the respiratory tract of man and other animals where they may cause diseases such as scarlet fever and tonsillitis. Other species are found in the intestinal tract of man and animals. *Strep. faecalis* is found in animal faeces and is used as an indicator organism for faecal contamination. This organism sometimes causes outbreaks of food poisoning. Some species ferment lactose (milk sugar) and are used in cheese production, e.g. *Strep. lactis.*

GRAM NEGATIVE BACTERIA

ACETOBACTER – Aerobic rods. Cause spoilage of fruits and vegetables. *A. aceti* oxidizes ethanol to acetic acid and is used industrially in the production of vinegar from wine.

ACHROMOBACTER – Short rods. Cause low-temperature spoilage of meats, poultry and seafoods.

AEROMONAS – Rods. Grow well at low temperatures. *A. hydrophila* and related species have been implicated as a cause of food-borne diarrhoea.

ALCALIGENES – Rods. Occur widely in nature. Cause spoilage of raw milk and poultry products. *Alcaligenes viscolactis* causes a type of spoilage known as ropiness in milk.

BACTEROIDES – Anaerobic rods, do not form spores and therefore are often overlooked in routine analyses of foods. Found in the intestinal tract of man and animals and may be transferred to meat where they cause spoilage.

BRUCELLA – *Brucella abortus* causes brucellosis in man and animals.

CAMPYLOBACTER – Curved rods. Live as a commensal in the intestinal tract of many animals. *C. jejuni* occurs worldwide in patients with diarrhoea and is a common cause of food-borne illness.

ERWINIA – Motile rods, grow well at low temperatures. Cause spoilage of fruits and vegetables, particularly soft rot of vegetables. Often produce characteristic red pigment.

ESCHERICHIA – Short rods. Main habitat is intestinal tract of man and animals. *E. coli* is used as an indicator organism since large numbers indicate faecal contamination of foods or water.

PROPIONIBACTERIUM – Small rods. Cause spoilage of alcoholic beverages and pickled foods, where they produce propionic acid. Used in the production of Swiss cheeses containing holes or 'eyes'.

PROTEUS – Aerobic motile rods. Cause spoilage of meat and eggs, when these foods are not stored in a refrigerator.

PSEUDOMONAS – Short aerobic rods. Grow well at low tempertures. Cause spoilage of a large range of refrigerated foods, e.g. meats, poultry, eggs, seafoods.

SALMONELLA – Short aerobic rods. Main habitat is the intestinal tract of man and animals. *S. typhi* causes typhoid fever. *S. typhimurium* and many other species cause food poisoning.

SERRATIA – Aerobic rods. Cause spoilage of unrefrigerated foods. Often produce red pigments, e.g. *Serratia marcescens* produces a red colour on mouldy bread.

SHIGELLA – Short, non-motile, aerobic rods. *Shigella sonnei* occurs in polluted waters and the intestinal tract of man. This organism causes bacillary dysentery.

VIBRIO – Curved rods. *V. cholerae* causes the disease cholera which can be contracted by drinking unchlorinated water or eating contaminated food. *V. parahaemolyticus* causes food poisoning.

YERSINIA – Rods. *Y. enterocolitica* is widespread and inhabits the intestines of animals, soil and water. It can grow at low temperatures and can cause food poisoning.

Factors affecting the growth of micro-organisms

All micro-organisms require certain environmental conditions for growth and multiplication. There are variations in the growth requirements of different species but it is possible to list six basic requirements and to indicate individual variations under these headings.

1 Time

The rate of multiplication of bacteria varies according to the species and to the conditions of growth. Under optimum conditions, most bacteria reproduce by binary fission once every 20 minutes. For some bacteria the **generation time**, i.e. the time between divisions, may be as short as 12 minutes. If the generation time is 20 minutes, under favourable conditions a single cell may produce several million cells in under seven hours. Table 15.2 shows how this can be calculated.

Fortunately, growth does not carry on at such a rapid rate for any great length of time. The life-cycle of a bacterial colony (a large number of bacteria grouped together) has been investigated and it has been found that when bacteria are placed on a fresh medium, there is no multiplication for about 30 minutes. During this **log phase** the cells are metabolizing rapidly, but this activity results in a slight increase in cell size rather than in cell numbers. Following this the cells multiply rapidly for a few hours or even days depending on the organism and the environment. This period of rapid multiplication is called the **log phase**, since the logarithm of the number of organisms varies directly with time. (After **x** minutes 10 cells produce 100 cells; after a further *x* minutes 100 cells produce 1000 cells.) The colony now enters a **stationary phase** of growth where the number of cells produced is equal to the number of cells dying. Finally, the growth rate decreases, usually due to shortage of a growth factor such as a vitamin or mineral element. The colony enters the **decline phase**, which is also logarithmic. The four phases of growth are illustrated by the graph shown in Figure 15.9.

Table 15.2 *Bacterial multiplication, assuming a generation time of 20 minutes*

Time in minutes	*Number of organisms*
0	1
20	2
40	4
60 (1 hour)	8
80	16
100	32
120 (2 hours)	64
140	128
160	256
180 (3 hours)	512
200	1024
220	2048
240 (4 hours)	4096
260	8192
280	16,384
300 (5 hours)	32,768
320	65,536
340	131,072
360 (6 hours)	262,144
380	524,288
400	1,048,576
420 (7 hours)	2,097,152

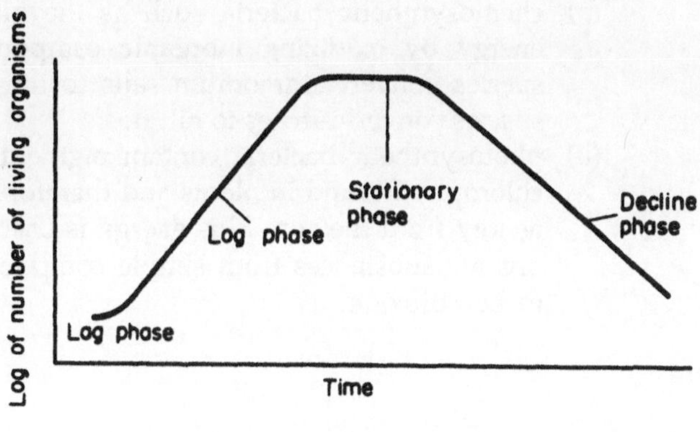

Figure 15.9 *Bacterial growth curve.*

2 Food

All micro-organisms require nutrients which will supply the following:

(a) energy, usually obtained from a substance containing carbon;
(b) nitrogen for protein synthesis;
(c) vitamins and related growth factors;
(d) minerals.

There are two basic types of nutrition. The organisms may be either heterotrophic or autotrophic.

Heterotrophic nutrition

Heterotrophic organisms resemble animals, since they require complex organic substances, such as protein and carbohydrate, for food. All moulds and yeasts and some bacteria, including most pathogens, are heterotrophic. Some can use a wide range of substances in order to obtain their food requirements, while others are more specific and will only grow on certain foods.

Some are able to synthesize vitamins themselves, e.g. bacteria in the intestinal tract, while others must have vitamins supplied by the substrate. It should be noted that the vitamin requirements of bacteria and other micro-organisms are not the same as those of humans.

Autotrophic nutrition

Autotrophic organisms resemble plants, since they are able to use simple inorganic substances as food. Many bacteria are autotrophic and there are very few substances that are not biodegradable, i.e. that cannot be broken down by a species of bacteria. Some bacteria can even live on concrete and others can grow in disinfectants such as carbolic acid.

Autotrophic bacteria obtain their energy in two ways:

(a) chemosynthetic bacteria such as the nitrifying bacteria obtain energy by oxidizing inorganic compounds. The *Nitrosomonas* species convert ammonium salts to nitrites and the *Nitrobacter* species convert nitrites to nitrates;
(b) photosynthetic bacteria contain pigments closely related to the chlorophyll found in plants and therefore they are able to utilize energy from the sun. This energy is used to synthesize complex organic substances from simple compounds such as water and carbon dioxide.

3 Moisture

Micro-organisms, like all other organisms, require water to maintain life. The amount of water available in a food can be described in terms of the water activity (A_w). Pure water has an $A_w = 1.0$. The water activity of most fresh foods is 0.99 but dissolved substances, such as sugar and salt, may lower this considerably. Dried foods have an A_w of 0.6 or less. Bacteria usually require more available moisture than yeasts and moulds. Some species of yeast are osmophilic, i.e. they can grow in an environment supplying very little available moisture. Table 15.3 shows the minimum water activity of some types of micro-organisms.

Table 15.3 *Minimum water activity of certain types of micro-organisms*

Organisms	*Minimum A_w*
Most spoilage bacteria	0.91
Most spoilage yeasts	0.88
Most spoilage moulds	0.80
Osmophilic yeasts	0.60

4 Temperature

Each micro-organism has:

(a) a maximum growth temperature;
(b) a minimum growth temperature;
(c) an optimum growth temperature, i.e. the temperature at which it grows best and multiplies most rapidly.

The optimum temperature is normally closer to the maximum than the minimum temperature.

Micro-organisms can be classified into three groups on the basis of their temperature requirements:

(a) **Psychrophiles** (cold-loving organisms) can grow well at temperatures below 20°C; optimum growth range is 10°C to 20°C;
(b) **Mesophiles** (organisms liking moderate temperatures) have an optimum growth temperature between 20°C and 45°C;
(c) **Thermophiles** (organisms liking higher temperatures) can grow well at temperatures above 45°C; optimum growth range is 50°C to 60°C.

This classification is very approximate and sometimes other terms may be used. For example, some organisms may be able to resist the effect of high temperatures even though they are not thermophilic; these are referred to as **thermoduric** (heat-resisting) micro-organisms. Similarly, organisms capable of surviving very low temperatures, although they are not psychrophilic are called **psychroduric** (cold-resisting) micro-organisms. Also, the term **psychrotrophs** is sometimes used to cover both psychrophiles and mesophiles, since some mesophiles have a low minimum growth temperature.

Psychrophiles may cause spoilage of refrigerated foods, e.g. members of the genera *Achromobacter* and *Pseudomonas*. The majority of bacteria are mesophilic. Bacteria which are pathogenic to man have an optimum temperature of 37°C (the temperature of the human body). Moulds and yeasts are usually mesophilic or psychrophilic; they do not grow well at higher temperatures. Thermophiles are particularly troublesome in the dairy industry since they may grow at pasteurization temperatures. Members of the genera *Bacillus* and *Clostridium* produce thermoduric spores and may cause spoilage of canned foods (see page 288).

5 Oxygen

The amount of oxygen available affects the growth of micro-organisms. Moulds are aerobic (i.e. require oxygen), while yeasts are either aerobic or anaerobic depending on the conditions. Bacteria are classified into four groups according to their oxygen requirements:

(a) **obligate aerobes** can only grow if there is a plentiful supply of oxygen available;
(b) **facultative aerobes** grow best if there is plenty of oxygen available but can grow anaerobically;
(c) **obligate anaerobes** can only grow if there is no oxygen present;
(d) **facultative anaerobes** grow best if there is no oxygen present but they can also grow aerobically.

Inorganic salts added to food can greatly affect the amount of oxygen available since they act as oxidizing or reducing agents, e.g. potassium nitrate, which is used as a meat preservative, increases the amount of oxygen available, since it is an oxidizing agent.

6 pH

Most micro-organisms grow best if the pH of the food is between 6.6 and 7.5 (i.e. if it is neutral). Bacteria, particularly pathogens, are less acid-tolerant than moulds and yeasts and there are no bacteria which can grow if the pH is below 3.5. Therefore, the spoilage of high acid foods such as fruit is usually caused by yeasts and moulds. Meat and sea foods are more susceptible to bacterial spoilage since the pH of these foods is nearer to 7.0. Very few foods are alkaline and, therefore, the maximum pH for growth is unimportant. Table 15.4 gives approximate values of the minimum pH for growth of some micro-organisms.

Control of growth of micro-organisms

In order to prevent food spoilage, the growth of micro-organisms must be prevented. This can be achieved by removing one or more of the conditions necessary for growth or by providing conditions which interfere with microbial metabolism. Many methods of food preservation rely on more than one method of controlling microbial growth. The six most important methods are outlined below.

Table 15.4 *Minimum pH for growth of certain micro-organisms*

Organism	*Minimum pH*
Salmonella typhi	4.5
Escherichia coli	4.4
Yeasts	2.5
Moulds	1.5–2.0

1 *Removal of moisture*

In order to prevent the growth of micro-organisms in a food the water activity of the food must be reduced to 0.6 or below. In the commercial production of dried foods this is achieved by applying heat and causing the water present in the food to evaporate. The addition of salt or sugar to the food has the same effect. The moisture available to the micro-organisms is reduced by osmosis (see Chapter 4). The salt or sugar solutions are more concentrated than the cytoplasm inside the cells of the micro-organism. Therefore, water passes out of the cell and the cell becomes dehydrated (see Figure 15.10).

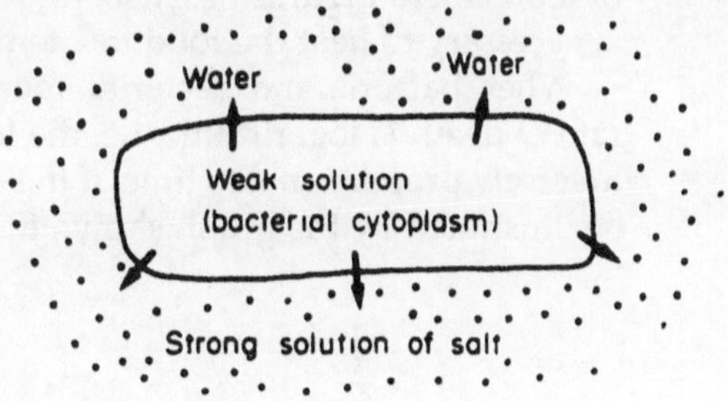

Figure 15.10 *Diagram illustrating the osmotic effect of a salt solution on a bacterial cell.*

2 *Altering temperature*

Microbial growth may be prevented by either decreasing or increasing the temperature.

(A) Lowering the temperature

There are two types of low-temperature preservation:

(i) *Refrigeration or chilling*. The food is placed at a temperature above the freezing point of water (i.e. above 0°C). The temperature inside a domestic refrigerator should be in the range 0–4°C. Slightly above this range *Listeria monocytogenes* is able to grow and multiply and this organism can cause a serious form of illness (see page 250). At temperatures in the range 0–4°C the growth of most species of micro-organisms is retarded and some may even be killed. However, many micro-organisms are still able to grow slowly at these temperatures and bacterial spores survive.

(ii) *Freezing*. The food is frozen and stored at –18°C or below. The freezing process has a killing effect and bacteria continue to die during storage. However, bacteria are only partially eliminated and spores are able to survive. When the food is thawed, the keeping time is shorter than that of fresh food, since the cellular structure of the food has been partially broken down by the freezing process, and bacteria are able to attack the cell contents more easily.

(B) Raising the temperature

It is possible to destroy both bacterial cells and spores by holding the food at a high temperature for a few hours or longer. The complete destruction of micro-organisms by heat is known as **sterilization**. Cooking may be regarded as a short-term means of food preservation since, if the food is cooked properly, the number of bacteria present will be reduced.

However, if food is to be preserved for longer periods of time, it must be heated in a sealed container, such as a can, to prevent the entry of more micro-organisms. Also, for foods other than high acid foods, it is necessary to heat the food to a temperature above 100°C.

When bacteria and bacterial spores are destroyed by heating, the rate of death is logarithmic, i.e. the log of the number of organisms is inversely proportional to time, if the temperature is constant. This may be illustrated by the graph shown in Figure 15.11.

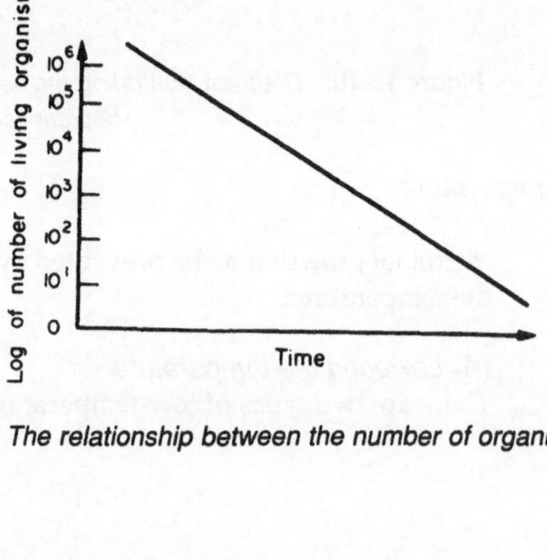

Figure 15.11 *The relationship between the number of organisms and time.*

The **Decimal Reduction Time** (DRT) is the time taken to reduce the number of organisms to one-tenth of the original value when heating at a constant temperature. If the DRT is plotted against temperature the relationship is again logarithmic as shown by Figure 15.12.

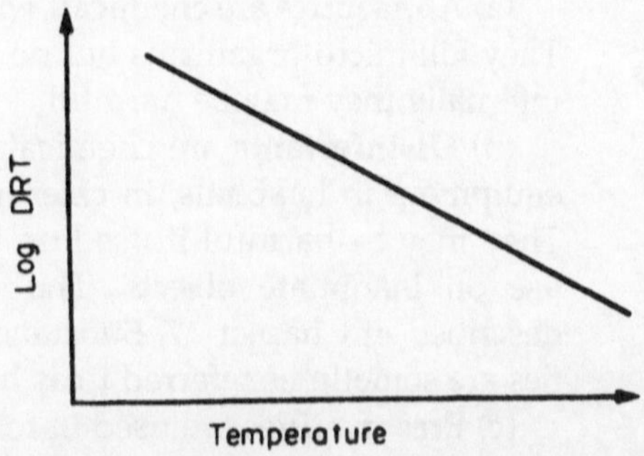

Figure 15.12 *The relationship between decimal reduction time (DRT) and temperature.*

The higher the temperature, the shorter the time necessary to reduce the numbers of micro-organisms, i.e. the greater the killing effect. Also, using a higher temperature for a shorter time has less effect on the appearance and nutritive value of the food.

3 Exclusion of oxygen

The exclusion of oxygen, e.g. by vacuum packing, prevents the growth of moulds and aerobic bacteria, but yeasts can respire anaerobically and many pathogenic bacteria are anaerobic. Therefore, this may only be used as a means of preservation, if other methods are also used, e.g. destruction by heat in canning.

4 Altering pH

The pH may be lowered so that the food becomes too acidic to allow micro-organisms to grow. The most common method is the use of vinegar (acetic acid) in pickling. In the manufacture of yoghurt, bacteria ferment lactose (milk sugar) producing lactic acid. The lactic acid lowers the pH and retards the growth of spoilage organisms.

5 Irradiation

It is possible to kill micro-organisms by the use of ionizing radiations, e.g. gamma rays. The use of irradiation as a means of food preservation is discussed in more detail in Chapter 18. Ultraviolet radiation also kills microbes, though it is less effective. It can be used, for example, to kill mould spores in bakeries.

A large range of chemicals can be used to check the growth of micro-organisms and they can be roughly classified as follows:

(a) **Antiseptics** are chemicals which are used externally on the body. They kill micro-organisms but do not harm the skin. If they are taken internally they may be harmful.

(b) **Disinfectants** are chemicals which are used to kill bacteria on equipment in hospitals, in catering establishments and in the home. They may be harmful if used on the body and are only intended for use on inanimate objects. The various types of disinfectants are described in Chapter 17. Substances which have disinfectant properties are sometimes referred to as **bactericides.**

(c) **Preservatives** are used in food preservation. They do not kill all micro-organisms but they retard growth and delay food spoilage (see page 301).

(e) **Antibiotics** and **sulphonamides** are used in medicine. These drugs circulate in the bloodstream and suppress the growth of pathogens in the body.

16 Food poisoning

Food poisoning is an illness caused by eating harmful or contaminated food. The most usual symptoms are stomach pains, vomiting and diarrhoea. Food which can cause food poisoning may appear harmless, i.e. the colour, taste and appearance are normal and there is no evidence of spoilage. If food spoilage occurs, the food is unpalatable because the colour, taste and appearance have been changed, although the food may be completely harmless.

There are three types of food poisoning:

1 Chemical
2 Biological
3 Bacterial

Chemical food poisoning

This is caused by the presence of toxic chemicals in food. A small proportion (less than 1%) of the food poisoning in the UK is caused by chemical poisons. Chemicals used in agriculture or industry may occasionally get into foods in error. In the 1950s, 52 people died in the Japanese town of Minamata and many others suffered brain damage as the result of eating fish containing high levels of methyl mercury. Investigations showed that the source of mercury was effluent from a local chemical factory. The effluent contained inorganic mercury but this was converted into methyl mercury by micro-organisms in the mud at the bottom of Minamata Bay. The methyl mercury accumulated in the fish and shellfish living in the bay.

Outbreaks of organic mercury poisoning have also occurred in Iraq and Guatemala where farmers who had received grain seeds treated with a mercury fungicide ate the seeds instead of planting them. Heavy metals such as lead, zinc, cadmium and copper may reach foods from containers. For example, if acid foods are stored in galvanized containers zinc poisoning can result.

In Spain during 1981 and 1982, over 350 people died and 20 000 were ill as a result of consuming cooking oil containing industrial rapeseed which was contaminated with the chemical aniline.

Biological food poisoning

Biological food poisoning is caused by eating foods containing naturally occurring poisons. There are many examples of this type of poisoning including:

(a) **Poisonous mushrooms**. There are species of poisonous mushrooms, such as *Amanita phalloides* and *A. virosa,* which have caused illness and in some cases death. These mushrooms are very similar in appearance to the edible variety and may easily be eaten by mistake.

(b) **Deadly nightshade**. This is a bushy plant which grows throughout Europe and Asia. All parts of the plant contain the drug belladonna, which is used in medicine to relieve illnesses such as asthma, bronchitis and heart disease. However, the drug may be lethal if taken in large doses and children have been poisoned by eating the berries of the plant.

(c) **Potatoes**. Potatoes are also members of the nightshade family and green potatoes contain a substance called solanine which causes illness or even death if eaten in large quantities. Therefore, green potatoes should always be discarded.

(d) **Rhubarb.** Oxalic acid occurs in the form of its salt, potassium oxalate, in the sap of plants such as rhubarb and spinach. It is also found in very small amounts in the human body. However, in large amounts it can be dangerous and the consumption of large quantities of spinach and rhubarb may be dangerous. In normal circumstances, there is no danger in eating moderate quantities of these foods as part of a well-balanced diet. However, rhubarb leaves should always be avoided, since they contain large amounts of oxalic acid.

(e) **Red kidney beans**. Raw kidney beans contain a toxic substance called haemagglutinin. A number of cases of poisoning have occurred as a result of cooking the beans in a slow cooker at an insufficiently high temperature. Boiling the beans for 10 minutes destroys the toxin. Canned kidney beans are heated sufficiently during processing and are therefore safe.

(f) **Scombrotoxic fish poisoning**. Scombroid fish (certain types of oily fish such as mackerel and tuna) contain the amino acid histidine. In stale fish this is converted, by bacterial action, into a histamine-containing compound which is toxic. Symptoms of the poisoning include vomiting, headache, swelling of the lips and tongue, itching and respiratory distress. Raw fish should, therefore, be stored correctly, i.e. in ice, refrigerated or frozen.

(g) **Paralytic shellfish poisoning (PSP)**. This is a rare but serious and sometimes fatal type of food poisoning. It has been caused by eating raw mussels or oysters which have fed on plankton containing the protozoa *Gonyaulax tamerensis*. Toxins accumulate in the shellfish which can cause paralysis of the heart and respiratory muscles.

(h) **Mycotoxins.** Some moulds produce toxic substances called mycotoxins (see page 217).

Bacterial food poisoning

Bacterial food poisoning is the most common cause of food poisoning and stringent hygiene precautions must be taken in order to prevent outbreaks of this type of illness. Since most food poisoning incidents occur as a result of unhygienic practices, this means that they are preventable. There has been a notable increase in the number of recorded incidents of food poisoning since the Second World War. In the 1960s in England and Wales between 4000 and 5000 cases of food poisoning were notified annually. This number increased steadily throughout the 1970s and early 1980s and showed a dramatic increase in the latter part of the 1980s. Figures on the number of cases of bacterial food poisoning occurring annually are available from a number of sources. Since the method of collecting the information varies, the figures vary according to the source. However, they all indicate that food poisoning is increasing and that this increase is a cause for concern. Table 16.1 shows the number of cases of bacterial food poisoning in England and Wales for the years 1982 to 1993. These figures include both formal notifications and those ascertained by other means.

Table 16.1 *Reported cases of food poisoning in England and Wales, 1982 to 1993*

Year	*Number of cases*
1982	14 253
1983	17 735
1984	20 702
1985	19 242
1986	23 948
1987	29 331
1988	39 713
1989	52 557
1990	52 145
1991	52 543
1992	63 347
1993	68 587

The real situation may be even more alarming than these figures suggest, since it is estimated that only about 10% or less of all cases are reported. The actual number of cases probably exceeds 700 000 per year. The increase in the number of cases in recent years is thought to be due to a number of factors. Some of these factors are as follows:

1 There has been an increase in the number of meals eaten away from home (in canteens, restaurants, etc.). If a single food in a catering establishment becomes contaminated with food poisoning bacteria, large numbers of people may be affected.

Catering establishments now produce more varied menus and this often involves keeping dishes warm until they are required. If food poisoning bacteria enter the food or are already present, they may be given ideal conditions in which to grow.

2 There has been an increase in the consumption of poultry. A significant proportion of bacterial food poisoning is due to chickens contaminated with *Salmonella*.

3 There has been a decline in formal meals and an increase in 'snacking' and 'take away' meals. Take away meals are often kept warm on the premises where they are being sold or are cooked earlier and then reheated. They may also be heated up again in the customers' homes. Both situations may provide conditions suitable for the growth of food poisoning bacteria.

4 There has been an increase in intensive farming. There is evidence that intensive farming methods result in more foods being contaminated with food poisoning bacteria, since the animals are reared in close quarters with one another.

5 There has been an increase in the use of convenience foods. Manufacturing processes are carried out under hygienic conditions and the whole operation is carefully monitored. However, mistakes do occur and one source of infection may lead to the contamination of thousands of items. In addition, the use of convenience foods, especially meat products, which are eaten cold or only warmed through, increases the risk of food poisoning.

6 Shopping habits have changed. Many customers now shop at supermarkets on a weekly basis. This means that food is stored for longer periods of time in the home. Prolonged storage increases the risk of food poisoning.

7 Public concern over the use of food additives has led to a decrease in the use of food preservatives.

8 Improvements have been made in the collection of data on food poisoning and in methods of identifying micro-organisms.

There are more food poisoning outbreaks during the summer months if the weather is hot. This is partly due to the increase in consumption of pre-packed meals, which may be kept at warm temperatures for several hours before they are eaten. Also, in the summer months foods may be stored incorrectly both in shops and in homes and catering establishments, especially if refrigeration is faulty.

The bacteria most frequently responsible for food poisoning are:

1 Organisms of the *Salmonella* group
2 *Clostridium perfringens*
3 *Staphylococcus aureus*

4 *Bacillus cereus*
5 *Campylobacter jejuni*

Other bacteria which have been responsible for outbreaks of food poisoning, particularly in recent years, are as follows:

1 *Listeria monocytogenes*
2 *Clostridium botulinum*
3 *Escherichia coli*
4 *Vibrio parahaemolyticus*
5 *Aeromonas* species

Table 16.2 shows the numbers of outbreaks and sporadic cases of food poisoning caused by the common food poisoning bacteria in England and Wales between 1989 and 1991.

A family outbreak affects two or more people in the same family, whereas a general outbreak involves two or more people in different families.

Table 16.2 *Causal agents of bacterial food poisoning in England and Wales, 1989–91.*

Causative agent	*General outbreaks*	*Family outbreaks*	*Sporadic cases*
Salmonella spp.	392	2374	51 845
Clostridium perfringens	146	6	12
Staphylococcus aureus	16	9	8
Bacillus cereus and other Bacillus spp.	57	16	37

Table 16.3 is a classification of food poisoning according to location of outbreak.

The home is the single most frequently recorded location and it is likely that many of these outbreaks resulted from cross-contamination and inappropriate handling practices in the domestic kitchen. Outbreaks involving meals at restaurants and receptions are the most frequently reported types of general outbreak.

There are three main types of bacterial food poisoning:

1 The *infective type* which is caused by eating food containing a large number of living bacteria. After being eaten the bacteria establish themselves in the alimentary canal and when they die they release an endotoxin (e.g. *Salmonella* poisoning).

2 The *toxin type* which is caused by eating food containing an exotoxin. The toxin is released into the food while the bacteria are growing and multiplying in the food. The bacteria themselves may be dead when the food is eaten (e.g. *Staphylococcal* poisoning).

Table 16.3 *Food poisoning outbreaks classified according to location of outbreak (England and Wales, 1989–91).*

Location	*Salmonella* spp.	*Clostridium perfringens*	*Staphylococcus aureus*	*Bacillus cereus and Bacilus* spp.
Private houses	2374	6	9	16
Restaurants/receptions	202	58	5	40
Hospitals	21	18	–	2
Institutions	52	35	1	1
Schools	9	7	–	1
Shops	32	1	1	1
Canteens	9	9	1	3
Farms	3	–	–	–
Infected abroad	12	–	–	–
Other	44	6	5	3
Unspecified	8	12	3	6

3 The third type is also caused by a toxin. The toxin is not produced in the food but is released into the intestines after the bacteria have been eaten and while they are growing in the intestinal tract (e.g. *Clostridium perfringens* poisoning).

The **incubation period** (i.e. the time between the contaminated food being eaten and the occurrence of the first symptoms) is longer for the infective type of food poisoning than the toxin type.

Salmonella

Salmonellae are aerobic bacilli which do not form spores. They cause an infective type of illness and, in healthy persons, about a million living organisms need to be ingested to cause food poisoning. The organisms most frequently responsible for outbreaks are *S. typhimurium* and *S. enteritidis*, but there are about 2000 different types of *Salmonella*. Sometimes the organism is named after the place where it was first recognized as the causative agent of food poisoning. Examples of such organisms are *S. newport* and *S. dublin*. The large increase in reported cases of *Salmonella* poisoning during the second half of the 1980s was largely due to an increase in *Salmonella enteritidis* phage type 4 (PT4).

Illness

Incubation period: 12–36 hours.
Symptoms: abdominal pains, diarrhoea, vomiting, headache, fever.
Duration of illness: 1–8 days (sometimes as long as 14 days).

The people most at risk from *Salmonella* poisoning are the very young, the old and the ill. A number of people die each year as a result of *Salmonella* poisoning (e.g. there were 62 deaths in 1991). The mortality rate is less than 1%.

Source

Salmonellae are found in the intestines of man and many animals and, consequently, are excreted in the faeces. There are two types of human carriers:

1 **Healthy carriers** (symptomless excreters). These people carry the organism in their intestines and excrete it in their faeces, but they do not suffer any symptoms of the illness.

2 **Convalescent carriers.** These are people who continue to excrete the organism after they have recovered from the illness. Some species of *Salmonella* may be excreted for months or even years, while others are excreted for only a few weeks.

Animals may suffer from *Salmonella* infections or may be symptomless excreters. Poultry, cattle, pigs, domestic pets (e.g. dogs and tortoises), rats and mice are among animals which are known to be occasional carriers.

Salmonellae are often present in meat and offal, particularly in poultry. Hens' eggs may have Salmonellae on the shell and inside the eggs. Ducks' eggs are frequently contaminated. Raw milk from cows carrying *Salmonella* may contain living organisms but they are destroyed during pasteurization.

Means of spread to food

Salmonellae may be spread to foods by insect pests, vermin and domestic pets. Occasionally, human carriers contaminate foods particularly if they do not wash their hands after using the toilet. Salmonellae in animal feeding stuffs, especially in imported fish meal, can introduce infection into farm animals. Chickens reared under battery conditions are more likely to be infected with *Salmonella* than free-range hens, since the birds are kept close together and cross-infection readily occurs between one bird and another.

One of the most common methods of spread of *Salmonella* is by cross-contamination from raw meat and poultry to cooked foods, during handling and preparation in the kitchen .

Foods commonly associated with outbreaks

The foods most frequently responsible for *Salmonella* poisoning are eggs and products containing eggs, especially where the eggs are raw (e.g. mayonnaise) or only lightly cooked. Poultry, including cold and reheated chicken and turkey, has also been responsible for many outbreaks. Other high risk foods include meat and meat products (e.g. meat pies) and cream.

Prevention

Salmonellae are readily killed by heat and they do not produce heat-resistant spores or toxins. In order to reduce the risk of *Salmonella* poisoning, food handlers should take the following precautions:

1 Frozen meat and poultry should be thawed thoroughly before cooking.

2 Foods should be cooked thoroughly. Eggs, in particular, should be boiled adequately.

3 Dishes containing raw or lightly cooked egg should be avoided, particularly for susceptible groups, such as young children and the elderly.

Pasteurized egg (frozen or dried) should be used in place of shell eggs, both in domestic cooking and catering.

4 Raw and cooked meats should be stored separately. Juices from raw meat must not be allowed to drip onto cooked meats.

5 Separate knives, chopping boards, meat slicers, etc., should be used for raw and cooked meats and poultry.

6 Foods likely to cause *Salmonella* poisoning should be stored in a refrigerator. This includes raw eggs which should be consumed within three weeks of being layed.

Example of an outbreak

One evening in May 1990 over 150 people attended a trade exhibition at a hotel. A buffet was provided which included chicken drumsticks (heated), sausage rolls, vol-au-vents, and various sandwiches. In the next few days 100 of the people who had the meal were found to be suffering from one or more symptoms of food poisoning and four were admitted to hospital. Sixty-two of those ill gave stool samples which were positive for *Salmonella enteritidis* PT4 (phage type 4). The same organism was also found in samples of chicken drumsticks which remained after the event. Investigations revealed an appalling catalogue of food handling faults which involved the chicken drumsticks being frozen (raw), thawed, heated, cooled, breadcrumbed, frozen, thawed, heated, cooled, refrigerated, heated and served, all over the course of four days.

The drumsticks (about 30 kg) were delivered partially frozen, placed in a refrigerator and cooked the next day in a fan-assisted oven at 200°C. They were cooled for about 2 hours, coated in egg and breadcrumbs and placed in a freezer. Two days later they were removed from the freezer, left to defrost in the kitchen for 3.5 hours, deep fried for 3–4 minutes to brown and left to cool. After about an hour they were placed on serving dishes and refrigerated for 3 hours. They were then removed from the fridge, reheated in four batches and served over the course of 3 hours.

It is unlikely that the 30 kg mass of partially frozen drumsticks would have defrosted in the refrigerator overnight. This would have resulted in them being inadequately cooked the next day and subsequent handling, storing and reheating procedures gave ample opportunity for the bacteria to multiply.

Clostridium perfringens

Clostridium perfringens is an anaerobic, spore-forming bacillus. The illness caused by this bacterium is due to the eating of food containing a large number of living bacteria which subsequently release a toxin in the intestines.

Illness

Incubation period: 8–22 hours.
Symptoms: nausea, abdominal pains, diarrhoea (vomiting is rare).
Duration of illness: 12–48 hours.

Source

Clostridium perfringens is frequently carried in human and animal intestines. Investigations have shown that about 25% of the human population excrete the bacterium in the faeces. The organism is also found in soil and its spores can survive for long periods in dust and dirt. Flies and bluebottles are often heavily infected with *Clostridium perfringens*.

Means of spread to food

Clostridium perfringens may be brought into the kitchen on raw meat and poultry. About 10% of samples of raw meat and poultry contain the organism. Bacteria from raw meat may be spread to cooked foods by cross-contamination in the kitchen. Food handlers excreting *Clostridium perfringens* can contaminate foods, particularly if they do not wash their hands after using the toilet. Insect pests may also contaminate foods.

Foods commonly associated with outbreaks

The majority of *Clostridium perfringens* outbreaks are caused by cold and reheated meat and poultry, and by dishes such as mince and stews. The anaerobic conditions required for the multiplication of the bacterium are found in foods cooked in bulk, e.g. at the bottom of a casserole or in the centre of a rolled joint. The bacteria are able to survive most cooking processes by forming spores, though the heat resistance of the spores varies depending on the particular strain of *Clostridium perfringens*. Some strains can survive for hours at boiling-point but others can survive for only a few minutes. Spores that survive germinate and start to multiply if the food is kept warm after cooking or if the food is cooled slowly and left unrefrigerated.

Prevention

Since *Clostridium perfringens* form heat-resistant spores it cannot be assumed that the bacteria are killed during cooking. In order to reduce the risk of *Clostridium perfringens* poisoning, food handlers should take the following precautions:

1 Joints of meat weighing more than 3 kg (6.5 lb) should be cut into smaller joints before cooking.

2 Cooked meat and poultry should be cooled rapidly and stored in a refrigerator. It may be necessary to divide large volumes of meat (e.g. mince) into smaller containers to facilitate cooling. Joints of meat should be removed from their cooking liquor immediately after cooking.

3 Raw and cooked meats should be stored separately.

4 Separate preparation areas and equipment (e.g. chopping boards) should be used for raw and cooked meats.

5 Reheating of meat should be avoided if possible. If it is necessary the meat should be heated quickly and thoroughly, and served as soon as possible.

Examples of outbreaks

1 Two outbreaks of *Clostridium perfringens* poisoning occurred in the same school within a year of each other. In the first outbreak, a large number of the children developed stomach pains and diarrhoea 9 to 12 hours after eating a school dinner which included cold salt beef. Beef joints had been delivered and cooked the previous afternoon. They were cooked in large boilers and left to cool overnight in the cooking liquor. The following day the joints were drained, sliced and eaten cold for lunch. The catering staff were told that cooking the meat the previous day and leaving it to cool slowly overnight was the likely cause of the outbreak. Almost a year later the second outbreak occurred, affecting about 200 children. This time it was caused by rolled joints of beef which were cooked in the afternoon, left overnight in the larder and sliced and eaten cold the next day. *Clostridium per-*

fringens was found in the meat and in the faeces of the patients. Following the first outbreak the kitchen staff made sure that meat was cooked and eaten on the same day, but in the few months before the second outbreak they had lapsed into their old habits.

2 An outbreak of *Clostridium perfringens* food poisoning occurred involving meals prepared for the 'Meals on Wheels' service. Minced beef in 2.7 kg (6 lb) frozen packs was incompletely thawed. It was then heated for two hours in chicken stock in a large pan. After heating it was placed in a poorly ventilated vegetable room at a temperature of 21°C for three hours to allow it to cool. The mince was reheated for 20 minutes before being served into foil containers for distribution in electrically-heated cabinets. The cabinets, which were designed to maintain food at a temperature of 63°C, had a highest temperature of 46°C at the beginning of the distribution and this temperature had fallen to 29°C when the last meals were being delivered. This outbreak could have been prevented if the meat had been thawed completely, cooked thoroughly, cooled quickly, stored at a low temperature and then reheated thoroughly and kept above 63°C during delivery.

Staphylococcus aureus

Staphylococci are facultative aerobes and, therefore, they are able to survive without oxygen. They do not form spores. They cause a toxin type of illness and the toxin is heat resistant. Therefore, although the bacteria themselves are easily destroyed by heat (heating for 10 minutes at 66°C is sufficient to kill them), the toxin may survive 100°C, i.e. the temperature of boiling water, for 30 minutes.

Illness

Incubation period: 2–6 hours.
Symptoms: severe vomiting, stomach cramps, diarrhoea – sometimes followed by collapse.
Duration of illness: 6–24 hours.

Source

As many as 70% of the population carry *Staph. aureus* in the nasopharyngeal region, i.e. the nose and throat. From here the organism is easily transferred to the skin, especially the hands, and to the hair. Also, *Staph. aureus* is the bacterium which usually infects wounds, boils and open sores. The organism is also found in animals, such as cows and goats, and may be present in raw milk.

Means of spread to food

Staph. aureus is spread by food handlers during the cooking and preparation of food. Handling food, rather than using the appropriate utensils, is perhaps the most common means of spread, particularly if the food handler has infected cuts or sores on his hands. Coughing and sneezing near food may cause contamination and hair falling into food or hanging down near food is also potentially dangerous.

Foods commonly associated with outbreaks

Many of the outbreaks of staphylococcal food poisoning are caused by cold meats, such as ham and tongue, and by cold meat pies. The use of nitrates and similar preservatives in these meats has little effect on the growth of *Staph. aureus*. Staphylococcal food poisoning may also be caused by other meat dishes, especially if the meat is used in rechauffé cookery (i.e. if the meat is reheated). Staphylococci have been shown to be present in as many as 38% of raw meat samples tested and cross-contamination from raw to cooked meats may occur.

Foods containing milk or cream, e.g. cakes, trifles, custards, are often responsible for outbreaks. Cheese prepared from raw or inadequately treated milk can also present a problem.

Prevention

Staphylococci are readily killed by heat but the exotoxin they release into foods is more heat resistant and can withstand up to 30 minutes at boiling-point. In order to reduce the risk of staphylococcal poisoning, food handlers should take the following precautions:

1 A high standard of personal hygiene must be maintained.

2 Foods should be handled as little as possible. Tongs or disposable plastic gloves should be used for cooked meats.

3 Foods likely to cause staphylococcal poisoning should be stored in a refrigerator.

Example of an outbreak

At a wedding reception 40 of the 139 guests became ill about two hours after eating a meal which included cold turkey and ham. Investigations showed that the strain of *Staphylococcus aureus* found in the turkey and ham was identical to that present in the nose and in septic spots on the hands of the person who prepared and cut the turkey and ham on the evening before the reception. Turkeys, chickens, hams, etc., should not be handled, jointed or sliced while still warm, since any staphylococci from the handler which contaminate the meat will have the opportunity to multiply.

Bacillus cereus

Bacillus cereus is a spore-forming, aerobic bacillus. It produces a heat-resistant exotoxin which is released into food. The toxin can survive for 1.5 hours at 121°C.

Illness

Incubation period: 1–6 hours.
Symptoms: vomiting, abdominal pains, some diarrhoea.
Duration of illness: 6–24 hours.

There is a second type of *Bacillus cereus* poisoning which is rare in the UK. It is caused by a second toxin which is not heat resistant. The incubation period is 9–18 hours and the main symptom is diarrhoea.

Source

Bacillus cereus is found in soil and dust and in water. It is frequently present in cereal foods, particularly in rice and cornflour.

Foods commonly associated with outbreaks

Rice dishes, cornflour sauce and milk puddings have all been responsible for *Bacillus cereus* outbreaks. In Britain the number of outbreaks has increased in recent years, the majority of outbreaks being caused by boiled and fried rice. This increase can be attributed to the greater popularity of rice dishes and to the increase in 'take away' establishments selling meals containing rice. The small numbers of *Bacillus cereus* found in raw rice are harmless, but if rice is cooked in advance and stored in warm conditions large numbers may be present. The heat-resistant spores can survive boiling and will germinate into vegetative bacteria which multiply if cooked rice is cooled slowly or stored at room temperature.

Prevention

In order to reduce the risk of *Bacillus cereus* poisoning, food handlers should take the following precautions:

1 Rice dishes, milk puddings and cornflour sauces should be cooled quickly (within 90 minutes) and stored in a refrigerator.

2 If reheating of the food is necessary, it should be heated up quickly and thoroughly and served as soon as possible.

Example of an outbreak

Five incidents at one Chinese restaurant affected 13 customers who all had fried rice with their meals. All those affected suffered from vomiting one to six hours after the meal and eight of the people also had diarrhoea. *Bacillus cereus* was isolated from the faeces of those affected and also from the fried rice. One sample of rice was found to contain 350 million *Bacillus cereus* per gram. It was common practice in the restaurant kitchen to boil rice intended for frying the day before and to leave it overnight at room temperature to dry off, and also to add old boiled rice left from the previous day to new batches of rice.

Clostridium botulinum

Clostridium botulinum is an anaerobic, spore-forming bacillus. It produces an exotoxin while growing in food. This exotoxin is one of the most lethal poisons known. The illness caused by this organism is called **botulism**.

Illness

Incubation period: 18–36 hours.
Symptoms: the toxin affects the central nervous system. Early symptoms include double vision, difficulty with speech and swallowing, headache and dizziness.
Duration of illness: the illness reaches its height in one to eight days and death often occurs as a result of paralysis of the respiratory centres; the fatality rate is about 50%. Life may be saved if botulism antitoxin is given in the early stages of the illness.

Source

Clostridium botulinum is found in soil, particularly in marine muds and on the beds of freshwater lakes. It is also found in some fish and on some vegetables.

Foods commonly associated with outbreaks

Since the organism is a strict anaerobe, it is only able to grow and multiply in an oxygen-free environment, such as is found in canned, bottled and vacuum-packed foods. It has also been found in the centre of large sausages and cheeses. In fact, its name is derived from the Latin word for sausage, botulus. *Clostridium botulinum* is not able to grow at a pH of less than 4.5 and, therefore, botulism is not caused by acid foods such as fruits. The spores of some strains can resist boiling for up to six hours but the botulinum toxin is destroyed by heat. Heating to 80°C for 15 minutes is sufficient to destroy the toxin. Commercially prepared foods are now a very rare source of the disease. Outbreaks of botulism in North America have been attributed to home-canned vegetables which were not heated sufficiently to destroy *Clostridium botulinum* spores. Vacuum-packed fish, which was eaten raw, was also responsible for a series of outbreaks in North America.

Examples of outbreaks

Outbreaks of botulism are very rare and there have been only two such incidents in the United Kingdom in the past 30 years.

1 In 1978 a can of salmon was responsible for an outbreak affecting four elderly people (two couples) in Birmingham. They ate canned salmon with salad for their Sunday tea. During the night one couple developed nausea, vomiting, dry mouths and blurred vision and were taken to hospital where their condition worsened. They had evidence of paralysis and difficulty breathing. After a while botulism was diagnosed and antitoxin was given to them. The other couple were visited and found to be very ill and so were also admitted to hospital and given antitoxin but eventually died. The first couple, who had the antitoxin earlier, survived. Examination of the empty can revealed a damaged rim and a small hole which could have allowed the organism to enter. The can was identified as the product of a cannery in Alaska. An emergency investigation of the cannery revealed a number of unsatisfactory practices. These could have led to damage to cans or even contamination of the contents of undamaged cans with botulinum spores, although it could not be shown definitely that the damage and contamination of the Birmingham can occurred at the cannery.

2 In June 1989 a series of cases of botulism occurred in the North West of England and in Wales. There were 27 cases but only one death. The outbreak was traced to hazelnut yoghurt manufactured by two Lancashire dairies. Both dairies used hazelnut conserve from the same supplier. The canned conserve (a low acid product) was insufficiently sterilized. Other similar cans were recalled, the yoghurts were withdrawn and the public were advised not to eat the yoghurt. Antitoxin was administered quickly to those with symptoms and the outbreak was contained.

Campylobacter jejuni

Campylobacter jejuni is the most common cause of reported gastroenteritis in the UK. The incubation period is usually 3–5 days and the symptoms include abdominal pains and fever followed by profuse diarrhoea (often bloody) which usually lasts from one to five days but can go on for weeks. The illness is relatively mild and deaths rarely occur. It may be possible to develop some immunity to the organism which would explain why the illness is most common in children and young adults.

Campylobacter infection is very common. In 1994 there were more than 44 000 recorded cases. (This is more than the reported cases of *Salmonella* poisoning). Most of these cases were sporadic cases; there were not very many general outbreaks. It appears that only small numbers of organisms are needed to cause infection (as few as 500) and there is some debate as to whether campylobacter infection should be regarded as food poisoning or a food-borne illness.

Campylobacter jejuni is found in the intestines of a variety of animals, including farm animals and domestic pets. It is found in foods such as poultry, meat, and shellfish. Surveys have showed that at least half of frozen chickens are contaminated. Campylobacter infection can result from eating undercooked infected poultry but also from handling contaminated carcases. It is important, therefore, to cook poultry thoroughly and that hands are washed after handling raw poultry.

Campylobacter jejuni has also been found in unpasteurized milk and in bird-pecked pasteurized milk. In some areas of the country more than half the cases of campylobacter infection are associated with doorstep delivered milk pecked by birds, especially magpies and crows. Some cases of campylobacter infection are not food-borne. The bacteria can be spread from person to person and by contact with farm animals and infected pets (particularly puppies and kittens with diarrhoea).

Listeria monocytogenes

Listeria monocytogenes causes **listeriosis**, a serious illness with a fatality rate of 30%. A toxic enzyme produced by the bacteria enters the bloodstream, causing flu-like symptoms, septicaemia or meningitis. Healthy adults are generally resistant to listeriosis but infants, the elderly and people whose immune systems have been suppressed by drugs or disease are all at risk. Pregnant women are also at risk, since the illness may cause miscarriage or stillbirth or it may give rise to meningitis or septicaemia in the newborn baby.

Listeriosis differs from other types of food poisoning since food may not be the only vehicle of infection. Also, it is not yet known whether large numbers of organisms are necessary to cause the illness. Therefore, it may be considered more like a food-borne illness than a type of food poisoning.

Listeria monocytogenes is a very common organism and is widely distributed in the environment. It is found in soil, water, the intestines of many animals and many foods. Raw chickens are commonly infected and it may also be present in untreated milk, dairy products made from raw milk, meat, salads, vegetables and seafoods. In the UK in 1989 incidents occurred in which soft cheeses made from untreated milk and imported liver pâté were both withdrawn from supermarket shelves after *L. monocytogenes* had been detected during routine sampling. Neither of these products would be cooked before they were eaten. The organism is normally destroyed at pasteurizing temperatures and by standard cooking procedures though it may survive in food that has been cooked or reheated in a microwave oven because of uneven heating. It is important, therefore, that high-risk food cooked in a microwave oven should be allowed to 'stand' after cooking to allow heat to diffuse to any cold spots.

Listeria bacteria can grow at low temperatures and will multiply to dangerous levels in chilled and refrigerated foods which are kept for too long or at too high a temperature. Refrigerators should be kept below 5°C and cook-chill food should not be stored for more than 5 days at 3°C.

Pregnant women are advised to avoid high-risk foods such as soft cheeses (e.g. Brie and Camembert), pâté, pre-packed coleslaw and other pre-prepared, chilled salads.

In England and Wales in 1988 there were 291 recorded cases of listeriosis and 26 unborn or newborn babies died. Since then there has been a decline in the number of cases. This is thought to be due to government health warnings and to improved temperature control of foods.

Escherichia coli

Escherichia coli is a gram-negative bacillus which can grow both aerobically and anaerobically. It is found in the intestines of people and animals and most forms of the organism are harmless. The presence of *E. coli* in food or water is used as an indication of faecal contamination.

There are many different strains of *E. coli*. Only some strains are pathogenic. Exposure to an unfamiliar strain can cause 'traveller's diarrhoea'.

Poisoning by one particular strain known as *E. coli* 0157 (also VTEC 0157) is much more common than it used to be and is causing considerable concern. The main worry is that in some people it develops into serious illness. The initial symptoms are abdominal cramps, vomiting and diarrhoea and in some people haemorrhagic colitis (bleeding of the bowel). Occasionally, particularly in young children, haemolytic uraemic syndrome (HUS) develops. This is a condition which leads to kidney failure and death in 5 –10% of cases.

Most cases of food poisoning caused by *E. coli* 0157 have been associated with the consumption of undercooked minced beef and beefburgers. Advice from the government states that beefburgers should be cooked until the juices run clear and there are no pink bits inside. There has been a steady increase in reported cases of *E. coli* 0157 since the mid-1980s. In 1992 there were 468 reported cases.

Vibrio parahaemolyticus

This organism has been isolated from fish, shellfish and other seafoods. In Japan, 50% of food poisoning incidents are caused by *Vibrio parahaemolyticus*. Outbreaks in Britain in recent years have been due to seafoods such as imported prawns.

Yersinia enterocolitica

This organism has been found in a variety of foods including milk, vegetables and meat. It causes enteritis (abdominal pains, fever and diarrhoea), mainly in children. Reported cases are particularly high in Norway and Sweden. Like *Listeria*, it can grow at low temperatures and may be of concern in cook-chill products.

Aeromonas

Some species, such as *Aeromonas hydrophila* and *A. sobria*, can cause food-borne or water-borne gastroenteritis and have been implicated in 'traveller's diarrhoea'. The organisms survive in chlorinated tap water and salt water and have been found in milk and seafoods.

Food- and water-borne diseases

Food-borne diseases differ from food poisoning in that the food acts merely as a means of transport for the organism and not as a medium for growth. The incubation period is normally longer and the symptoms are different and more varied. In addition, food-borne diseases may be transmitted by other means; for example, many are transmitted by water.

Bacterial diseases

Bacillary dysentery

Dysentery is an infection of the large intestine which may be spread by food or water.

Bacillary dysentery is caused by bacteria of the genus *Shigella*; most notably *Shigella sonnei*. About 5000 cases occur in England and Wales every year (in 1993 there were 6841 cases). Most outbreaks occur in institutions such as schools. The incubation period for the disease is normally two to four days and the main symptom is acute diarrhoea which may persist for several days. Cross-infection plays a major part in the spread of the disease. Affected people may infect their own hands or, by way of toilet seats, etc., the hands of others. Correct personal hygiene and, particularly, washing the hands after using the toilet are essential if spread of the disease is to be prevented.

Typhoid and paratyphoid fevers

The term 'enteric fever' is used to describe both typhoid and paratyphoid fevers, although there are several differences between the two diseases. Typhoid fever is caused by *Salmonella typhi*, whereas paratyphoid fever is usually caused by *S. paratyphi B*. Both organisms are excreted in the faeces and urine of patients suffering from the diseases or are excreted by healthy carriers. In the past, healthy carriers of *S. typhi* have been responsible for several serious outbreaks of typhoid fever. Outbreaks of both diseases have been caused by water contaminated by sewage.

The typhoid outbreak which occurred in Aberdeen in 1964 was traced to contaminated water used for cooling cans of corned beef. The water had not been chlorinated in order to kill pathogens. *Salmonella typhi* entered one of the cans through a faulty seam, which later sealed on cooling. When the can was opened the bacteria rapidly spread to other foods by cross-contamination and caused a serious outbreak of typhoid fever.

Outbreaks have also been caused by milk, cream and ice cream contaminated by food handlers who were either convalescent or healthy carriers of the organism. Typhoid and paratyphoid bacteria may also be transferred to uncovered food substances by flies and vermin which have been in contact with contaminated excreta.

The incubation period for typhoid fever is usually 7 to 21 days; for paratyphoid fever it is shorter, being between 7 and 10 days. The main symptoms of enteric fever are weakness, fever and diarrhoea. The fatality rate is fairly low, although the illness may still cause death in severe or untreated cases. There were 175 notifications of typhoid fever in England and Wales during 1993; in 122 of these cases the infection had been acquired abroad.

Cholera

Cholera is caused by the bacterium *Vibrio cholerae*. The disease is usually water-borne and is rarely spread by food or from person to person. It does not, therefore, present an important public health problem to countries with high standards of hygiene in the provision of water supplies and in sewage disposal. The chlorination of mains water supplies has been of great importance in the elimination of cholera outbreaks in Britain. However, cases of cholera do occur which have been contracted in other countries.

The disease has a short incubation period (one to six days), during which the bacteria multiply rapidly in the small intestine. Then violent, watery diarrhoea sets in. This gives rise to severe dehydration, together with a serious loss from the body of alkali and potassium salts. Recovery can be aided by the use of antibiotics but treatment mainly depends on replacing lost water and mineral salts and maintaining the balance of body fluids.

Brucellosis

Brucellosis, or undulant fever, is caused by the bacterium *Brucella abortus*. It was an endemic infection in cattle in the United Kingdom until eradication began in the early 1970s. The disease may be spread from cattle to humans by the consumption of contaminated, untreated milk or by direct physical contact with infected animals. The illness gives rise to prolonged ill health. The main symptoms are the gradual onset of recurrent fever, sweating and pain in the joints and the muscles.

The incubation period varies from one to four weeks. The disease is difficult to recognize, since the symptoms are relatively mild and are often confused with those of other diseases, such as influenza. However, the illness can be diagnosed either bacteriologically or by means of blood tests. The transmission of brucellosis via cows' milk is now rare in Britain, since pasteurization destroys *Brucella abortus*. In addition, a programme of vaccination of dairy herds was introduced in the early 1970s. Before 1970 laboratory reports indicated that there were at least 400 human cases per year in England and Wales. Most of these cases were due to drinking contaminated raw milk. By 1985 the disease had almost been eliminated. There are now about 15 cases a year, mostly contracted abroad.

Brucella melitensis is a similar organism which infects goats and goats' milk, particularly in Mediterranean countries.

Tuberculosis

Tuberculosis is caused by the bacterium *Mycobacterium tuberculosis*. At one time, tuberculosis was very common in Britain, particularly in urban areas. One of the main sources of the organism was untreated cows' milk, but the introduction of pasteurization eliminated the chances of contracting tuberculosis through drinking milk, since the organism is destroyed by pasteurization. In addition, all dairy herds in Britain are inspected regularly to ensure that they are tuberculosis-free. The introduction of the BCG vaccine and the immunization of school children in the late 1950s have helped to prevent the spread of tuberculosis by other means.

Protozoan diseases

Amoebic dysentery

This is caused by the protozoan *Entamoeba histolytica*. It is rare in Europe but more common in tropical countries. Cases that occur in Britain are usually among people who contract the illness abroad.

Giardiasis

Giardiasis is caused by the protozoan *Giardia lamblia*. It is common in parts of the world with poor sanitation and water supplies. The main symptom is profuse, watery diarrhoea. Outbreaks in the UK have sometimes been traced to food handlers returning from abroad.

Cryptosporidiosis

Cryptosporidium lives in the intestines of farm animals, wild animals and domestic pets. It can be spread to humans in a variety of ways including through contaminated food and water, by person-to-person contact and by direct contact with animals or with slurry spread on agricultural land. Foods which have caused cryptosporidiosis include sausages, pâté and untreated milk. The main symptom of the disease is diarrhoea which may last for 10 or more days.

Viral diseases

Viruses cannot multiply in food but food may act as a means of transport for some viruses. They are destroyed by most cooking processes but some present in uncooked foods or foods infected after cooking can cause poisoning.

Hepatitis A

Hepatitis is inflammation of the liver. There are two main types: hepatitis A (infective hepatitis) which is usually transmitted by contaminated food or water and hepatitis B which is spread by blood. Hepatitis A is more likely to be contracted in the Middle or Far East than in the UK. It can be spread by infected food handlers though many outbreaks have been caused by shellfish collected from sewage-contaminated water.

Rotaviruses

These viruses can cause severe diarrhoea in young children. Large numbers of the virus are excreted in the faeces (up to 10^{10} per g of faeces). The infection can be spread, for example, by inadequate hand-washing between nappy changing and handling food.

SRSVs

Small round structured viruses (SRSVs), also referred to as Norwalk-like agents, are considered to be the commonest cause of food-borne viral gastroenteritis in the UK. There were 710 reported cases in 1991. The viruses cause an illness sometimes called 'winter vomiting disease'. The symptoms begin suddenly and include abdominal pain, vomiting (which may be projectile) and diarrhoea. The viruses can be spread by infected food handlers, person-to-person contact and by eating shellfish from sewage-contaminated water.

There are two types of parasitic worms which may be transmitted to humans by food in Britain. There are, of course, many other types of parasitic worms common in other countries.

1 The Trichina worm (Trichinella spiralis)

This is a non-segmented roundworm which infests the small intestine of a variety of hosts, such as man, pigs and rats. The female worm is fertilized within the intestine and burrows its way into the intestinal wall where it lays its larvae. The larvae are carried throughout the body of the host and undergo further development within the muscles. In the case of the pig, if the infected flesh is inadequately cooked and consumed by man, it will cause a disease known as **trichinosis.** Early symptoms of the disease include nausea and fever but later the disease is characterized by muscular aches and pains. In Britain, all carcases in slaughterhouses are inspected by an Environmental Health Officer. If infection by *Trichinella* is suspected, the carcase is placed in cold storage. A period of 20 days at –15°C is normally sufficient to kill the larvae, but progressively longer times may be needed for larger pieces of meat.

2 Tapeworms

Tapeworms are flat worms consisting of a head and a chain of flat, oblong segments arising from the head-piece. The species most often responsible for disease in man are *Taenia saginata,* which occurs in beef, and *T. solium,* which occurs in pork. Both parasites have a stage-two life-cycle. The larval stage occurs in the intermediate host, i.e. the cow or the pig, and the adult stage occurs in man.

When animals eat the eggs, the eggs hatch into larvae which are carried by the bloodstream to the muscle of the animal where they form cysts. The cysts are visible in the meat, e.g. "measly" pork. If undercooked, infected meat is eaten, the cysts survive and develop into an adult tapeworm. Tapeworm infections are now very rare in Britain but are still common in tropical countries. In the UK meat inspection and hygiene standards are such that cattle rarely eat eggs shed by humans which means that the life-cycle is unlikely to be completed.

17 Food hygiene

In order to prevent food poisoning, strict standards of hygiene must be maintained. It is also aesthetically pleasing if food is prepared under hygienic conditions. The main aims of food hygiene are:

1 to prevent food becoming contaminated with food poisoning bacteria;
2 to prevent the multiplication of any food poisoning bacteria which do get into food;
3 to destroy any food poisoning bacteria which may be present by thorough cooking.

Food poisoning bacteria come from three sources:

1 The food handlers

Staphylococcus aureus, *Salmonella* and *Clostridium perfringens* may all be carried by personnel involved in food preparation.

2 The environment

The spores of *Clostridium perfringens* and *Bacillus cereus* may be found in dust in food-preparation rooms. Also, most types of food-poisoning bacteria may be spread by cross-contamination in the kitchen and by pests.

3 The food

The food itself may contain food-poisoning bacteria when it is brought into the kitchen or the bacteria may enter the food due to faulty handling during preparation.

It follows that measures to prevent food poisoning can be divided into three categories:

1 Personal hygiene.
2 Hygiene in the kitchen.
3 Hygienic food handling.

Personal hygiene

Personal hygiene is aimed at preventing the spread of food poisoning bacteria from the body or clothing to food. It is the responsibility of the individual and all food handlers should have an elementary knowledge and understanding of its importance,

The following list covers the main points of personal hygiene.

1 Hands

Hands should be washed frequently, especially:

(a) before handling food in the kitchen. This is important since bacteria will be present on the surface of the skin. Handwashing usually removes most Gram negative bacteria but Gram positive bacteria (such as *Staph. aureus*) may remain, as they rise to the surface of the skin from the pores. For this reason cooked, high-risk foods should not be touched with the bare hands;
(b) between food-handling operations. This is necessary to prevent cross-contamination of all types of food poisoning bacteria from raw to cooked food;
(c) after using the toilet and before leaving the washroom. This reduces the risk of the transfer of bacteria, such as *Salmonella* and *Clostridium perfringens*, from faeces and door handles to food;
(d) after smoking, coughing and sneezing and after using a handkerchief. This reduces the risk of the transfer of *Staph. aureus* to food;
(e) after handling waste food or refuse. A large number of a wide variety of bacteria will be present in waste.

The hands should be washed with plenty of warm water and soap and the nails scrubbed with a brush. They should then be rinsed under running water and dried. Hot air driers or paper towels are more hygienic than cloth towels which allow transfer of bacteria from person to person. The use of barrier creams helps to keep hands smooth and free from cracks and crevices which may harbour bacteria.

The tasting of food with the fingers, biting nails, etc., should be avoided in food preparation areas as these habits can spread bacteria such as *Staph. aureus* from the mouth to hands to food.

2 Coughing and sneezing

Coughing and sneezing may be responsible for the spread of Staphylococci on to food or working surfaces and should therefore be avoided wherever open food is handled. Handkerchiefs or tissues should be used at all times. Disposable paper tissues are preferable since they can be discarded. In addition, the hands should be washed after using a tissue or handkerchief.

3 *Smoking*

It is against the law to smoke in a food-preparation area. Smoking involves contact between the hand and mouth and can be responsible for the spread of *Staph. aureus*. It also encourages coughing.

4 *Outdoor clothing*

Outdoor clothing should be placed in lockers outside food rooms, since it is frequently contaminated by bacteria such as *Staphylococcus* and *Streptococcus*. This contamination is particularly high in congested areas, especially where people make frequent use of public transport .

5. *Protective clothing*

Protective clothing should be worn by all food handlers. This should be clean and it should cover all parts of the body liable to contaminate food. The clothing must be laundered regularly. Otherwise, if it is worn continuously, it may harbour harmful bacteria. Protective headwear should be designed so as to retain the hair in position, since hair and dandruff are a potential source of contamination by bacteria, particularly *Staph. aureus*. If hair is long it should be tied back. Hair should not be touched or combed in the vicinity of food. The main danger is the transfer of bacteria from the hair to the hands and thence to food.

6 *Cuts, grazes, boils and septic spots*

Open cuts, grazes, boils and septic lesions frequently harbour Staphylococci and therefore should be covered with a clean, waterproof dressing wherever food is handled. These dressings should be brightly coloured so that they will be readily seen if they fall into food. Those used in food premises are normally blue. A well-equipped first-aid box containing these dressings and other equipment, such as bandages and cotton wool, should be kept on the premises.

7 *Nails*

Long, dirty nails harbour dirt and bacteria. Therefore, fingernails must be kept clean and short. Nail varnish should not be worn by food handlers, since, if it becomes chipped, it may provide crevices which can harbour bacteria. In addition chips of nail varnish may enter food and this is neither hygienic nor aesthetically pleasing.

8 *Jewellery*

Personal jewellery may harbour bacteria or may fall into food and, therefore, jewellery, other than wedding rings, should not be worn by food handlers.

9 *Health*

Any food handler who is suffering from diarrhoea, vomiting, septic cuts, boils or other skin infection should notify his/her employer and should not handle food. This is because any of these conditions indicates that the food handler is a potential source of food poisoning organisms.

Hygiene in the kitchen

Premises and equipment

The premises

Food premises should be designed so that they are easy to clean. In older buildings alterations should be made to facilitate cleaning. Large pieces of equipment such as refrigeration units should be placed where they can be cleaned all around, or else be movable or built into a continuous surface. A common layout in kitchens is to have preparation equipment round the edges and island cooking equipment in the centre with extractor fans above for ventilation. Preparation areas for raw and cooked foods should be well separated to prevent cross-contamination and there should be a 'flow' of food from delivery, to storage, to preparation, to cooking, to final preparation, to service, with no back tracking. The 'dirty' area is where raw meat, fish and vegetables are prepared and should be near to the exit to the outside and the delivery area. The 'clean' area of the kitchen is for the preparation of cooked meats and desserts and should be near to the servery or door to the restaurant.

Floors

Floors should be hard-wearing, non-absorbent, non-slip and easy to clean. Quarry tiles are often used in kitchens. These should be laid close together and the junction between the floor and the wall should be coved (curved) to aid cleaning. There are now many more modern materials that can be used. For example, epoxy resin which can be laid as a continuous layer with no joints.

Walls

Walls should be smooth, non-absorbent and light in colour. Glazed ceramic tiles are often used and are hygienic if in good condition. Other suitable materials include stainless steel sheeting, rigid plastic sheeting and a washable hard gloss paint on a sound plaster base.

Lighting

Good lighting is essential in a kitchen to facilitate cleaning and for safety reasons. Good natural lighting is desirable and should be supplemented by artificial lighting, such as fluorescent tubes with diffusers.

Ventilation

Efficient ventilation and extraction systems are essential in kitchens to control humidity and temperature and to remove cooking odours. As a result of cooking processes and washing up, large amounts of steam and water vapour are produced in kitchens. This will increase relative humidity to a level unpleasant to work in unless ventilation is good. If windows are used for ventilation they should be covered with a mesh screen to prevent entry of birds, insects, etc. In many kitchens, stoves and cooking equipment are sited centrally with canopies and an extraction system above. Regular cleaning of canopies, fans, filters and ducts must be carried out.

Toilets and washing facilities

Adequate toilets and washing facilities should be provided for the staff in food businesses. Toilets should be kept clean and in working order and should be separated from any food room by at least two doors and a ventilated space. 'Wash Your Hands' notices should be clearly displayed. Wash-hand basins must be placed in food preparation areas as well as next to the toilets. They should have hot and cold water, soap, nail brush and a hygienic means of drying the hands and should not be used for washing food or equipment. Staff should also be provided with suitable changing rooms, lockers for leaving outside clothes and rest rooms away from the food preparation area.

Equipment and surfaces

Equipment should be designed and positioned so that it can be easily cleaned. It should be kept in good repair and be made of material that is non-absorbent and non-reactive to foods or cleaning chemicals. Stainless steel is ideal for both equipment and work surfaces. Plastics are suitable for some purposes. Wood is not suitable in food areas as it is absorbent and is difficult to clean and disinfect. Chopping boards should be made of a hard plastic e.g. polypropylene or synthetic rubber. They should be colour-coded for use with separate foods (e.g. red for raw meat, blue for fish, green for vegetables, brown for cooked meat) to avoid the risk of cross-contamination when raw and cooked foods are prepared in the same area. Equipment such as mincers, slicers and mixing machines which may be used for both raw and cooked foods can also be responsible for cross-contamination. Slicers and mixers should never be used for both raw and cooked foods without being thoroughly cleaned in between. The use of mincers for both types of food should be discouraged because of the difficulty of thorough cleaning.

Cloths should be used with discretion in kitchens as they too can be a cause of cross-contamination (e.g. used to mop up drip from a defrosting chicken and then used to wipe a surface to be used for cooked foods). They should either be colour-coded for different uses or ideally single-use disposable wipes should be used.

Cleanliness in the kitchen is fundamental to good hygiene. Cleaning involves the removal of 'soil', i.e. dirt and/or food particles which can harbour bacteria, attract pests and lead to both food poisoning and food spoilage. The effectiveness of cleaning depends on the choice of cleaning agents, the choice of cleaning tools and the physical effort exerted by the person doing the cleaning.

Detergents

Most cleaning operations in food areas require the use of a detergent in water. As described in Chapter 4, detergent molecules have a 'head' which is hydrophilic (water-loving) and a 'tail' which is hydrophobic (water-hating). Detergents aid cleaning by:

1 *Lowering the surface tension of water.* Pure water is not a good 'wetting' agent, because it has a high surface tension. Due to hydrogen bonding (see page 51) molecules of water are strongly attracted to one another. For molecules at the centre of a body of water these forces are acting in all directions and there is no net pull in any particular direction. However, for molecules near the surface of the water the net force is a pull inwards. This causes the body of water to tend to assume a shape with the minimum surface area, i.e. a sphere. This explains why water dripping from a tap tends to form spherical droplets. The effect is illustrated in Figure 17.1

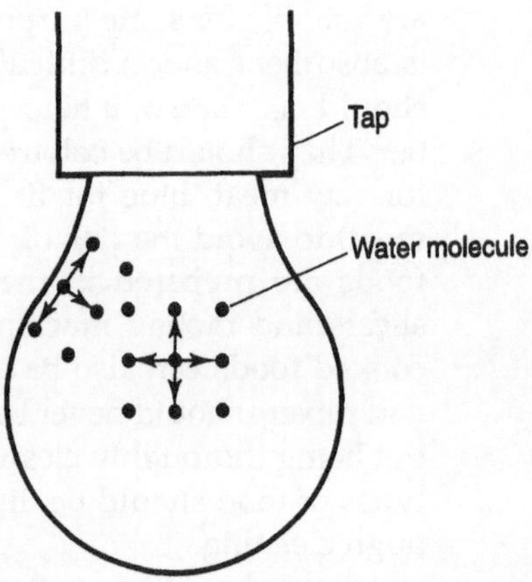

Figure 17.1 *Diagram illustrating the high surface tension of water.*

Because of this high surface tension, water will not easily 'wet' a solid surface. However, if a detergent is added, the detergent will go preferentially to the surface of the water and will therefore lower the surface tension. This is illustrated in Figure 17.2.

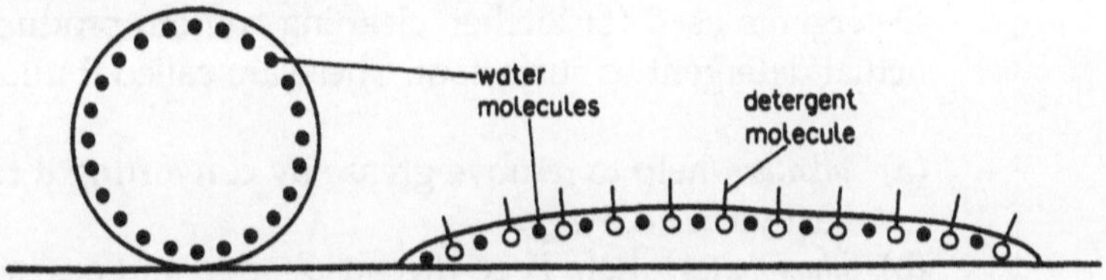

Figure 17.2 *The action of a detergent in lowering the surface tension of water.*

2 *Emulsifying grease.* As explained in Chapter 4, soaps and detergents emulsify grease because the hydrophobic tails dissolve in the grease leaving the water-loving heads in the water. Detergent molecules surround particles of fat and grease lifting it off the greasy surface, as shown in Figure 17.3.

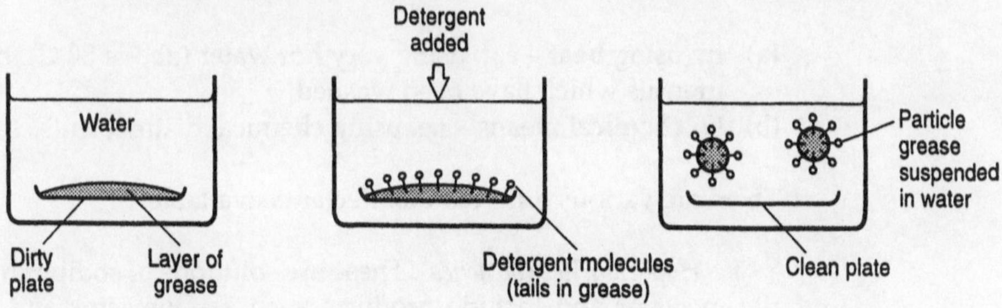

Figure 17.3 *The action of a detergent in emulsifying grease.*

3 *Keeping dirt and grease suspended in water.* The electrostatic charges on the head of the molecules repel each other and keep the particles of grease and dirt suspended in the water and prevent them from coalescing (joining together) and being redeposited on the item being washed. There are various types of detergents:

(a) **anionic** – negatively charged. The most common. Used in washing up liquids and general cleaners.
(b) **cationic** – positively charged. Lower cleaning ability. Some have disinfectant activity e.g. quats.
(c) **non-ionic** – no charge. Low foaming. More expensive than anionics.
(d) **amphoteric** – charge depends on the pH of the solution. They show properties of cationic detergents in acid conditions, non-ionic detergents in neutral conditions and anionic detergents in alkaline conditions. Used in some oven cleaners.

NB Anionic and cationic detergents should not be mixed as they will inactivate each other.

Detergents used for kitchen cleaning contain products other than the actual detergent or surfactant. These are called 'builders' and include:

(a) *alkalis* – help to remove grease by converting it to a soap which is easily rinsed away;
(b) *phosphates* – help keep dirt suspended and also soften hard water;
(c) *bleaching agents* – help remove stains such as tannin from tea.

Disinfection

Disinfection is a process which kills micro-organisms, reducing their number to a safe level. This differs from sterilization which is a process which kills all microbes including bacterial spores. In a food preparation area it is not practical or necessary to sterilize but it is important to disinfect, especially those surfaces which come into contact with high risk foods. Disinfection can be brought about in two main ways:

(a) by using **heat** – e.g. using very hot water (above 80 C) for rinsing utensils which have been washed;
(b) by **chemical** means – i.e. using chemical disinfectants.

There are various different disinfectants available:

1 *Hypochlorites (bleaches)*. These are solutions of sodium hypochlorite in water and include products such as Domestos and Chloros. Until recently these were very widely used in the food industry. They are cheap and effective in killing bacteria. They have a distinct smell but this disappears rapidly and they do not taint food. Concentrated solutions need careful handling and diluted solutions are unstable. They cause corrosion of some metals. **NB** NEVER MIX HYPOCHLORITES WITH ACIDS OR ACID CLEANERS (E.G. TOILET CLEANERS). CHLORINE GAS WILL BE RELEASED WHICH IS HIGHLY TOXIC.

2 *Quaternary ammonium compounds (quats)*. These are cationic detergents and include products such as Savlon. They are odourless, stable to heat and easy to use, being suitable for most surfaces including steel and plastic. However, they are inactivated by organic matter and are more expensive than hypochlorites. They are now widely used in the food industry.

3 *Iodophors*. These iodine-based disinfectants are sometimes used in food premises. They kill a wide range of microbes and are stable during storage but they are relatively expensive and corrode some metals.

4 *Phenols*. These products, e.g. Dettol, are not suitable for food premises as they have a strong smell and will taint food.

Sanitizers are combined detergents and disinfectants, i.e. they clean and disinfect.

Cleaning procedures

There are four basic stages in cleaning:

1 Physically removing excess dirt or food by sweeping, wiping, pre-rinsing, etc.
2 Washing with hot water and detergent.
3 Rinsing and/or disinfecting.
4 Drying.

These four stages can be applied to cleaning floors, equipment, crockery, etc., but not all stages will always be needed, for example when cleaning a kitchen floor:

1 Sweep to remove excess dirt.
2 Wash with hot water and detergent using either a mop or a floor-cleaning machine.
3 Rinsing and disinfection are not needed.
4 Leave to air dry.

Washing up

This is the most common cleaning process in kitchens. Ideally there should be two areas in the kitchen, the pan-wash for the washing of pots, pans, utensils, etc., and the wash-up area for crockery, cutlery, glasses, etc., used by customers. It is desirable to keep these two operations separate from each other and both should be well separated from any food preparation area. There are two main methods of washing up:

(a) **Two-sink method** (for washing up by hand). This follows the four stages of the standard cleaning procedure as follows:

1 Scrape or rinse off excess food residues.
2 Wash in the first sink with hot water (45–50°C) and detergent using a cloth or brush.
3 Rinse in racks in the second sink with very hot water (80°C+) or cooler water with a chemical disinfectant. Both wash and rinse waters should be changed as soon as they become too dirty or lose temperature.
4 Leave in racks to air dry. This is more hygienic than using a cloth.

(b) **Dish-washing machine**. These are needed in all but the smallest of catering establishments and operate as follows:

1 A pre-rinse softens and removes food particles. When using small machines this may need to be done by hand.
2 A detergent wash using water at 60°C. The correct type of detergent must be used.
3 A rinse using water at 82°C+. A chemical rinse additive may be needed.

4 Air drying by residual heat from the rinse.

After washing, tableware, etc. should be stacked and stored in a clean place.

Dish-washing machines should be serviced and maintained regularly.

Cleaning schedules

Efficient cleaning is an important part of the running of any catering establishment. Cleaning schedules are a means of ensuring that cleaning is carried effectively and sufficiently frequently.

A cleaning schedule should include some or all of the following details:

(a) the item to be cleaned;
(b) the cleaning tools and cleaning agents needed;
(c) the method;
(d) the person responsible for carrying out the cleaning;
(e) the frequency of cleaning, e.g. daily, weekly;
(f) the supervisor's signature when the work has been carried out and checked.

Table 17.1 shows part of a typical cleaning schedule.

Table 17.1 *Part of a typical cleaning schedule*

Item	*Frequency*	*Method and equipment*	*Staff*	*Checked by*
Floor	Daily	Sweep. Wash with mop using hot water and heavy duty detergent.	Mr X	.....
Work tops	Daily	Wash with hot water and detergent. Spray with disinfectant. Wipe.	Ms Y	.....
Fryer	Weekly	Drain. Fill with water and heavy duty detergent Boil. Wash, rinse, dry and refill.	Mr Z	.....

Use and storage of cleaning products

Cleaning agents. Many cleaning agents are potentially dangerous and should be used and stored correctly. Most neutral and slightly alkaline detergents (such as washing-up liquids, general-purpose cleaners and non-bleach sanitizers) are normally safe but there are hazards involved in many other products. Acid products (e.g. descaling liquids) are corrosive to the skin. Some cleaning agents, e.g. those designed for cleaning ovens and fryers, are highly caustic (alkaline) and should be used only in a well-ventilated area with rubber gloves, overalls and face protection. Some cleaning fluids contain solvents which ignite at low temperatures; these should be stored in a cool place and must not be used near naked flames. Different types of cleaning agents must never be mixed together as dangerous reactions can occur. For example, if an ammonia based cleaner is mixed with hypochlorite solution chloramine fumes are produced which cause choking. Manufacturer's instructions should always be followed regarding use and storage.

Cleaning agents must not be stored in any food room. They should be kept in a separate store which should be cool, dry, well-ventilated and fitted with slatted shelves.

Employers are legally obliged to minimize risks of using hazardous chemicals. This is laid down in the **Control of Substances Hazardous to Health Regulations 1988 (COSHH).** Employers must:

1 Assess the risk to workers of any substance they handle in the course of their work.
2 Introduce measures to prevent or control the risk of handling hazardous chemicals.
3 Inform employees of the risk of hazardous substances.
4 Train employees to work safely.
5 Ensure that hazardous chemicals are used and stored correctly.

Cleaning equipment. Mops, cloths, brushes, etc., are in contact with many different surfaces and are an ideal means of spreading bacteria. They should be washed and disinfected (preferably with heat) regularly and stored dry in an area away from any food room.

Waste disposal

Food waste is ideal for the growth of bacteria and unless it is stored correctly it will attract flies, rats and other pests. Waste must be separated from fresh food and removed from the kitchen regularly.

In the kitchen

Waste should be collected in bins with plastic liners and lids, preferably pedal-operated. Alternatively, stands with lids which hold disposable paper or plastic sacks may be used. These should be replaced regularly and never be allowed to overflow.

Waste disposal units which grind up food and wash it into the drainage system can be used in food preparation areas for the disposal of waste food.

Outside the kitchen

There should be a properly designed refuse storage area outside the building with steel or plastic bins. Bins should have well-fitting lids to discourage flies and other pests and be placed on a stand 250–300 mm (10–12 ins) above a drained and concreted area which should be washed down frequently. Bins should be emptied regularly and washed out.

Pest control

Many living creatures are attracted to food premises in search of food, warmth and shelter. The main pests include rats, mice, insects and birds. They are undesirable because:

(a) they carry pathogens which can contaminate food and so spread disease;
(b) they spoil food and cause an economic loss;
(c) some pests, e.g. rats, will cause damage to buildings.

Rodents

Rats and mice are rodents, a group of mammals whose teeth and jaws are adapted for gnawing hard materials. They can do considerable damage to buildings, e.g. chewing through skirting boards, electric cables and even water pipes. They are also a health hazard as they often carry pathogens in their intestines and droppings as well as on their feet and fur and can contaminate open food and work surfaces. Rats in particular have been implicated in spreading many diseases including *Salmonella* poisoning and Weil's disease. There are two species of rat which infest food premises: the brown rat which is the most common and the black rat or ship rat which is smaller. The house mouse is a lot smaller but breeds more prolifically.

Signs of an infestation. The animals themselves are not often seen but they will leave signs of their presence including:

(a) droppings;
(b) damage to food and containers (nibbled packets of food, etc.);
(c) gnawing marks on woodwork, etc.;
(d) smear marks where they have brushed against walls or other surfaces;
(e) characteristic odour left on contaminated food.

Prevention. The two main ways of preventing infestation are:

(a) Physically denying access, i.e. rodent proofing the building.
(b) Discouraging them from entering food premises by good housekeeping.

Rodent-proofing measures include:

(a) Keep building in good repair, e.g. cover disused drains, mend holes in walls, floors etc.

(b) Doors and windows should fit tightly and external doors should be fitted with metal kick plates.

(c) Holes in walls around pipes or cables should be sealed.

(d) Drains should be kept in good repair and should have effective water seals. Drainpipes should be fitted with wire balloons inside and cone guards on the outside, to prevent access to buildings.

(e) Air bricks and ventilation gratings should be fitted with metal mesh if the holes are more than 6 mm across.

Good housekeeping measures include:

(a) Keep premises clean; wipe up spillages immediately.

(b) Store food in bins or other vermin-proof containers.

(c) Store rooms should be kept clean. Store foods off the floor and use in rotation.

(d) Deliveries of raw materials should be checked for signs of infestation.

(e) Inspect buildings for signs of infestation, particularly lift shafts, cellars and 'dead' space such as above false ceilings. Check also outside the buildings and remove any food debris or rubbish.

Eradication. If an infestation is suspected expert advice should be sought from a specialist control firm or the local Environmental Health Department. Poisons can be used to kill both rats and mice. These are called rodenticides and are put down as baits in places where there are signs of infestation. Warfarin was the first widely used rodenticide but some rats are now resistant to it and other poisons are used such as difenacoum.

Traps can be effective in dealing with a mouse-infested area.

Flies

Both houseflies and blowflies may be a problem in food premises. They breed rapidly and may contaminate food with pathogenic bacteria. Flies are attracted to waste food, animal droppings, etc., and may carry pathogens on their legs and excreta which can contaminate food when they land on it. They feed by regurgitating previously eaten food and sucking up the liquid mixture. They also excrete on food when they land on it.

Control. It is almost impossible to prevent flies getting into buildings but some fly-proofing measures can be used:

(a) outside opening windows should be covered by a mesh screen;

(b) external doors should be self-closing.

In addition, good housekeeping measures are important including:

(a) foods should be covered and stored correctly;
(b) premises should be kept clean;
(c) bins should be kept covered and waste disposed of correctly.

Eradication. There are two main ways of killing flies:

(a) Ultraviolet 'insectocutor'. Ultraviolet light attracts flying insects which are killed when they touch an electrified metal grid. The electrocuted flies fall into a collecting tray underneath.

(b) Insecticides. Chemicals such as pyrethrins can be used to kill flies in food premises. They can be used in the form of an aerosol spray but deposits of the insecticide on food or equipment must be avoided.

Cockroaches

There are many different types of cockroach but only two are commonly found in the UK:

(a) The oriental cockroach or 'black beetle', found in warm, moist parts of kitchens e.g. behind ovens and hot water pipes.

(b) The German cockroach or 'steam-fly', yellow-brown and smaller, usually found in cooler parts of food premises, e.g. basements and store rooms.

They often carry pathogenic bacteria and may spread food-poisoning bacteria (as well as those responsible for typhoid, cholera and dysentery) as they walk over food, work surfaces and equipment. An infestation can be recognized by droppings and a characteristic smell, though the insects themselves, being nocturnal, may not be seen. They are most likely to be present in premises which are dirty and where food is left out at night.

Control. Control measures involve good housekeeping. Premises should be kept clean, foods covered and stored correctly and waste stored and disposed of properly. Hiding places, e.g. behind cupboards and hot water pipes, should be checked and eliminated if possible.

Eradication. Infestations can be treated with various insecticides in the form of sprays, lacquers or dusts but expert advice and guidance should be sought about their use in food premises.

Other pests

Ants. Red Pharoah's ants may be a problem in food premises and may carry pathogens. They should not be attracted into clean, well-maintained buildings but if an infestation occurs it may take a considerable time to get rid of all the ants.

Birds. Birds are sometimes a problem in food premises, especially in large buildings such as food warehouses and manufacturing premises. They often carry *Salmonella* and their droppings may contaminate food. Screens over windows will help to keep birds out.

Beetles, moths and mites. There are many species of these insects which infest stored food products. Flour beetles are common pests of flour and cereal products, and grain weevils (also a type of beetle) have long snouts used for boring into cereal grains. Moths such as the warehouse moth and mill moth spin silky threads which form a webbing which causes clumping of grains and flours and can block milling machinery. Mites are very small and produce a minty smell and a fine dust in the foods they infest e.g. flour and cereal products.

The main means of control of these pests involve inspecting deliveries, destroying infested food, cleaning food stores thoroughly and using insecticidal lacquers.

Hygienic food handling

Hygienic preparation, cooking and storage of food is of prime importance if food poisoning is to be prevented.

High risk foods

Many foods are likely to be contaminated when they are bought and others may become contaminated in the kitchen. Those foods which are most likely to cause food poisoning are described as high risk foods. They require particular care when being handled or cooked.

Meat and poultry

Meat and poultry together account for about 80% of all food-poisoning cases in the UK.

Poultry. Poultry often carries *Salmonella* and *Campylobacter*. Care should be taken to prevent cross-contamination. It is estimated that 70% of raw chickens carry *Salmonella*. Frozen poultry should be properly thawed and then thoroughly cooked.

Rolled meats. Rolled joints of meat can be responsible for *Clostridium perfringens* poisoning because spores from the outside are rolled into the centre where they are likely to survive cooking. They should be cooked thoroughly and eaten immediately. Slow cooling must be avoided.

Sausages, burgers, mince, etc. These often have a high bacterial count as they are finely divided, have a large surface area and pick up bacteria from equipment and the environment. They must be thoroughly cooked to prevent *Salmonella, E. coli* and other types of food poisoning.

Cold cooked meats. Cold cooked meats such as ham and tongue are subject to handling and therefore to contamination by *Staphylococcus aureus*. They must be stored correctly and should be handled using tongs or disposable gloves.

Stocks and gravies. Stocks and gravies provide an ideal medium for bacterial growth. Once made they should be used straight away or cooled quickly and refrigerated. Stocks should never be left to 'cool' overnight in the kitchen. When required they should be brought to the boil quickly and held above 70°C.

Eggs

Shell eggs (both hens' and ducks') may be contaminated with *Salmonella*. They should be thoroughly cooked i.e. hard boiled or used only in well-cooked dishes, especially if they are to be eaten by very young, elderly or ill people. For dishes which are uncooked or only lightly cooked, such as mayonnaise, mousses and omelettes, pasteurized egg should be used. Eggs and egg dishes should be stored in a refrigerator.

Milk and cream dishes

Cold desserts such as trifles and custards are easily contaminated, particularly by *Staphylococcus aureus*, and are an ideal medium for bacterial growth. They must be kept refrigerated. In restaurants cold desserts should be displayed in a refrigerated sweet trolley or cabinet.

Cooked rice

Rice, once cooked, should either be eaten straight away, kept hot (above 63°C) for service or cooled within 90 minutes and refrigerated. Rice which is cooled slowly or stored at room temperature is a potential cause of *Bacillus cereus* poisoning.

Seafoods

Shellfish and other seafoods should be bought only from a reputable supplier. Care is needed with frozen prawns. They should be stored below 5°C after thawing until required.

Reheated (rechauffé) dishes

When foods are reheated any bacteria present have a further opportunity to multiply. Reheating therefore requires special care. Foods should be cooled quickly (within 90 mins) after cooking and be stored in a refrigerator until ready to be reheated. They should then be heated up quickly and thoroughly. Liquid or semi-liquid foods (sauces, gravies, stews, etc.) should be brought to boiling point. More solid foods (pieces of meat, rice, etc.) should be heated so the centre temperature is over 70°C.

Hot and cold food must never be mixed together. Foods should never be reheated more than once.

Preventing contamination

It is essential to prevent the contamination of food by bacteria carried by food handlers or by bacteria from raw foods. The direct handling of food should be avoided where possible. Food should be handled with utensils, such as tongs. Food handlers should wear disposable plastic gloves when handling high risk foods, such as cooked meats.

Cross-contamination is the spread of bacteria from raw foods to cooked or ready-to-eat foods. In kitchens it is essential to keep raw and cooked foods separate in order to prevent cross-contamination. This means having separate preparation areas for the two types of food, which are often referred to as 'dirty' and 'clean' zones. Raw food has a much higher bacterial load than cooked food and raw meats in particular, are very likely to contain food-poisoning bacteria. Separate equipment should be used for the preparation of raw and cooked foods. Items such as knives and chopping boards can be colour-coded for different uses, e.g. for raw meat, raw vegetables, cooked foods. Equipment such as meat slicers and mincers, which cannot be duplicated, should be thoroughly cleaned and disinfected after being used for raw meat.

Cloths used in kitchens for wiping and drying harbour bacteria. Disposable paper towels should be used.

Temperature control

It is essential to control the temperature of food during preparation, processing, cooking and storage in order to prevent the multiplication of pathogenic bacteria. Good temperature control is probably the single most important factor in the prevention of food poisoning. It is thought that a breakdown in temperature control is a major factor in at least 75% of food-poisoning outbreaks.

Food handlers must avoid keeping high risk foods, such as meat and poultry, egg and milk dishes, cream cakes and desserts, in the danger zone (5–63°C) for longer than necessary. Consideration should be given to the following processes:

Preparation

Food should be kept in preparation areas for the minimum time.

Preparation areas should be well ventilated and not too hot. When preparation is finished, foods should be either cooked, refrigerated or frozen.

Defrosting

Some frozen foods, such as chickens and joints of meat, must be defrosted before cooking. This should be carried out at a low temperature, i.e. in a refrigerator, or quickly, e.g. in a microwave oven. Care is needed to ensure that food is completely defrosted before cooking. Otherwise, at the end of the cooking time, the centre of the food may not be hot enough to kill bacteria. Small items of meat, such as chops, sausages and burgers can be cooked from frozen, because, during cooking, the heat reaches the centre quickly.

Cooking

Foods, particularly meat and poultry, should be cooked thoroughly, so that the centre temperature is 70°C, i.e. high enough to kill most bacteria. This is particularly important for products such as burgers, sausages and rolled joints of meat, where bacteria originally present on the outside of the meat may be transferred to the centre. Stews and gravies should be heated to boiling point (100°C) . Centre temperatures can be checked using a probe thermometer. This must be cleaned between being used for different products.

After cooking, foods should be served immediately, kept hot or cooled quickly.

Hot holding

If food is to be kept hot, it should be kept at 70°C or more in preheated hot cabinets or bain-maries (water baths). For food on display (e.g. in a self-service canteen) hot lamps may be used.

Chilling

Cooked foods should be cooled quickly and within 1.5 hours. They are best cooled at a temperature of 10°C or below. Cooling may be carried out in a well-ventilated cooling room or larder on the north side of the building or in a special cabinet. Blast chillers are used in many establishments. They use a blast of cold air to cool foods quickly and steadily. Large bulks of food, such as joints, stews, rice, etc., should be divided or spread out to speed the cooling process. Once cold, foods should be stored in a refrigerator.

Reheating

Reheating is best avoided but, if it is carried out, foods should be heated up quickly and heated through thoroughly (see page 272). Small portions may be heated in a microwave oven, though care is needed to ensure even cooking and the absence of 'cold spots'. Forced convection ovens are suitable for larger quantities. Stews, gravies, etc., should be heated in pans, brought up quickly to boiling point (100°C) and then simmered for 15 minutes.

Storage of food

All foods should be stored in suitable containers and in clean conditions to prevent contamination. A good system of **stock rotation** is essential. This involves using the oldest food first, i.e. using a 'first in, first out (FIFO)' system. When refilling shelves with newly delivered stock, the old stock must be brought forward and the new stock placed behind it.

Dry food storage

Foods such as flour, pulses, dried fruit and canned products should be stored in a dry food store which should be clean, cool, dry, well lit and well ventilated. Foods, unless already suitably packaged, should be stored in vermin-proof containers with tight fitting lids. They should be placed on shelves, preferably stainless steel and mobile, at least 40 cm above floor level to allow for cleaning.

Vegetables should be stored in a cool, dry area away from direct sunlight. They should be placed in racks or bins raised off the floor, e.g. on pallets.

Chilled storage

Refrigerators can be used for the short-term storage of a wide variety of foods. Since most pathogenic bacteria are unable to multiply at refrigeration temperatures (1–4°C), food storage in a refrigerator is reasonably safe. However, the temperature should not exceed 4°C as *Listeria monocytogenes* and *Yersinia enterocolitica* can grow and multiply at temperatures just above this. Many spoilage organisms can grow fairly well at low temperatures and spoilage will eventually occur, even within a refrigerator.

In order for a refrigerator to function efficiently, air must be able to circulate freely around the food. Therefore, refrigerators should not be overloaded.

It is imperative that raw foods should be well separated from cooked foods to prevent cross-contamination by food-poisoning bacteria. In catering establishments there should, ideally, be separate refrigerators for raw and cooked foods. If they are stored in the same refrigerator, cooked foods should be above raw foods. With large walk-in refrigerators, different foods should be properly separated so that, for example, raw meat cannot drip on to cooked foods.

Strong smelling foods, such as fish, should be stored in air-tight containers. The use of such containers for other foods prevents dehydration, since moisture evaporates from uncovered food.

Refrigerators with automatic defrosting are recommended, as they keep the ice layer inside the refrigerator to a minimum. For other refrigerators defrosting must be carried out at regular intervals. The operating temperature of refrigerators should be checked at least once a day and records kept of the temperatures.

There are many types of refrigeration units used in catering and retailing. In catering establishments refrigerated sweet trolleys and salad bars are used, as well as standard refrigerators and large walk-in units. Refrigerators are available with glass doors which can be used for displaying products such as cream cakes or wine. Open refrigerated display cabinets are used in supermarkets and other retail outlets. These usually operate at 1° to 3°C and foods must be kept below the load line. In butchers shops refrigerated counters are used.

Deep freeze storage

Deep freeze cabinets used for long-term food storage should be maintained at a temperature of –18°C or below. The freezing of food kills some bacteria but spores and some vegetative cells survive. Meat and fish may be stored for up to six months and fruits and vegetables for up to one year. When frozen food is thawed, the bacteria which have survived start to grow and multiply again. Foods should not, therefore, be thawed and refrozen.

However, if foods are partially thawed, as occurs, for example, while shopping or as a result of a power cut, it may be safe to refreeze the food if the central core of the food is still frozen and the food is cold.

Once food is completely thawed, it should be used straight away. It is normally safe to cook raw, thawed food and refreeze it as a cooked dish.

Freezers should be defrosted when necessary (usually about every six months) and operating temperatures should be checked daily with a freezer thermometer and recorded.

HACCP system of quality control

The Hazard Analysis Critical Control Point (HACCP) system is a method of quality control being used increasingly in the catering and food manufacturing industries. It is an approach which aims to assess the potential hazards in a food operation, decide which areas are critical to the safety of the consumer and devise ways of ensuring microbiological food safety. Each food product requires a separate HACCP system.

There are five main stages to the system:

1 **Flow chart**

A flow chart is produced which shows all the steps or processes in the operation e.g. storage, defrosting, cooking, cooling.

2 Identifying and assessing the hazards

A hazard is anything that may cause harm to the consumer. It may be microbiological, e.g. presence of food-poisoning bacteria, or chemical, e.g. the presence of toxic cleaning agents, or physical e.g. the presence of foreign bodies. The following should be considered:

(a) microbiological aspects of the food itself. Bacteria will grow in a food if the food is moist, has a neutral pH and is not protected by chemical or heat preservation, i.e. high risk foods;
(b) intended process and effects on bacteria;
(c) intended use, e.g. susceptibility of the consumer.

3 Identifying the critical control points (CCPs)

A critical control point is a step in the operation which has to be carried out correctly to make sure the hazard is removed (or reduced to a safe level). For example, defrosting of frozen chickens is a step which if carried out incorrectly could allow Salmonellae present to multiply. Defrosting is, therefore, a critical control point.

4 Specifying control procedures

This involves establishing safe food handling routines at the CCPs to control the hazards. For example, the time and temperature for defrosting frozen chickens is specified.

5 Monitoring control procedures

Unless the control procedures are implemented and monitored the HACCP system does not work. Microbiological testing, e.g. testing for the presence of Salmonellae in cooked chickens, is expensive and time-consuming. It may be practical for food manufacturing operations but not for catering. However, there are many other methods of monitoring including:

(a) temperature checks on foods, e.g. after defrosting or cooking;
(b) temperature checks on equipment such as refrigerators and freezers;
(c) visual checks by staff, e.g. for cleanliness of equipment, ingredients within 'use by' date.

Results of monitoring should always be recorded.

Table 17.2 gives an example of a flow diagram of the defrosting, cooking and service of turkey showing the hazards, control procedures and monitoring.

Table 17.2 *HACCP system for the production of cooked chicken*

Step	*Hazards*	*Control Procedures*	*Monitoring*
Frozen storage CCP ↓	If freezer is not cold enough bacteria will mutliply	Store in freezer at –18°C or below	Check freezer temperature
Defrosting CCP ↓	If insufficiently defrosted bacteria will survive cooking If defrosted above 5°C bacteria will multiply If drips are not retained cross-contamination can occur	Defrost for at least 15 hours per kg in a refrigerator at 1–5°C Retain drip in a tray	Check refrigerator temperature Check final internal temperature of bird is 1–5°C Check no ice in body cavity Visual check of drip tray
Cooking CCP ↓	If cooking time and/or temperature are insufficient bacteria will survive	Cook to ensure an internal temperature of 70°C+	Record cooking time and temperature Check internal temperature Check juices are clear
Slicing CCP ↓	If touched by dirty knives/utensils or by bare hands contamination may occur	Use cleaned and disinfected knives and utensils Avoid touching with bare hands	Visual check on cleanliness Visual checks on handling procedures
Hot-holding CCP ↓	If held below 63°C bacteria will multiply	Hold in hot cupboard at 65°C+ for no more than 2 hours	Check temperature of hot cupboard Record hot-holding time and temperature Spot check chicken temperature
Service			

CCP = critical control point

Legislation

Legislation controlling food has two main aims:

(a) the protection of the health of the consumer;
(b) the prevention of fraud.

The Food Safety Act 1990

This is the primary piece of legislation in Great Britain dealing with food safety. It covers the whole of the human food chain from the farm to the consumer and is wider-ranging than the previous **Food Act 1984**. The term 'food' now includes dietary supplements and water after it leaves the tap. Food premises covered under the act include stalls and vehicles (hot dog vans, etc.) as well as food manufacturing, retailing and catering premises.

The main provisions of the act are:

Offences

It is an offence to:

(a) render food injurious to health;
(b) sell or possess food which fails to comply with food safety requirements by being injurious to health, unfit for human consumption or contaminated;
(c) sell food which is not of the nature, substance or quality demanded by the purchaser.

Enforcement

The act is enforced by both central and local government. The local authority enforcement officers are:

(a) **trading standards officers** who deal with matters involving the composition, labelling and chemical contamination of food;
(b) **environmental health officers (EHOs)** who deal with hygiene matters including microbiological contamination, extraneous matter in food and food which is unfit for human consumption.

Powers of enforcement officers

Local authority officers have powers to:

(a) enter food premises at any reasonable time to inspect premises, processes and records;
(b) detain suspect food or seize it and take it before a Justice of the Peace to be condemned.

Improvement notices

EHOs can serve an **Improvement Notice** if there is a breach of hygiene regulations. The proprietor of the food business will be required to take measures within a given period of time (not less than 14 days) to comply with the Notice.

Prohibition orders

If a business is convicted of a breach of hygiene regulations and the court feels that public health is at risk, the court can impose a Prohibition Order which will prohibit the use of a particular process or piece of equipment, or the whole or part of the premises.

Emergency prohibition notices and orders

When a food business presents an imminent risk to health, enforcement officers can serve an **Emergency Prohibition Notice**. The premises are then closed immediately and the enforcement officer must take the matter before a court within three days. If the court agrees that there is an imminent risk of injury to health it will make an Emergency Prohibition Order. This can only be lifted if the local authority is satisfied improvements have been made and issues a certificate.

Penalties

Penalties for offences under the main provisions of the Act are up to £20 000 per offence.

For other offences fines of up to £5000 and a prison sentence of up to 6 months can be imposed by a magistrates' court.

Crown courts can give unlimited fines and up to 2 years in prison.

Due diligence

The legal defence of 'due diligence' enables someone to be acquitted of an offence if they can show that they took all reasonable precautions and exercised due diligence. This means that food businesses need to look carefully at their quality control arrangements and the checks they make on foods and food processes.

The Food Safety Act also gives government ministers powers to issue regulations laying down detailed rules on a wide range of food matters such as the control of food composition, labelling, additives and hygiene. The main regulations involving the catering industry are:

The Food Premises (Registration) Regulations 1991

Under these regulations any new food business must register with their local authority at least 28 days before it opens. There is no charge for registration and registration cannot be refused. The purpose of registration is to enable authorities to be aware of all the food premises in their area so that they are able to plan their inspection programmes effectively. Premises that are not regularly used as a food business do not need to be registered. Only premises used for five or more days in any five consecutive weeks require registration.

The Food Safety (General Food Hygiene) Regulations 1995

These regulations have replaced the **Food Hygiene (General) Regulations 1970**

They came into force in September 1995 and they aim to ensure that food hygiene in Britain is in line with elsewhere in Europe, as set out in the Food Hygiene Directive (93/43/EEC). They apply to anyone who owns, runs or works in a food business (except manufacturers and processors of animal products such as meat, milk and eggs who are covered by product specific regulations). The regulations set out basic hygiene principles which are not new but which have a different emphasis from previous regulations. They require food businesses to take responsibility for applying food safety standards which are appropriate to their particular circumstances. Rather than having just a long list of rules these regulations make the proprietor of a food business responsible for assessing the risks to food safety and ensuring that appropriate controls are in place.

The proprietor must:

1 Ensure that food operations (including preparation, processing, manufacturing, storing, transporting and selling) are carried out in a hygienic way.

2 Identify steps which are critical to food safety and implement safety procedures by:

(a) analysing the potential hazards in the food operations;
(b) identifying the points where hazards may occur;
(c) deciding which points are critical to food safety ('critical points');
(d) identifying and implementing control and monitoring procedures at these points.

3 Ensure that the following rules of hygiene are complied with.

Food premises

Food premises should:

(a) be kept clean and in good repair;
(b) be designed and constructed to permit adequate cleaning and/or disinfection, protection against cross-contamination and suitable temperature conditions for processing and storage;

(c) have adequate wash-hand basins with hot and cold water, materials for washing hands and for hygienic drying;
(d) have sufficient well-ventilated toilets which do not lead directly into food rooms;
(e) have sufficient natural or mechanical ventilation;
(f) have sufficient natural and/or artificial lighting;
(g) have adequate drainage facilities;
(h) have adequate staff changing facilities.

Rooms where food is prepared, treated or processed should also have:

(i) surface finishes (e.g. walls, floors, doors and surfaces which come into contact with food) which are easy to clean and, where necessary, disinfect;
(j) windows which can be opened fitted with insect-proof screens where necessary;
(k) adequate facilities for washing food and equipment.

Equipment
All equipment which comes into contact with food should be kept clean and in such condition to minimize any risk of food contamination.

Food waste
Waste must not be allowed to accumulate in food rooms but be deposited in closable containers. Adequate provision must be made for the removal and storage of food waste and other refuse.

Water supply
There must be an adequate supply of wholesome water, to be used whenever necessary to ensure food is not contaminated.

Personal hygiene
All food handlers must:

(a) maintain a high degree of personal cleanliness;
(b) wear suitable clean and, where appropriate, protective clothing;
(c) not be permitted to work while afflicted with infected wounds, skin infections, sores, diarrhoea etc.;
(d) inform their employer if they are known or suspected to be suffering from, or be a carrier of, a disease likely to be transmitted through food.

Foods
(a) Foods or raw materials must not be accepted by a food business if they are known or suspected to be so contaminated they would be unfit for human consumption.

(b) All food which is handled, stored, packaged, displayed and transported must be protected against contamination.

(c) Adequate procedures must be in place to ensure pests are controlled.

Training

The proprietor of a food business must ensure that food handlers are supervised and instructed and/or trained in food hygiene matters appropriate to their work activities.

The Food Safety (Temperature Control) Regulations 1995

These regulations set out temperature controls for high-risk foods by keeping these foods outside the Danger Zone (8°C–63°C).

Chill holding

Cold high risk foods must not be kept above 8°C. This applies to food which is likely to support the growth of pathogens or the formation of toxins. It does not apply to food which is kept for service or on display for sale for up to 4 hours. Nor does it apply to raw food which is to be cooked.

Hot holding

Foods which are kept hot must not be kept below 63°C. This applies to foods which have been cooked or reheated, are for service or on display for sale and need to be kept hot to control the growth of pathogens or the formation of toxins.

Cooling of food

Foods which need to be kept at a temperature below ambient temperatures must be cooled as quickly as possible after cooking.

18 Food preservation

All food was once living tissue and is of organic origin. Some foods, such as meat and fish, are killed before being distributed to the consumer. Other foods, such as fruits and vegetables, may be stored and distributed in the living state. Because of its organic nature, food is susceptible to deterioration or spoilage by saprophytic and parasitic micro-organisms.

When food spoilage takes place, two distinct processes are involved.

1 Autolysis

The word autolysis means self-destruction and is used to describe the cellular breakdown caused by enzymes contained within the food itself. This breakdown starts immediately after slaughter or harvest. In many instances a limited amount of enzyme activity may be beneficial; for example, in the ripening of fruit and the tenderization of meat. However, in most instances it is detrimental.

2 Microbial spoilage

Once the cellular structure becomes disorganized, the food is vulnerable to attack by micro-organisms. The main agents of microbial spoilage are bacteria, moulds and yeasts. These organisms break down the complex organic components of the food into simpler compounds and so cause alterations in the flavour, texture, colour and smell of the food. Examples of bacteria which are responsible for food spoilage are given in Chapter 15.

Food preservation

The main aims of food preservation are to prevent autolysis and microbial growth. The growth requirements of micro-organisms and the principles of the control of microbial growth have been covered in Chapter 15. Preservation may be short term or long term and may be achieved in a variety of ways. Blanching food in order to inactivate enzymes and prevent autolysis may be regarded as a short-term means of preservation. All methods of cooking, including the use of microwaves, will have the same effect and also destroy some of the micro-organisms present in the food; therefore they are also short-term methods. In any method of preservation involving the use of heat to destroy micro-organisms, it can usually be assumed that most enzymes will be inactivated. Long-term methods of preservation usually involve the removal of more than one of the requirements necessary for growth. Also a method of destruction of micro-organisms, e.g. heating, is sometimes involved in the process.

Heat treatment

The two main methods of preservation involving the use of heat are heat sterilization and pasteurization.

1 Heat sterilization

Sterilization involves the use of heat to bring about the total destruction of all micro-organisms and their spores. The sterilized food must be placed in an airtight container to prevent the entry of further spoilage organisms. A steel can coated with a thin layer of tin is the most common type of container. For some products the inside of the can may be coated with lacquer as a further protection against corrosion. Glass bottles and jars are used as containers for some products, particularly jams and preserves. In recent years, flexible plastic containers have been used for a variety of liquid products, particularly milk and cream.

The canning process

The modern canning process usually involves the following operations:

1 *Cleaning and preparation*. All inedible parts are removed from the food and the food is graded and washed.

2 *Blanching*. Most vegetable foods are blanched, either by being immersed in boiling water or by being exposed to steam. This is often a continuous process in which the food is passed through a tunnel into which the steam is injected. The period of exposure may vary from two to ten minutes. Blanching inactivates enzymes which may affect the stability of the food while it awaits further processing. In addition, the blanching process helps to drive out air bubbles trapped within the food, thus allowing a better 'fill'. If too much air remains in the cans the desired temperature may not be reached during sterilization and micro-organisms may survive inside some of the cans.

3 *Filling and exhausting*. The washed, open cans are filled automatically with a weighed amount of the food. For vegetables, fruits and some other foods the cans are topped up to within 1 cm of the top with liquor. The liquor is normally brine in the case of vegetables and

sugar syrup in the case of fruits. After filling, the cans are usually passed to an exhaust box in which they are exposed to hot water or steam and the contents heated to about 95°C so that, when the lid is sealed on, a partial vacuum will form in the can.

4 *Sealing.* Lids are placed on the cans and they are passed to an automatic sealing machine, which bends the edge of the lid and the flange on the can body into a roll. The roll is then flattened forming a hermetic, i.e. airtight, seal.

5 *Sterilization.* The amount of heat required for adequate sterilization depends on the following factors:

(a) The size of the can and the nature of its contents. Heat takes longer to penetrate into a large can. Also, heat penetration is faster in convection packs, such as soups, than in conduction packs, such as corned beef.

(b) The pH of the food.

The sterilization process is designed to eliminate *Clostridium botulinum* and its spores, since this is the most dangerous and most heat-resistant micro-organism likely to be present in canned foods. Therefore, foods are classified into groups depending on the heat treatment necessary to eliminate this micro-organism.

Foods may be classified into three groups:

(i) High acid foods which have a pH below 3.7. Very few bacteria can survive conditions of such high acidity. Consequently, only a mild heat treatment is necessary to eliminate yeasts and moulds which may be present, since they are less heat resistant than bacteria. For most can sizes heating to 100°C for eight to 16 minutes is sufficient. Bacterial spores may survive but they are unable to germinate and, therefore, cannot cause spoilage.

(ii) Medium acid foods which have a pH between 3.7 and 4.5. Many spoilage bacteria are able to grow in this pH range and, therefore, the heat treatment required is more severe than for high acid foods. However, the pH is still too low to allow the growth of *Clostridium botulinum.*

(iii) Low acid foods which have a pH above 4.5. These foods include meat, fish and most vegetables. In order to ensure complete destruction of bacteria, especially *Clostridium botulinum* spores, it is essential that these products are subjected to a severe heat treatment. The temperature required depends on the time of exposure to heat.

Most cans of low acid food are heated so that all the food reaches 121°C for 3 minutes and this is referred to as an F_0 value of 3. (The F value of a process is the number of minutes at 121°C which will have a sterilizing effect, i.e. kill all bacteria including spores of

Clostridium botulinum. The symbol F_0 is used to express the F value under certain conditions.) This heat treatment is accepted as the minimum degree of sterilization to be safe and is also known as the **'botulinum cook'**.

Some catering size cans of ham (e.g. 6 kg or more) may not be sterilized but only given a pasteurizing treatment which kills vegetative bacteria but not spores. This is because excessive heating would cause unacceptable shrinkage of the meat. The salts used in curing inhibit the growth of *Clostridium botulinum* but, even so, these cans are not shelf-stable and must be kept refrigerated.

6 *Cooling*. The can must be cooled slowly by gradually reducing the pressure of the steam used for heating and thus bringing about a gradual reduction in temperature. If the pressure was reduced suddenly, the cans would buckle. The cans are then cooled further using water. Since temporary leakage may occur at this point, it is imperative that the cooling water is clean and sterile. Sterilization of the water is achieved by chlorination; the usual level of chlorine in the cooling water is between 3 and 5 ppm (parts per million) of chlorine. Cooling is only continued until the cans reach a temperature of 38°C and then the warmth of the can is sufficient to allow the cans to be dried in the air. This avoids rusting and also reduces the danger of micro-organisms present in water on the surface being drawn into the can through a temporary leak.

Modern canning processes are completely automated and are run on a continuous system rather than using batch processes.

Asceptic canning

There are many variations on the standard canning process. One of the most common is the use of aseptic filling, in which the bulked product and the containers are sterilized separately. The containers are then filled aseptically, i.e. under conditions where the entry of micro-organisms is prevented, before being sealed.

Aseptic canning is mainly used for liquid foods which are heat sensitive and therefore likely to be overcooked in the standard canning process (e.g. dairy custards). Changes in flavour and colour and reduction in nutritive value are minimized if these products are sterilized using a multi-plate heat exchanger, such as is used in the pasteurization of milk.

Spoilage of canned foods

The main reasons for spoilage of canned foods are:

1 Insufficient sterilization, which means that spores of anaerobic bacteria may survive and germinate.

2 Leakage, which is due to either a badly made can or a can which has been improperly sealed.

3 Corrosion of the can, which may be due to attack by the con-

tents, particularly acid foods, or damage due to storage in unsatisfactory conditions, i.e. storage in a warm, humid atmosphere.

There are a large variety of different types of spoilage which may occur but the following are the most common:

1 *Thermophilic gas spoilage*. This is usually caused by anaerobic spore-forming bacteria, such as the genus *Clostridium*. This type of spoilage occurs in cans of low acid foods which have been insufficiently sterilized. Usually, large amounts of hydrogen are produced and this gas causes the ends of the cans to bulge. This is known as a **'blown can'**.

2 *Carbon dioxide gas spoilage*. Non-spore-forming bacteria may enter the can after sterilization, either through leakage of cooling water or through unsatisfactory sealing. In this case the contents of the can often appear slimy and frothy.

3 *Flat sour spoilage*. Some species of bacteria which produce heat-resistant spores, such as members of the genus *Bacillus*, may survive if the heat treatment is not sufficient. These bacteria may grow anaerobically in low acid foods. They do not produce any marked change in the appearance of the food but they ferment the food producing acid which gives the food a disagreeable taste. Since these organisms do not produce gas, this type of spoilage is not detected until the food is eaten.

'Blown', rusty or badly dented cans should not be used.

Sterilization of milk

Milk may be sterilized in two ways:

1 *The in-bottle and continuous flow sterilization processes*. In these processes the milk is heat treated to destroy all microbial cells and the majority of their spores. The milk will keep for at least a week (usually longer) without refrigeration. The milk is first homogenized, i.e. the fat globules are reduced in size so that they are evenly distributed throughout the milk and do not form a cream layer on the surface. This is achieved by heating the milk to about 60°C and forcing it through fine holes under high pressure. The milk is then filtered.

In the in-bottle process the milk is placed in glass or plastic bottles, the bottles are sealed and then heated to sterilizing temperature, i.e. at least 100°C. Various time and temperature combinations can be used but usually higher temperatures and shorter times are chosen, for example 112°C for 15 minutes.

In the continuous flow process the milk is sterilized in bulk in a multi-plate heat exchanger using similar temperatures and times and it is then aseptically filled into containers which have been sterilized previously.

The main disadvantages of sterilized milk are:

(a) the flavour is altered and the milk has a cooked taste;
(b) the colour of the milk is altered due to caramelization of sugars and to the Maillard browning reaction which takes place between the sugars and amino acids;
(c) the vitamin content is reduced; thiamin and ascorbic acid are the vitamins which are most affected. However, the loss of ascorbic acid is not of great practical significance since milk is not one of the most important sources of vitamin C.

2 *The UHT (ultra heat treatment) process.* In this process the milk is heated to a very high temperature for a very short time. Such a process kills all micro-organisms and their spores without producing such a marked effect on the flavour, colour and nutritive value of the milk. According to the **Dairy Products (Hygiene) Regulations 1995**, UHT milk must be heated to not less than 135°C for not less than one second. It must then be placed immediately into aseptic opaque containers. The heating stage is carried out in a multi-plate heat exchanger. UHT milk is free from micro-organisms and should keep unopened for six months or more.

Both sterilized and UHT milk must comply with certain standards. After being kept in a closed container for 15 days at 30°C it must taste normal, not show any sign of deterioration and have a satisfactory plate count.

2 Pasteurization

Pasteurization is a mild heat treatment which kills pathogens and therefore makes foods safe to eat. In the case of milk, for example, the pasteurization process destroys organisms such as *Mycobacterium tuberculosis*, *Brucella abortus* and *Listeria monocytogenes*. Food manufacturers regard pasteurization also as a means of extending the shelf-life of a food, since the heat greatly reduces the number of spoilage organisms present.

Milk is normally pasteurized by the **HTST (high temperature short time) process.** In this process the milk is heated to a temperature of at least 71.7°C, held there for 15 seconds, then immediately cooled to below 10°C. Different time and temperature combinations may be used to give an equivalent effect.

The **Dairy Products (Hygiene) Regulations 1995** state that pasteurized milk must give a negative reaction to the phosphatase test. Phosphatase is an enzyme which is slightly more heat resistant than pathogens such as *Mycobacterium tuberculosis*. A heat treatment which destroys phosphatase will also destroy these pathogens.

Liquid milk to be pasteurized is transported from the farm to the dairy in large chilled tanks. According to the **Dairy Products (Hygiene) Regulations 1995**, the temperature of the milk during transport must be kept at 10°C or below. At the dairy the milk must be cooled to 6°C (unless it is treated within 4 hours of acceptance). Before pasteurization the milk is filtered and, in some cases, homogenized. The milk is then passed through a multi-plate heat exchanger and heated to 71.7C for 15 seconds. The process is outlined in Figure 18.1.

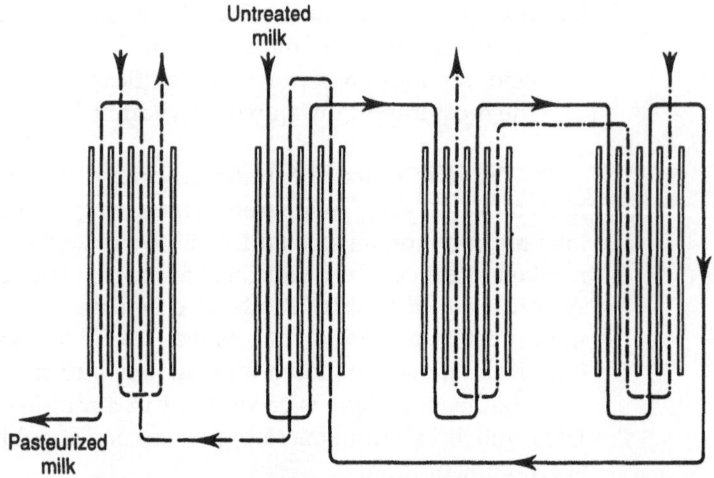

Stage 1 The incoming milk is being heated by milk which has already been pasteurized.

Stage 2 The temperature of the milk is raised to the temperature required for pasteurization by means of hot water.

Stage 3 The milk is held at 72°C for 15 seconds in order to achieve adequate pasteurization.

Stage 4 The milk is partially cooled by giving up some of its heat to the cold incoming milk.

Stage 5 The milk is cooled to 10°C or below by cooling water.

Figure 18.1 *Simplified diagram of the HTST pasteurization process.*

The sale of raw, untreated milk is still permitted in England and Wales but it must be labelled 'raw milk'. In addition, according to the **Food Labelling Regulations 1984** (as amended), it must also be marked or labelled with the words 'This milk has not been heat-treated and may therefore contain organisms harmful to health'.

Both liquid egg and ice cream mix are pasteurized in order to eliminate possible pathogens, especially Salmonellae. According to the **Egg Products Regulations 1993**, all whole egg and yolk must be pasteurized by being held at a minimum of 64.4°C for at least 2.5 minutes and then immediately cooled to below 4°C. Egg products for freezing must be frozen immediately after pasteurization and cooling.

The **Ice Cream (Heat Treatment etc.) Regulations 1959 and 1963** stipulate that where a complete cold mix is reconstituted using wholesome drinking water the mixture must be converted to ice cream within one hour of preparation. Otherwise (unless the pH is 4.5 or less) the following must be observed:

1 The mixture should be kept for no longer than one hour at any temperature over 7.2°C before being pasteurized or sterilized.

2 The following times and temperatures may be used for pasteurization:

(i) a minimum temperature of 65.6°C for a minimum of 30 minutes;
(ii) a minimum temperature of 71.1°C for a minimum of 10 minutes;
(iii) a minimum temperature of 79.5°C for a minimum of 15 seconds.

3 The required process for sterilization is heating to a minimum of 148.9°C for a minimum of 2 seconds.

4 After pasteurization or sterilization the temperature of the mix must be reduced to 7.2°C within 1.5 hours and the mix must be held at this temperature until freezing begins.

Once it has been manufactured ice cream must be held at or below –2.2°C until it is sold.

Freezing

The preservation of foods by freezing involves two methods of control of the growth of micro-organisms:

1 The growth rate of micro-organisms is reduced by the low temperature. Also the rate of undesirable chemical changes is reduced considerably at low temperatures.

2 A large percentage of the water present in the food is converted to ice and is therefore unavailable to micro-organisms.

Quick-freezing processes, in which the food passes through the range of maximum ice-crystal formation in the shortest time possible, are preferable, since the formation of large ice crystals causes undesirable changes in the texture and appearance of the food. Quick freezing has been defined as that process in which the food passes through this zone (0°C to –4°C) in 30 minutes or less. The small ice crystals formed by such a process do not disrupt the texture of the food.

Most foods can be frozen successfully and, in general, frozen food products are superior to canned foods, since the product bears a closer resemblance to the fresh food. Also, the nutritive value of the food is not as seriously affected by the freezing process. In some cases the vitamin content of fresh frozen foods may be higher than that of fresh foods, since foods such as fruits and vegetables often lose ascorbic acid during transportation and storage. Foods containing fat dispersed in a colloidal form, i.e. as an emulsion, may not freeze successfully. The reason for this is that as freezing takes place, the removal of water causes an increase in the concentration of salts in the food which may cause irreversible changes in the colloidal structure.

Before freezing all inedible parts of the food are removed. Most foods, particularly fruits and vegetables, are blanched in order to inactivate enzymes. Blanching also reduces the number of bacteria present by as much as 90%. Before freezing, substances such as ascorbic acid, which reduces browning of some fruits and vegetables, or antioxidants, which prevent undesirable changes in any fat present, may be added to the food.

There various methods of freezing including:

1 *Plate freezing*. In this method the refrigerant passes through a number of hollow plates. The food is placed between the plates.

2 *Immersion freezing*. In this method the food is placed directly into the refrigerant. The refrigerant used depends on the food being frozen. Brine is sometimes used, especially for fish, whereas invert sugar solutions are often used for fruits and vegetables. In more modern processes liquid nitrogen (boiling point –196°C) makes an excellent refrigerant.

3 *Blast freezing*. In this method a blast of very cold air is blown directly on to the food.

4 *Fluidized bed freezing*. This method is very successful for freezing foods which are of small particle size, such as peas. It is an adaptation of blast freezing in which the air is blown upwards through mesh over which the food is passing. The air speed is controlled so that the solid particles of food flow as if they were liquid. In this method the rate of heat exchange from the food to the air may be very rapid and this is desirable for a quick freezing process.

Dehydration

The traditional method of drying foods was simply to lay the foods in the sun. This method is still used for the drying of foods in some countries. Some traditional methods involve the use of other means of control of growth in addition to the removal of moisture. For example, both smoking and salting have been used in the traditional methods used for drying meat and fish.

The modern process of dehydration consists of the removal of moisture from the food by the application of heat usually in the presence of a controlled flow of air. It is important that the temperature used should not be too high, since this will cause undesirable changes in the food. Also, excessive heat may cause 'case hardening', where the outside of the food becomes brittle and hard while moisture is trapped in the centre and is unable to pass through the food by the normal processes of diffusion and capillary action.

Before drying, food undergoes a variety of treatments. In the case of vegetables this includes washing, grading and blanching (to destroy enzymes). Sodium sulphite is usually added to the blanching water; this improves the colour of the product, aids vitamin C retention and destroys many of the micro-organisms. Other foods, such as meats, may be cooked prior to dehydration.

There are many types of equipment used for dehydrating foods. Some of the more usual methods of drying are:

1 *Tunnel drying*. In this method the food is placed on conveyor belts or perforated trays and passed through a warm-air tunnel. A more modern development is fluidized bed drying, in which warm air is blown upwards and the particles of food are kept in motion This method is used particularly for vegetables.

2 *Spray drying*. This method is used for drying fairly liquid foods such as milk and eggs. The food enters the top of a large drying chamber as a fine spray. The spray mixes with warm air, the water evaporates and a fine powder is produced which is removed from the bottom of the chamber.

3 *Roller drying*. In this method the food is applied in paste form as a thin film to the surface of a revolving heated roller or drum. As the drum rotates the food dries and the dried product is removed from the drum by a scraper knife. Products dried by this method include instant breakfast cereals and potatoes.

4 *Freeze drying*. In this method of drying the food is first of all frozen and then subjected to a mild heating process in a vacuum cabinet. The ice crystals which form during the freezing stage sublime when heated under reduced pressure, i.e. they change directly from ice to water vapour without passing through the liquid phase. This results in a product which is porous and very little changed in size and shape from the original food. Since little heat is required there is little heat damage and the colour, flavour and nutrient content affected less than in some other methods of drying. The product, being porous, can be rapidly rehydrated (reconstituted) in cold water. A wide variety of foods can be dried by this method, e.g. meat, shellfish, fruits and vegetables.

Addition of chemical inhibitors

Many methods of preservation, including many of the traditional methods, depend on the addition of antimicrobial substances to foods. Some of these methods are outlined below:

1 *Curing*. The curing of meats such as bacon involves using a brine solution composed of sodium chloride (25%), potassium nitrate (1%) and sodium nitrite (0.1%). The meat may be soaked in the brine or the brine may be injected into the meat by hollow needles. The salt content inhibits microbial growth and the meat develops a characteristic colour and flavour.

Some cured products, e.g. herring and bacon, are also smoked, by exposing them to smoke from a wood fire. The smoke contains anti-microbial substances which reduce spoilage. It also gives the food a characteristic taste.

2 *Preserving with sugar*. Many fruit products, such as jams and crystallized fruits, are preserved with sugar. Sugar reduces microbial activity due to its dehydrating effect (see page 231).

3 *Addition of acid*. This may be carried out in one of two ways. The food may be pickled, i.e. soaked in an acid solution such as vinegar (acetic acid). This is used for a variety of foods, particularly vegetables. Another method is to inoculate the food with a culture of selected bacteria and to rely on acid produced by the activities of these bacteria. Foods such as yoghurt and sauerkraut (fermented cabbage) are produced in this way.

4 *Other chemical preservatives*. The chemicals which may be added to food in controlled amounts for use as preservatives are discussed in more detail in Chapter 19.

Irradiation

It has been known for many years that various types of radiation can be used to inhibit microbial growth. Ultraviolet (UV) light does not penetrate deeply but has certain uses, for example disinfecting cleaned surfaces in bakeries and treating water used for cleaning shellfish. Ionizing radiation in the form of gamma (Υ) rays is very effective in killing micro-organisms. Gamma rays penetrate deeply and can be used for preserving food. The rays are emitted by the radioactive isotopes cobalt-60 and caesium-137 which are by-products of the nuclear power industry.

Since gamma rays are highly penetrating they are able to pass through large containers of food and thus food can be treated in bulk or in its final packaging. The food passes along a conveyor and is briefly exposed to the radioactive isotope. Low levels of irradiation have no effect on the flavour and texture of food but with higher levels various chemical changes occur which can affect the food.

The unit of radiation dose is the **Gray** (Gy). One Gray is the dose of radiation received by one kilogram of matter when it absorbs one joule of radiation energy.

$$1 \text{ kiloGray (kGy)} = 1000 \text{ Gray (Gy)}$$

Uses of irradiation

Irradiation is used mainly to extend the storage life of food by inactivating enzymes and destroying spoilage microbes. It also inhibits sprouting and kills insects and other pests. Higher doses can be used to destroy or reduce the number of pathogens in foods, such as *Salmonella* and *Campylobacter* in raw poultry. Doses high enough to sterilize foods, i.e. kill all microbes including bacterial spores, are not widely used since they are likely to produce unacceptable changes to the taste of the foods. The World Health Organization has declared irradiation to be 'a powerful tool against preventable food losses and food-borne illness'.

There are three levels of radiation treatment known (from the lowest to the highest) as radurization, radicidation and radappertization. Table 18.1 shows the doses together with their particular uses.

Table 18.1 *Food irradiation levels and uses*

Level	*Uses*	*Products*
Radurization Low dose (up to 1 kGy)	Inhibition of sprouting	Potatoes, onion, garlic
	Killing insects	Cereals and pulses, dried fruit, spices
	Delay of ripening	Fresh fruit e.g. bananas
Radicidation Medium dose (1 – 10 kGy)	Extension of shelf life	Fresh fish, strawberries
	Killing vegetative pathogens e.g. *Salmonella*	Fresh and frozen meat, poultry, seafood, animal feedstuffs
Radappertization High dose (10 – 50 kGy)	Commercial sterilization	Meat, poultry, sterilized hospital diets
	Decontamination of ingredients	Spices, enzyme preparations, gums

Legislation

In Britain only certain types of irradiated food may be sold and the treatment must be carried out under licence. The **Food (Control of Irradiation) Regulations 1990** specify the types of food which may be treated and the maximum permitted overall dosage. These foods and the maximum dosages are shown in Table 18.2.

Table 18.2 *Permitted foods and maximum irradiation dosages*

Food	*Maximum permitted dosage*
Fruit	2 kGy
Vegetables	1 kGy
Cereals	1 kGy
Bulbs and tubers (potatoes, onions, etc.)	0.2 kGy
Spices and condiments	10 kGy
Fish and shellfish	3 kGy
Poultry	7 kGy

The **Food Labelling (Amendment) (Irradiated Foods) Regulations 1990** require the fact that food has been irradiated to be stated on a label. There is still some consumer resistance to irradiated food and in 1995 there was only one licensed food irradiation premises in the UK.

Short-term preservation

The following can all be considered as means of short-term preservation of food:

Cooking

Conventional methods of cooking using heat (e.g. grilling, roasting, stewing, braising), will, if adequate, reduce the number of micro-organisms and kill pathogens. The useful life of the food will therefore be extended.

The use of microwaves

Microwaves are very short electromagnetic waves that move with the speed of light and have a wavelength of between 1 mm and 30 cm. They are produced by a magnetron and are able to penetrate foods and cause an increase in temperature. The mechanism for this action is as follows: Water is a polar molecule (see page 51), this means that water molecules will behave like small magnets. When microwaves are directed at them, they will align themselves in a certain direction in the magnetic field which has been set up. As the current reverses, the direction of the field is changed and the molecules change their direction and turn through 180 degrees. This happens millions of times in a second. This continual movement sets up friction which generates heat.

Microwaves preserve food in two ways:

(a) the internal generation of heat which will reduce the numbers of micro-organisms present;

(b) the microwaves themselves also have a lethal effect on micro-organisms.

Chilling

The temperatures used for chilling vary considerably. The term 'chilled storage' can apply to any reduction in the normal temperature of food. The temperature used depends on the nature of the product and the storage atmosphere. Bananas, for example, are best stored at 15°C, whereas meat is stored at –1 to 2°C.

Cook–chill system

This is a system of food production widely used in some areas of catering, e.g. hospitals, school meals, welfare services and other large scale catering organizations. The food is prepared, cooked and chilled in a central production kitchen and then distributed in the chilled state to the satellite kitchen (regeneration unit) for final heating and service. It is an ideal system where food needs to be transported, where there is a high volume of demand and where the demand is fairly static.

The main stages in the process are as follows:

1 *Preparation*. Foods should be of high quality and should be stored at suitable temperature and humidity levels. All foods must be prepared under strict standards of hygiene. Raw foods should be prepared in a separate area from the cooking area. Separate utensils and machines should be used for raw and cooked foods. Joints of meat should not be larger than 2.5 kg.

2 *Cooking*. The food should be cooked so that all non-sporing pathogens are killed, i.e. the centre temperature should reach 70°C. The temperature should be checked with a probe thermometer.

3 *Portioning*. Food must be portioned within 30 minutes of the end of cooking. This should be carried out in a cool room at 10°C. Foods should be spread evenly into clean containers (e.g. stainless steel) to a depth of no more than 50 mm.

4 *Chilling*. Chilling must start within 30 minutes of cooking and foods should be chilled to between 0°C and +3°C within a further 90 minutes. Specially designed rapid chillers are used with automatic controls and an accurate thermometer.

5 *Storage*. The chilled food should be held in a refrigerated store designed for the purpose which maintains the foods at 0°C to 3°C. Stores should be fitted with accurate temperature recording devices and an alarm (if the temperature rises too high). All products must be labelled and strict stock control and rotation must be enforced. Foods can be stored for up to 5 days including the day of cooking.

6 *Distribution*. The chilled food should be maintained at or below 3°C. For short distribution distances insulated containers may be used but for longer journeys refrigerated vehicles are needed.

7 *Reheating* (regeneration). Foods may be reheated in a variety of

reheating equipment including infra-red units, forced air convection ovens and steamer ovens. The centre temperature of the food should reach 70°C and be held at 70°C for at least 2 minutes.

In hospitals, chilled foods may be distributed from the central kitchen to the wards in specially designed trolleys which maintain the low temperatures. On the ward the trolleys are plugged in to the electricity supply which heats the food up to 70°C.

Cook–freeze system

This is similar to the cook–chill system but food is frozen rather than merely being chilled. The procedures are similar to cook–chill with the exception of temperature and storage times. After cooking and portioning, the foods are blast frozen. The temperature must reach –5°C within 90 minutes and subsequently reach a storage temperature of –18°C. The frozen food may be stored for up to 8 weeks without significant loss of nutrients or palatability.

There are many advantages of cook–chill and cook–freeze systems. They give increased flexibility in the preparation and service of meals. They make more efficient use of space, staff and equipment. Staff can work normal office hours rather than conventional, unsocial catering hours. Hot cooked meals do not need to be transported and nutritional quality compares favourably with conventional catering.

Sous-vide system

The sous-vide method of cookery was developed in France in the mid-1970s by the chef Georges Pralus. It is a system which combines vacuum packing with cook–chill and is particularly suited to the hotel and restaurant sector of the catering industry. Pralus cooked pâté de foie gras in plastic pouches (an extension of the classical method of cooking 'en papillote' – steam cooking in an envelope) and found the pâté had improved yield, flavour and palatability. In the basic sous-vide process, raw or par-cooked food is put into high-barrier plastic bags or pouches from which the air is then extracted. The pouches are then heat sealed. After gentle cooking, often at pasteurization temperatures, the pouches are chilled to 0 – 3°C, stored for up to 21 days, reheated and the bags then opened and the food served.

There are potential hazards with the system. It is essential that these are understood and proper production controls are enforced. The heating process does not kill all organisms and the vacuum packing creates conditions in which anaerobic spore-formers can multiply. Low temperature storage is needed to prevent growth of these organisms. Of particular concern is the anaerobic organism *Clostridium botulinum*. In France sous-vide systems have developed greatly and there are several large companies supplying supermarkets.

Controlled atmosphere storage

This involves controlling the humidity and composition of the atmosphere and is normally used in conjunction with chilling. The optimum humidity depends on the food stored and the temperature of storage. Too high a humidity encourages microbial growth, while too low a humidity results in loss of moisture and, in vegetables, wilting. The composition of the atmosphere affects storage. If the level of carbon dioxide in the air is increased the rate of spoilage is reduced. The optimum concentration of carbon dioxide depends on the food stored. For meat, concentrations of 10% are used, while between 5% and 10% is best for vegetables and 2.5% for eggs.

19 Food additives and food labelling

Food additives are substances which are added to food for one or more of the following purposes:

(a) to maintain the nutritional quality of food;
(b) to improve the keeping quality of food;
(c) to make food more attractive;
(d) as an essential aid to food processing.

Food additives should not be used if they disguise faulty processing, deceive the consumer or substantially reduce the nutritional value of the food.

The term 'food additive' is defined legally in the **Food Labelling Regulations 1984** as:

> any substance not commonly regarded or used as a food, which is added to or used in or on food at any stage to affect its keeping qualities, texture, consistency, appearance, taste, odour, alkalinity or acidity or to serve any other technological function in relation to food.

Additives may be:

1 *Natural substances,* which have been produced biologically and have been extracted from natural products. For example, lecithin, which is used as an emulsifier, is extracted from soya beans.

2 *Synthetic compounds,* which are 'nature identical'. These have been synthesized either chemically or biologically to match naturally occurring counterparts. For example, L-ascorbic acid (vitamin C), which is used as an antioxidant, can be made synthetically.

3 *Artificial compounds,* which are synthesized chemically and have no naturally occurring counterpart. For example, azodicarbonamide, which is used as a flour improver, does not occur naturally and is synthesized by chemical methods.

Under law, for purposes of control, additives are classified into the following categories:

1 Preservatives	4 Colours
2 Antioxidants	5 Sweeteners
3 Emulsifiers and stabilizers	6 Miscellaneous additives

For each category lists of permitted additives have been drawn up. Of the permitted additives, 280 have been given a number. When the additive has also been approved by the European Community (EC), it has an 'E' in front of it.

The safety of additives

There is widespread concern over the use of additives in foods. Many people feel that the addition of chemicals to food, especially those with 'E' numbers is highly undesirable. Tartrazine (E102), a yellow colour used widely in soft drinks and manufactured foods, has a reputation for causing hyperactivity in children but it is only a very small number of people who are affected. There are many 'natural' substances in ordinary foods such as wheat and strawberries that adversely affect many more people. It is impossible to prove that additives are absolutely safe but the risks need to be weighed against their benefits. The risk of possible ill effects must be insignificant compared to the benefits gained. Some additives actually ensure that food is safe to eat while others ensure that perishable foods keep in good condition and increase the variety of foods available.

Other risks associated with food and diet are considerably greater than the risk from the consumption of certain additives. For example, the high fat, high sugar, low fibre diet of many of the population in UK is associated with obesity, high blood pressure and coronary heart disease and is a much greater threat to health and even life itself.

New additives are rigorously tested and the government are advised by the COT (Committee on Toxicity of Chemicals in Food, Consumer Products and the Environment) and the Food Advisory Committee before permitting a new additive. The COT sets an Acceptable Daily Intake (ADI) for each additive. This is the amount which, the committee believes, can be eaten every day for a lifetime without risk to health.

Preservatives

Preservatives prevent or reduce the growth of micro-organisms in food. There are 36 preservatives which are permitted in the UK. All of these except one, nisin, are also permitted in the EC. A list of these permitted preservatives and some examples of where they are used in foods is given in Table 19.1. The serial numbers of the preservatives fall in the range 200 to 290.

The use of chemicals to preserve food is controlled by the **Preservatives in Food Regulations 1989.** Many of the preservatives which are permitted are chemically similar and they can be conveniently placed into groups according to their chemical structure.

Table 19.1 *Permitted preservatives and examples of use*

Preservative		*Example of use*
E200	sorbic acid	Soft drinks, fruit yoghurt, fat spreads
E201	sodium sorbate	Frozen pizza, flour confectionery
E202	potassium sorbate	
E203	calcium sorbate	
E210	benzoic acid	Beer, jam, salad cream, soft drinks, fruit-based pie fillings, marinated herring and mackerel
E211	sodium benzoate	
E212	potassium benzoate	
E213	calcium benzoate	
E214	ethyl-4-hydroxybenzoate	
E215	sodium ethyl 4-hydroxybenzoate	
E216	propyl 4-hydroxybenzoate	
E217	sodium propyl 4-hydroxybenzoate	
E218	methyl 4-hydroxybenzoate	
E219	sodium methyl 4-hydroybenzoate	
E220	sulphur dioxide	Dried fruit, dehydrated vegetables, fruit juices, prawns, sausages, cider, beer and wine. Also used to prevent browning of raw peeled potatoes
E221	sodium sulphite	
E222	sodium hydrogen sulphite	
E223	sodium metabisulphite	
E224	potassium metabisulphite	
E226	calcium sulphite	
E227	calcium hydrogen sulphite	
E228	potassium bisulphite	
E230	biphenyl	Surface treatment of citrus fruit
E231	2-hydroxybiphenyl	
E232	sodium 2-ohenylphenate	
E233	thiabendazole	Surface treatment of bananas
234	nisin	Cheese, clotted cream
E239	hexamine	Marinated herring and mackerel
E249	potassium nitrite	Bacon, ham, cured meats, meat pastes, corned beef
E250	sodium nitrite	
E251	sodium nitrate	
E252	potassium nitrate	
E280	propionic acid	Bread and flour confectionery, Christmas pudding
E281	sodium propionate	
E282	calcium propionate	
E283	potassium propionate	

Sorbic acid and its salts (E200–E203) are used to inhibit the growth of moulds and yeasts. Sorbic acid is a short-chain unsaturated acid. It is non-toxic and is probably metabolized in the body in the same way as naturally occurring unsaturated fatty acids.

$$CH_3{-}CH{=}CH{-}CH{=}CH{-}COOH$$

Sorbic acid

Benzoic acid, C_6H_5COOH, and its derivatives (E210–E219) form a group of widely used preservatives. Benzoic acid occurs naturally in some foods. It is non-toxic. During metabolism it combines with glycine and is excreted as hippuric acid. The derivatives of benzoic acid are metabolized in the same way.

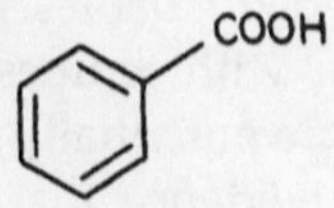

Benzoic acid

Sulphur dioxide and sulphites and metabisulphites (E220–E228) are widely used as preservatives. Sulphur dioxide, SO_2, is a gas which was used traditionally to preserve fruit pulp and wine. Nowadays, it is more common for the salts of sulphur dioxide to be used since they are more convenient. All of these compounds have a drawback in that they impart an unpleasant taste to food and leave an unpleasant after-taste which can be detected at low concentrations. Therefore, their use is restricted to foods which are boiled or cooked in some way. The heating drives off the sulphur dioxide and the taste of the food is not affected. Another drawback of the use of these compounds is that they cause destruction of thiamin.

Diphenyl and its derivatives (E230–E232) and thiabendazole (E233) are used to prevent the growth of moulds on the peel of citrus fruits and bananas. They are often applied by treating the paper in which the fruits are wrapped with the compounds.

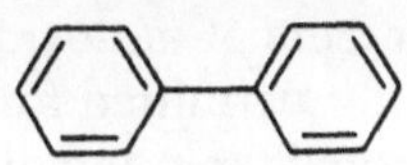

Diphenyl

Nisin (234) is an antibiotic. It is produced by certain strains of *Streptococcus lactis* and it occurs naturally in some cheeses. Nisin is only effective against a limited range of organisms, namely certain species of Gram-positive bacteria. Therefore, its use is limited to certain specialist uses, such as the preservation of cheese, where it prevents spoilage due to gas-forming bacteria. Nisin is not used in medicine. Therefore, the possibility of the development of resistant strains of bacteria does not present a problem. It is a polypeptide and is metabolized in the same manner as other polypeptides in the body.

Hexamine (E239) is manufactured from formaldehyde and ammonia. It has limited use.

Sodium and potassium nitrites and nitrates (E249–E252) are used in the preservation of meats and cheeses. Nitrates are capable of being converted to nitrites either when food spoils or by bacteria in the stomach (especially in tiny babies). Nitrites are able to enter the bloodstream and react with the haemoglobin in the red blood cells. Haemoglobin is responsible for oxygen transport and when the ability to transport oxygen is impaired there may be difficulty in breathing and pallor, dizziness and headaches. Infants are far more susceptible to this condition than adults and nitrites and nitrates are not permitted in foods intended for babies under six months. Nitrates are also capable of reacting with amines present in the stomach to form nitrosamines which are potentially carcinogenic (cancer-producing). However, there is also evidence that intakes of vitamins A, C and E are protective against some forms of cancer. In addition, nitrites inhibit the growth of *Clostridium botulinum* bacteria which are responsible for botulism (see page 248). Without the use of nitrites and nitrates it is possible that there would be many more cases of botulism.

Propionic acid, CH_3CH_2COOH, and its salts (E280–E283) are used in bread and other baked goods as mould suppressants. These compounds occur naturally in fermented foods and they are easily metabolized by the body in the same way as any other fatty acid and its salts.

Antioxidants

Antioxidants are used to prevent the oxidative rancidity of fats and oils. There are some naturally occurring antioxidants, such as vitamin E (tocoferols) which is found in the nuts and seeds from which we obtain vegetable oils, but they do not occur naturally in sufficient quantity to prevent oxidative changes. There are 15 permitted antioxidants. All but one of them (ethoxyquin) are permitted in the EC. The serial numbers of antioxidants are in the range 300 to 322. BHA and BHT are not permitted for use in baby foods. Table 19.2 lists the permitted antioxidants and gives some examples of their uses. The use of antioxidants is controlled by the **Antioxidants in food Regulations 1978.**

Emulsifiers and stabilizers

Emulsifiers are used to disperse oils and fats in water in foods or, conversely, to disperse water in oil or fat (see page 54). They also may be used in baked goods to slow down the rate of staling. Stabilizers are used to improve the stability of emulsions and to prevent the breakdown of emulsions into two separate layers. There are over 50 permitted emulsifiers and stabilizers. Most of them have E numbers and are permitted in the EC. Table 19.3 lists the emulsifiers and stabilizers which are permitted for use in the UK and gives examples of their uses. The use of emulsifiers and stabilizers is controlled by the **Emulsifiers and Stabilizers in Food Regulations 1989.**

Table 19.2 *Permitted antioxidants and examples of use*

	Antioxidant	*Example of use*
E300	L-ascorbic acid	Fruit drinks, also used to improve flour and bread dough
E301	sodium L-ascorbate	
E302	calcium L-ascorbate	
E304	L-ascorbyl palmitate	Chicken stock cubes
E306	extracts of natural origin rich in tocopherols	Vegetable oils
E307	synthetic alpha-tocopherol	Cereal-based baby foods
E308	synthetic gamma-tocopherol	
E309	synthetic delta-tocopherol	
E310	propyl gallate	Vegetable oils, chewing gum
E311	octyl gallate	
E312	dodecyl gallate	
E320	butylated hydroxyanisole (BHA)	Beef stock cubes, cheese spread
E321	butylated hydroxytoluene (BHT)	Chewing gum, dried potato products
E322	lecithins	Fat spreads (also used as an emulsifier)
	ethoxyquin	Used to prevent 'scald' (a discoloration on apples and pears)

Table 19.3 *Permitted emulsifiers and stabilizers and examples of use*

	Emulsifier or stabilizer	*Example of use*
E400	alginic acid	Ice cream, soft cheese
E401	sodium alginate	Cake mixes
E402	potassium alginate	
E403	ammonium alginate	
E404	calcium alginate	
E405	propylene glycol alginate	Salad dressings, cottage cheese
E406	agar	Ice cream
E407	carrageenan	Quick setting jelly mixes, milk shakes
E410	locust bean gum (carob gum)	Salad cream
E412	guar gum	Packet soups and meringue mixes
E413	tragacanth	Salad dressings, processed cheese
E414	gum arabic (acacia)	Confectionery
E415	xanthan gum	Sweet pickle, coleslaw
416	karaya gum	Soft cheese, brown sauce

Table 19.3 *Continued*

	Emulsifier or stabilizer	*Example of use*
432	Polysorbate 20	
433	Polysorbate 80	
434	Polysorbate 40	Frozen bakery products, confectionery creams
435	Polysorbate 60	
436	Polysorbate 65	
E440(a)	pectin	
E440(b)	amidated pectin	Jams and preserves
	pectin extract	
442	ammonium phosphatides	Cocoa and chocolate products
E460	powdered cellulose	High-fibre bread, grated cheese
E461	methylcellulose	Low fat spreads, whipped toppings
E463	hydroxypropylcellulose	
E464	hydroxypropylmethylcellulose	Edible ices
E465	ethylmethylcellulose	Gateaux
E466	sodium carboxymethylcellulose	Jelly, sterilized whipping cream
E470	sodium, potassium and calcium salts of fatty acids	Cake mixes
E471	mono- and di-glycerides of fatty acids	Flour confectionery, margarine, frozen desserts
E472(a)	acetic acid esters of mono- and di-glycerides of fatty acids	Mousse mixes
E472(b)	lactic acid esters of mono- and di-glycerides of fatty acids	Dessert topping
E472(c)	citric acid esters of mono- and di-glycerides of fatty acids	Continental sausages
E472(e)	derivatives of tartaric acid and mono- and di-glycerides of fatty acids	Bread, frozen pizza
E473	sucrose esters of fatty acids	Edible ices
E474	sucroglycerides	
E475	polyglycerol esters of fatty acids	Cake mixes
476	polyglycerol polyricinoleate	Chocolate-flavour coatings for cakes and biscuits
E477	propane-1,2-diol esters of fatty acids	Instant desserts
E481	sodium stearoyl-2-lactylate	Bread, cakes and biscuits
E482	calcium stearoyl-2-lactylate	Gravy granules
E483	stearyl tartrate	
491	sorbitan monostearate	
492	sorbitan tristearate	
493	sorbitan monolaurate	Cake mixes
494	sorbitan mono-oleate	
495	sorbitan monopalmitate	
	extract of quillaia	Used in soft drinks to promote foam
	derivatives of soya bean oil	Emulsions used to grease bakery tins

Colours

Colours are added to food to make it more attractive or to replace colour lost during processing. Many canned fruits and vegetables have a very unappealing colour if colour is not added to replace that lost during processing. The addition of colours to food is controlled by the **Colouring Matter in Food Regulations 1973.** Only 50 permitted colours may be used. Their serial numbers are in the range 100 to 180 and about two-thirds of them have 'E' numbers and are permitted in the EC.

One of the commonest food colourings is caramel (E150) which is made by heating sugar until it turns brown (see page 63). Many colours are of natural origin and are extracted from plants. For example, curcumin (E100) is a yellow extract obtained from turmeric roots and beta-carotene (E160a) can be extracted from carrots. There are 15 permitted artificial colours. Some of these are known as the azo dyes. An example is tartrazine (E102).

Table 19.4 lists the permitted colours and some examples of their use.

Table 19.4 *Permitted colours and examples of use*

	Colour	*Example of use*
E100	curcumin	Flour confectionery, margarine
E101	riboflavin	Sauces
E101(a)	riboflavin-5-phosphate	Sauces
E102	tartrazine	Soft drinks, cake mixes, instant puddings
E104	quinoline yellow	Biscuits, jellies
E110	sunset yellow FCF	Biscuits, jellies
E120	cochineal, carminic acid	Alcoholic drinks, home food colour
E122	carmoisine	Jams, jellies
E123	amaranth	Packet soups, cake and trifle mixes
E124	ponceau 4R	Dessert mixes, jams, jellies
E127	erythrosine BS	Glacé cherries
128	red 2G	Sausages
E131	patent blue V	Scotch eggs
E132	indigo carmine	Blancmange, sweets
133	brilliant blue FCF	Canned vegetables
E140	chlorophyll	Soups, canned vegetables, confectionery
E141	copper complexes of chlorophyll and chlorophyllins	Parsley sauce, soups
E142	green S	Boiled sweets
E150	caramel	Beer, soft drinks, sauces, gravy browning and granules
E151	black PN	Brown sauce, chocolate mousse
E153	carbon black	Liquorice
154	brown FK	Kippers
155	chocolate brown HT	Chocolate cake

Table 19.4 *Continued*

	Colour	*Example of use*
E160(a)	alpha-carotene, beta-carotene, gamma-carotene	Margarine, soft drinks
E160(b)	annatto, bixin, norbixin	Crisps, margarine, cheese
E160(c)	capsanthin, capsorubin	Processed cheese slices
E160(d)	lycopene	
E160(e)	beta-apo-8-carotenal	Cheese slices
E160(f)	ethyl esters of beta-apo-8-carotenoic acid	
E161(a)	flavoxanthin	
E161(b)	lutein	Poultry feed (to deepen colour of egg yolks)
E161(c)	cryptoxanthin	
E161(d)	rubixanthin	
E161(e)	violoxanthin	
E161(f)	rhodoxanthin	
E161(g)	canthaxanthin	Preserves, confectionery, dessert mixes
E162	beetroot red (betanin)	Ice cream, jellies, yoghurt
E163	anthocyanins	Yoghurt, soft drinks
E171	titanium dioxide	Sweets
E172	iron oxides and hydroxides	Cake mixes, meat paste
E173	aluminium	Sugar-coated confectionery for cake decoration
E174	silver	Sugar-coated confectionery for cake decoration
E175	gold	Sugar-coated confectionery for cake decoration
E180	pigment rubine	Colouring the rind of hard cheese
	methyl violet	
	paprika	Canned vegetables
	saffron, crocin	Rice
	sandalwood, santolin	
	turmeric	Soups

Sweeteners

There are two types of sweetening agents or sweeteners:

(a) *intense sweeteners* which are many times sweeter than sucrose and are used in small amounts;
(b) *bulk sweeteners* which have a sweetening power roughly equivalent to that of sucrose and are used in larger quantities.

The use of sweeteners in foods is controlled by the **Sweeteners in Food Regulations 1983**. Only two sweeteners have been given serial numbers and the prefix 'E'. They are mannitol and sorbitol. None of the permitted intense sweeteners have been given serial numbers and they are not approved for use throughout the EC. Table 19.5 lists the permitted sweeteners and gives examples of their use.

Table 19.5 *Permitted sweeteners and examples of use*

	Sweetener	Example of use
	Intense sweeteners	
	acesulfame potassium	Canned foods, soft drinks, table-top sweeteners
	aspartame	Soft drinks, yoghurts, dessert and drink mixes, sweetening tablets
	saccharin sodium saccharin calcium saccharin	Soft drinks, cider, sweetening tablets, table-top sweeteners
	thaumatin	Table-top sweeteners, yoghurt
	Bulk sweeteners	
E420	sorbitol, sorbitol syrup	Sugar-free confectionery, jams for diabetics
	hydrogenated glucose syrup isomalt lactitol	Sugar-free confectionery, low sugar jams
E421	mannitol	
	xylitol	Sugar-free chewing gum

Aspartame (which is sold under the brand name Nutrasweet) is a dipeptide made up from the amino acids aspartic acid and phenylalanine. It is metabolized in the body in the same way that any other dipeptide is broken down. Concern has been expressed about whether aspartame is suitable for people suffering from phenylketonuria (PKU). PKU is a genetic disease and people who suffer from it are unable to metabolize phenylalanine. However, a government committee has concluded that aspartame can safely be used by those with PKU.

Miscellaneous food additives

In addition to the five main categories outlined above there are many other types of additives. The use of these substances is controlled by the **Miscellaneous Additives in Food Regulations 1980**. Under this legislation, over 120 miscellaneous additives have been approved for use in foods. It is not possible in this text to give a comprehensive list of all these additives and their uses but some examples of the type of substances considered in this category are given below.

(A) Flavour enhancers

These are not flavourings but they are substances which enhance existing flavours and make them seem stronger, although they themselves are practically tasteless. The most widely used flavour enhancer is monosodium glutamate or MSG (621). It is the sodium salt of glutamic acid, an amino acid which is commonly found in proteins (see page 93). Therefore, MSG is readily metabolized in the body. However, the consumption of large amounts of MSG may cause an unfavourable reaction in some people. The disorder has become known as the 'Chinese Restaurant Syndrome' and the symptoms include palpitations, chest or neck pain and dizziness. These effects are short-lived and on the whole MSG is not thought to be harmful. MSG occurs naturally in soy sauce, which is made by fermenting soya beans. Commercially, it can be made from seaweed, but it is more usually obtained from sugar beet or wheat.

Other flavour enhancers used in manufactured foods, include sodium 5′-ribonucleotide and sodium inosinate.

(B) Acids, buffers and bases

These substances are added to food in order to adjust or control its pH.

(C) Humectants

These substances absorb water and, therefore, help to prevent the food from drying out. Glycerol (E422) is added to sweets for this purpose.

(D) Firming and crisping agents

These substances are added to foods such as canned fruits and vegetables in order to keep them firm. Calcium chloride (509) is used in this way.

(E) Flour improvers

These substances are used to strengthen doughs, e.g. azodicarbonamide (927).

(F) Flour bleaching agents

These substances are added to flour in order to whiten it, e.g. chlorine dioxide (926).

Extraction solvents

Many flavourings and colourings are dissolved in other substances before being added to foods. Solvents may also be used to facilitate the addition of other ingredients. The use of solvents is controlled by the **Extraction Solvents in Food Regulations 1993** and only ten are permitted. These permitted solvents are listed in Table 19.6.

Mineral hydrocarbons

Mineral hydrocarbons are mineral oils and waxes of fairly high molecular weight. They are not metabolized and hence have no nutritive value. They interfere with the absorption of vitamins A and D, therefore, their presence in food is not desirable. Their use is controlled by the **Mineral Hydrocarbons in Food Regulations 1966**. Their main uses are as follows:

(a) as a coating for dried fruits, such as currants, raisins and sultanas to prevent them sticking together during storage (maximum 0.5% by weight);
(b) as a coating for citrus fruits to replace the natural oils which are lost during cleaning (maximum 0.1% by weight);
(c) as a coating for cheeses to minimize drying out during storage.

Table 19.6 *Permitted solvents*

Ethanol (ethyl alcohol)
Ethyl acetate (ethyl ethanoate)
Diethyl ether
Glycerol
Glyceryl monoacetate
Glyceryl diacetate
Glyceryl triacetate
Propan-2-ol (isopropyl alcohol)
Propan-1,2-diol (propylene glycol)
Cyclohexane

Flavourings

There are several thousand flavouring agents available to the food industry including both natural and synthetic flavours. Natural flavouring agents include essential oils (see page 75) which are volatile substances extracted from plants e.g. oil of cloves, oil of lemon. Herbs and spices contain many essential oils and other flavouring compounds and are widely used as flavouring agents. Synthetic flavours are usually copies of natural components and include substances such as acids, aldehydes, esters and ketones. Many of the simpler artificial fruit flavours are based on esters (see page 42). Natural flavours are usually mixtures of many different chemical compounds and so a large number of compounds need to be blended together to obtain a good artificial flavour.

There are so many flavouring agents that there is no permitted list although the **Flavourings in Food Regulations 1992** lists specified substances which are permitted only in limited amounts. These regulations also give details of labelling e.g. 'natural flavouring substances' must refer only to substances obtained by physical, enzymatic or microbiological processes from material of animal or vegetable origin.

The labelling of packaged food is controlled by the **Food Labelling Regulations 1984**. These regulations state that the label must show the following:

1 The name of the food

This name must be:

(a) the legal name (where a legal name exists). For example, chocolate and honey are legal names;
(b) the customary name (where no legal name exists). For example, pizza and muesli are both customary names;
(c) a descriptive name (where no legal or customary name exists). This name must be sufficiently precise to inform the purchaser of the true nature of the contents and to avoid confusion. 'Malted milk drink' is an example of a descriptive name.

2 A list of ingredients

Most foods must have a list of ingredients, including water if the water content is more than 5% by weight. The list of ingredients must be arranged in descending order by weight. The heading of the list must be the word 'Ingredients' or must include the word 'ingredients'. The name of the ingredient must be the name which would be used if the ingredient was sold as a food, where this is applicable. An additive must be listed by the principal function it serves, followed by its name and/or serial number.

3 Special emphasis

Where a food is characterized by a particular ingredient, and special emphasis is given to it on the label, the minimum percentage of the ingredient must be shown. Similarly, for a product with a low content of a particular ingredient, the maximum percentage should be given.

4 'Best before'/'use by' date

For most packaged foods the label should give an indication of durability with either:

(a) 'best before' followed by the date in the form of day/month/year. (Day/month if date is within 3 months and month/year for 3 to 18 months).
(b) 'use by' followed by the date (day/month or day/month/year) up to which the food, if properly stored, is recommended for use.

5 Manufacturer's address

The name and address of the manufacturer or packer must be included so that the consumer knows who to contact if further information is required or a complaint is to be made. The place of origin of the food should also be included if necessary.

6 Instructions for use

In the case of a dry mix, concentrate or similar food (except custard powder and blancmange powder), the instructions must specify every substance (other than water) required. This must appear next to the name of the food.

Nutrition labelling

Nutrition labelling is compulsory when a nutritional claim (e.g. 'low fat', 'high fibre') is made. Otherwise nutritional labelling is voluntary. Nutrition labels must, at the minimum, show the 'Group 1' foods, i.e. the amount of energy (kJ and kcal), protein, carbohydrate and fat per 100 g or 100 ml of the food. Most labels also show amounts per portion or per serving. The other standard format for labels is a 'Group 2' format which also includes sugars (as part of carbohydrates), saturates (as part of fat), fibre and sodium. These have to be added to the basic list if a claim is made about any of them. In addition, the amounts of polyols, starch, monounsaturates, polyunsaturates and cholesterol can be shown. The amount and percentage of the RDA (Recommended Daily Amount) of certain vitamins and minerals present in significant amounts may also be shown. Amounts must be declared when a claim is made. 'Significant' amounts mean 15% of the RDA per 100 g (or per package if the package contains only a single portion).

Full details of the requirements for nutrition labelling are given in the **Food Labelling (Amendment) Regulations 1994**.

Appendix I

Percentage contribution of different foods to the nutrient content of the average household diet

	Energy	*Protein*	*Fat*	*Carbohydrate*	*Vitamin A (retinol equivalent)*
Milk, including cream	9.9	16.9	10.8	7.5	11.5
Cheese	3.1	5.8	5.7	–	4.6
Total milk, cream and cheese	13.1	22.8	16.5	7.6	16.1
Meat, carcase	5.0	10.1	9.2	–	0.2
Poultry	1.7	5.6	2.5	–	0.5
Bacon	1.4	2.3	2.9	–	–
Other meat, including liver	6.3	10.5	9.9	2.1	37.5
Total meat	14.4	28.5	24.5	2.1	38.2
Fish	1.5	5.0	1.8	0.3	0.1
Eggs	1.1	3.0	1.9	–	2.5
Butter	2.2	–	5.5	–	4.5
Margarine	4.2	–	10.6	–	8.6
Other fats	6.2	0.5	15.2	0.1	6.3
Total fats	12.6	0.6	31.2	0.2	19.3
Sugar, preserves and confectionery	7.0	6.8	1.4	13.8	–
Potatoes	3.8	3.1	0.2	7.2	–
Green vetetables	0.5	1.4	0.2	0.5	0.8
Root vegetables	0.3	0.2	0.1	0.6	13.1
Other vegetables	5.1	4.9	4.2	6.0	6.6
Total vegetables	9.8	9.5	4.9	14.3	20.6
Fresh fruit	1.8	0.8	0.3	3.4	0.4
Other fruit and fruit juices	1.9	1.0	1.4	2.7	0.1
Total fruit	3.7	1.7	1.6	6.1	0.5
White bread	6.0	6.5	0.9	10.4	–
Other bread	6.6	7.9	1.8	10.7	0.1
Breakfast cereals	3.4	2.7	0.5	6.1	–
Cakes, pastries and biscuits	8.1	3.8	7.8	9.7	0.5
Flour and other cereals	6.6	4.8	2.9	10.4	0.8
Total cereals	30.6	25.7	13.9	47.3	1.4
Beverages, alcoholic and soft drinks	3.9	0.8	0.1	5.7	0.4
Other foods	2.3	1.4	2.3	2.7	0.7

Thiamin	Riboflavin	Niacin equivalent	Vitamin C	Vitamin D	Calcium	Iron
9.6	35.4	11.0	4.8	7.2	45.6	2.1
0.4	3.8	3.5	–	1.2	11.7	0.4
10.0	39.1	14.5	4.8	8.5	57.3	2.6
3.5	4.8	11.2	–	–	0.4	5.9
1.2	1.6	6.8	–	–	0.1	1.3
2.5	1.0	2.6	–	–	0.1	0.8
5.7	8.6	11.3	1.6	0.7	2.0	9.5
12.8	16.0	31.9	1.6	0.7	2.6	17.6
0.7	1.5	5.2	–	22.0	1.8	2.1
0.9	4.3	2.2	–	8.9	1.0	2.8
–	0.1	–	–	1.5	0.1	0.1
–	–	–	–	30.3	0.2	0.3
–	0.3	0.3	0.1	17.0	0.2	–
–	0.4	0.4	0.1	48.8	0.5	0.5
0.4	0.9	0.3	0.9	–	1.5	1.6
10.2	1.6	3.8	12.3	–	0.5	3.8
3.3	0.9	1.4	6.2	–	1.3	2.5
1.1	0.1	0.3	1.6	–	0.7	0.4
6.9	3.1	6.9	19.2	0.1	3.2	9.3
21.4	5.8	12.4	39.3	0.1	5.8	16.2
2.4	1.4	1.3	22.3	–	1.2	1.2
2.5	0.8	1.7	21.6	–	0.9	2.1
4.9	2.1	2.9	43.8	–	2.1	3.2
8.5	1.6	4.4	–	–	6.4	7.4
14.3	2.6	5.0	–	0.2	6.7	12.9
12.5	12.8	7.0	0.7	7.6	0.9	13.8
3.6	2.5	2.7	0.1	1.1	4.0	6.8
6.5	1.7	3.3	0.5	1.4	5.6	5.9
45.5	21.1	22.4	1.3	10.2	23.7	47.1
1.2	6.0	5.9	6.9	0.6	1.6	3.2
2.1	2.7	1.9	1.4	0.2	1.9	3.2

Appendix II

Dietary reference values for food energy and nutrients for the United Kingdom (Department of Health, 1991)

DRV = Dietary Reference Value. A term used to cover both EAR and RNI.

EAR = Estimated Average Requirement of a group of people. About half will need more than the EAR and half less.

RNI = Reference Nutrient Intake. An amount of the nutrient that is enough, or more than enough, for about 97% of people in a group.

Estimated Average Requirements (EARs) for energy

	Males		*Females*	
Age	*MJ/day*	*kcal/day*	*MJ/day*	*kcal/day*
0–3 months	2.28	545	2.16	515
4–6 months	2.89	690	2.69	645
7–9 months	3.44	825	3.20	765
10–12 months	3.85	920	3.61	865
1–3 years	5.15	1230	4.86	1165
4–6 years	7.16	1715	6.46	1545
7–10 years	8.24	1970	7.28	1740
11–14 years	9.27	2220	7.92	1845
15–18 years	11.51	2755	8.83	2110
19–50 years	10.60	2550	8.10	1940
51–59 years	10.60	2550	8.00	1900
60–64 years	9.93	2380	7.99	1900
65–74 years	9.71	2330	7.96	1900
75+ years	8.77	2100	7.61	1810
Pregnancy			+0.80*	+200*
Lactation			+1.90–2.40	+450–570

* = for last three months only

Reference Nutrient Intakes (RNIs) for protein, vitamins and minerals

Age	*Protein g/day*	*Vitamin A µg/day*	*Thiamin mg/day*	*Riboflavin mg/day*	*Niacin mg/day*	*Folate µg/day*	*Vitamin C mg/day*	*Vitamin D µg/day*	*Calcium mg/day*	*Iron mg/day*
0–3 months	12.5	350	0.2	0.4	3	50	25	8.5	525	1.7
4–6 months	12.7	350	0.2	0.4	3	50	25	8.5	525	4.3
7–9 months	13.7	350	0.2	0.4	4	50	25	7	525	7.8
10–12 months	14.9	350	0.3	0.4	5	50	25	7	525	7.8
1–3 years	14.5	400	0.5	0.6	8	70	30	7	350	6.9
4–6 years	19.7	500	0.7	0.8	11	100	30	–	450	6.1
7–10 years	28.3	500	0.7	1.0	12	150	30	–	550	8.7
Males										
11–14 years	42.1	600	0.9	1.2	15	200	35	–	1000	11.3
15–18 years	55.2	700	1.1	1.3	18	200	40	–	1000	11.3
19–50 years	55.5	700	1.0	1.3	17	200	40	–	700	8.7
50+ years	53.3	700	0.9	1.3	16	200	40	**	700	8.7
Females										
11–14 years	41.2	600	0.7	1.1	12	200	35	–	800	14.8
15–18 years	45.0	600	0.8	1.1	14	200	40	–	800	14.8
19–50 years	45.0	600	0.8	1.1	13	200	40	–	700	14.8
50+ years	46.5	600	0.8	1.1	12	200	40	**	700	8.7
Pregnancy	+6	+100	+0.1*	+0.3	+0	+100	+10	10	+0	+0
Lactation	+11	+350	+0.2	+0.5	+2	+60	+30	10	+550	+0

* = for last three months only
** = 10 µg/day after age 65 years

Further reading

Coultate, T.P. (1989). *Food: The Chemistry of Its Components*, 2nd edition. The Royal Society of Chemistry.

Davies, J. and Hammond, B. (1988). *Cooking Explained*, 3rd edition. Longman.

Davis, B. (1987). *Food Commodities*, 2nd edition. Butterworth-Heinemann.

Department of Health (1991). *Dietary Reference Values for Food Energy and Nutrients for the United Kingdom*. Report on Health and Social Subjects No. 41. HMSO.

Department of Health (1994). *Nutritional Aspects of Cardiovascular Disease*. Report on Health and Social Subjects No. 46. HMSO.

Fox, B.A. and Cameron, A.G. (1995). *Food Science, Nutrition and Health*, 6th edition. Edward Arnold.

Garrow, J.S. and James, W.P.T. (1993). *Human Nutrition and Dietetics*, 9th edition. Churchill Livingstone.

Hobbs, B.C. and Roberts, D. (1993). *Food Poisoning and Food Hygiene*, 6th edition. Edward Arnold.

Jay, J.M. (1986). *Modern Food Microbiology*, 3rd edition. Van Nostrand, Reinhold and Co.

Jukes, D.J. (1993). *Food Legislation of the UK*, 3rd edition. Butterworth-Heinemann.

Holland, B., Welch, A.A., Unwin, I.D. *et al.* (1991). *McCance and Widdowson's The Composition of Foods*, 5th edition. The Royal Society of Chemistry and Ministry of Agriculture, Fisheries and Food.

Kent, N.L. (1993). *Technology of Cereals*, 4th edition. Butterworth-Heinemann.

Lawrie, R.A. (1991). *Meat Science*, 5th edition. Butterworth-Heinemann.

McGee, H. (1986). *On Food and Cooking*. Allen and Unwin.

Ministry of Agriculture, Fisheries and Food (1995). *Manual of Nutrition*, 10th edition. HMSO.

Parry, T.J. and Pawsey, R.K. (1984). *Principles of Microbiology*, 2nd edition. Hutchinson Educational.

Stretch, J.A. and Southgate, H.A. (1991). *Food Hygiene, Health and Safety*. Pitman.

Trickett, J. (1992). *The Prevention of Food Poisoning*, 3rd edition. Stanley Thornes.

Index

Page numbers in *italics* refer to tables.

9 780750 623735